AF539499

GOVERNANCE OF HOSPITALS

GOVERNANCE OF HOSPITALS

(Encyclopaedia of Hospital Management—1)

DR. S.L. GOEL
Professor of Public Administration (Retd.),
Panjab University, Chandigarh
Editor, Indian Journal of Public Administration, IIPA, New Delhi
Former Member, UGC, Former Member Distance Education Council
Former Member All India Board of Management, AICTE
Member, Executive Council, IIPA, New Delhi.
Former Vice-President, IIPA, New Delhi.
Emeritus Fellow, University Grants Commission
Former Director, State Bank of India (Local Board) Chandigarh
Former Director, National Horticulture Board, Ministry of Agriculture,
Government of India, New Delhi.

and

DR. R. KUMAR
MBBS, MS, Ex. PGI
President, Chandigarh Ophthalmological Society, 2000-01,
Columnist on Health Education and Management,
Advisor on Health Care and Medical Tourism,
Member Tourism Advisory Forum,
Chandigarh Administration, Chandigarh

DEEP & DEEP PUBLICATIONS PVT. LTD.
F-159, Rajouri Garden, New Delhi-110027

GOVERNANCE OF HOSPITALS
(Encyclopaedia of Hospital Management—1)

ISBN 978-81-8450-216-9

Typeset by S.S. COMPOSERS
3190, Mohindra Park, Shakur Basti, Delhi-110034.

Printed in India at MAYUR ENTERPRISES
WZ Plot No. 3, Gujjar Market, Tihar Village, New Delhi-110018.

Published by DEEP & DEEP PUBLICATIONS PVT. LTD.
F-159, Rajouri Garden, New Delhi-110027.
Phones: 25435369, 25440916
E-mail: ddpbooks@yahoo.co.in • ddpubs@gmail.com
Showroom:
2/13, Ansari Road, Daryaganj, New Delhi-110002 • Telefax: 23245122

Contents

Contents

Preface

"A patient coming to the hospital gives us an opportunity to serve. By treating a patient we are not doing a favour to him, the patient is doing a favour to us by giving us an opportunity to serve the humanity."

—*Mahatma Gandhi*

Good Governance is an essential ingredient for socio-economic development of the country. The Government of India and State Governments come out with new ideas and approaches but these do not succeed when put to action because of lack of good governance. Good Governance is of paramount importance in these times of far reaching changes. In this backdrop of major changes, we need to re-orient ourselves to deliver ways and means to promote good governance. No government of course can hope to survive without a strong and effective good governance nor can an administrative system exist without the support of those it was established to serve.

S.G. Barve feels that Good Governance is more an art than a science and there can be very few esoteric principles about it. It is a question of performance rather than theory or action. There are no sensational short-cuts to good governance. There are no spectacular solutions. What is wanted is a long and patient siege. Another outstanding deficiency is failure to locate definite responsibility at different points and levels of the administrative hierarchy. This location if responsibility has to be finally carried down to the level of the individual functionary.

The issue of good governance has, in recent times, emerged at the forefront of the agenda for sustainable human development. It is imperative that this process while being sustainable in terms of resources over generations and across space, recognizes the legitimate claim of each person in a society to be an active and a productive participant. Empowering people for meaningful participation in this development process is one of the key interventions of the Government of India in its attempt to usher in sustainable development.

Good governance implies utmost concern for people's welfare wherein the government and its bureaucracy follow policies and discharge their duties with a deep sense of commitment; respect of law in a manner which is transparent, ensuring human rights and dignity, probity and public accountability.

In the new millennium, the greatest challenge before the largest democracy of the world, is to steer the overall growth in the country along the lines of fairness, equality, equity, justice and sustainability especially when the role of the Government itself is being redefined. Good Governance is of paramount significance in these times of far reaching changes and ushering in an era of globalization, liberalization and privatization.

The fact that India is the second most populous country that survives on just 2.4% of world's landmass, creates its own population resource tension. Combined with the colonial legacy of systems that sub-served the exploitative objectives of the then colonial administration, has made the task of change much more difficult. Thus, despite the creation of an enabling framework for sustainable development, India continues to face enormous challenges in search of options for development that are environmentally sound and suitable to its specific social conditions through good governance.

Combating poverty and its eventual eradication has been the central theme of all the major policies and programmes of the Government of India since Independence. In the decades of the 90's, the focused intervention of the Government on various social development sectors bore fruit. At the beginning of the 90's, an estimated 320 million people, or 36% of the total population, were below the poverty line. However, by the end of the decade, India succeeded in bringing down the number of people living below the poverty line by 18.75% to 260 million. In absolute numbers, a huge 60 million people were brought above the poverty line in 10 year's time.

Despite the impressive statistics, the nation is aware that the absolute number of people still living below the poverty line is huge. The proportions of poor people in rural and urban areas are 27% and 23.62% respectively.

Notwithstanding the significant progress in the areas of poverty eradication, improvement of literacy rates and health standards, etc. and the emergence of an enabling framework for sustainable development, India continues to face enormous challenges in achieving sustainable development. There still remains a disparity between India and the rest of the world on various social development indicators. India has taken it as a challenge to reduce the poverty ratio, ensure attendance of children in schools, reduce gender gaps in literacy and wage rates by 50%, reduce population growth, attain at least 75% literacy, reduce infant mortality to 45 per 1000 live births, reduce maternal mortality rate to 2 per 1000 live births, increase forest cover to 25%, provide sustained access to drinking water in rural areas and to clean up major stretches of polluted rivers.

The Ministers of Health of countries of the South-East Asia Region adopted the Declaration on Health Development in the South-East Asia Region in the 21st Century at their 15th meeting in Bangkok, Thailand in August 1997. This Regional Health Declaration serves as the basis for future health development in Member-states and is the Region's contribution to the World Health Declaration and the global health policy.

It is a statement of commitment on health development and a pledge to ensure health for all by mobilizing all for health. It is also resolve to strengthen national capacity and regional solidarity to further this aim.

The Declaration is founded on the principles of human rights, equity, social justice, and the centrality of health to sustainable development. It identifies the challenges of addressing inequities in health, creating an enabling environment for health, and ensuring basic health services to all—particularly to the poor, to women and to other vulnerable groups. It enunciates policy actions to meet these challenges.

The World Health Report 2000, 'Health Systems: Improving Performance by WHO' rightly states that:

> "From the safe delivery of the healthy baby to the care with dignity of the frail-elderly, health systems have a vital and continuing responsibility to people throughout the life span. They are crucial to the healthy development of individuals, families and societies everywhere."

Health systems are defined as comprising all the organizations, institutions and resources that are devoted to producing health actions. A health action is defined as any effort, whether in personal health care, public health services or through intersectoral initiatives, whose primary purpose is to improve health.

The ultimate responsibility for the overall performance of a country's health system is with government, which in turn should involve all sectors of society in its stewardship. The careful and responsible management of the well-being of the population is the very essence of good government. For every country it means establishing the best and fairest health system possible with available resources. The health of the people is always a national priority; government responsibility for it is continuous and permanent. Ministers of health must therefore take on a large part of the stewardship of health systems.

Hospital administration at tertiary, secondary, community and primary level as well as specialized hospitals are facing a large number of problems to cope with new and emerging developments in the 21st century.

The Director General of WHO, Gro Harlem Brundland rightly observes that the way health systems are designed, managed and financed affects people's lives and livelihoods. The difference between a well performing health system and one that is failing can be measured in death, disability, impoverishment, humiliation and despair.

If policy-makers are to act on measures of performance, they need a clear understanding of the key functions that health systems have to undertake. The report defines four key functions providing services, generating the human and physical resources that makes service delivery possible; raising and pooling the resources used to pay for health care, and, most critically, the function of stewardship—setting and enforcing the rules of the game and providing strategic direction for all the different actors involved.

Science and Technology advancements have provided many opportunities for diagnosis and treatment but the escalating cost of medical services is a cause of concern. Besides, there has been deterioration of quality in all the areas. Prolongation of life has put great pressure on hospital resources and many new life style diseases like heart, diabetes caused by sedative life, alcoholism, accidents, etc. Besides AIDS, HIV, Cancer are also cause of concern.

Declines in crude birth and death rates and increases in life expectancy have resulted in a progressive aging of the population. These demographic changes, as well as the emergence of an increasingly affluent middle class, have brought with them the attendant problems of cardiovascular diseases, cancers, neurological and metabolic disorders, and other chronic conditions. We are therefore facing not only the burden of communicable diseases, but also an increasing burden of non-communicable diseases. They can no longer address these problems sequentially, but must face them simultaneously. This double burden of diseases imposes a tremendous strain on national health budgets.

The health sector alone is not able to cope with such problems. Hence there is an urgent need for close interaction with other social sectors, such as education, housing and environment. Another critical issue which governments now face is that of the sustainability of their health programmes. In response, countries are taking steps to develop and strengthen international partnerships for health development, and geopolitical associations such as the South Asian Association for Regional Cooperation (SAARC) and the Association of South East Asian Nations (ASEAN) are contributing substantially to strengthen cooperation among countries of the Region.

World Health Report 2000 states that health systems are valuable and important, but they could accomplish much more with the available understanding of how to improve health. The failings which limit performance do not result primarily from lack of knowledge but from not fully applying what is already known: that is, from systemic rather than technical failures. This is true even of most medical errors, because "the problem is not bad people; the problem is that the system needs to be made safer." How to measure current performance and how to achieve the potential improvements in it are subject of this report. Research to expand knowledge is crucial in the long-run, as progress over the last two centuries shows; in the short-run, much could be accomplished by the wider and better application of existing knowledge. This can improve health more quickly than continued and more equality distributed socio-economic progress, important as that is. The next sections discuss how modern health systems arose, and how they have been repeatedly subjected to reforms intended to make them work better in one way or another.

Providing health care efficiently requires financial resources to be properly balanced among the many inputs used to deliver health services. Large numbers of physicians, nurses and other staff are useless without adequately built, equipped and supplied facilities. Available resources should be allocated to both the investments in the new skills, facilities and equipment, and to maintenance of the existing infrastructure. Moreover, these delicate balances must be maintained both over time and across different geographical areas. In practice, imbalances between investment and recurrent expenditures and among the different categories of inputs are frequent, and create barriers to satisfactory performance. New investment choices must be made carefully to reduce the risk of future imbalance, and the existing mix of inputs needs to be monitored on a regular basis. Clear policy guidance and incentives for purchasers and providers are necessary if they are to adopt efficient practices in response to health needs and expectations.

The real work of doctor . . . is not an affair of health centres, or public clinics, or operating theatres, or laboratories, or hospital beds.

These techniques have their place in medicine, but they are not medicine. The essential unit of medical practice is the occasion when, in the intimacy of the consulting room or sick room, a person who is ill, or believes himself to be ill, seeks the advice of a doctor whom he trusts. This is consultation and else in the practice of medicine dervies from it. (Sir James Calvert Spence)

Hospital care is mutidimensional. It is a service provided by a coordinated group of professional, technical, supportive, and other workers under the direction of a physician. The quality of the care received by patients is affected by the adequacy of the hospital facilities and their maintenance, by the administrative and professional organizations of the hospital, by the competence of the personnel, and by the interpersonal relations among the staff as well as between the staff and the patients.

In these Volumes, we have been able to provide material on all issues to make the hospitals effective and efficient. Besides us (Editors), many scholars of eminence have contributed Articles in the volumes, some of them are awardees of B.C. Roy award and others. We are extremely grateful to them to join us in providing literature on Hospital Administration which is not available at one place. The joint wisdom would help the policy-makers, planners, decision-makers and hospital administrators in shaping and executive implementation of health services in 21st century.

Today, a hospital is a place for the definition and treatment of human ills and restoration of health and well-being of those temporarily deprived of these. A large number of professionally and technically skilled people apply their knowledge and skill with the help of complicated equipment and appliances to produce quality care for patient. The excellence of the product—the *raison 'd etre* for a hospital, therefore, depends on how well the human and material resources are applied to promote patient care.

In the dynamic society, the hospital occupies a unique place to accommodate explosion of science into medicine and the whole galaxy of new treatment techniques, new equipment and proliferation of services which have made profound impact on the provision of care facilities and services. Besides this, the development of socio-politico, cultural and educational systems have made the people conscious of their rights and they demand that modern and best means of medical and health care be made available to them; not only within the four walls of the hospital but at their doorstep or in the vicinity of living places. These impacts have made hospital a complex organization.

Management of such a complex organization requires blending of technical and administrative competence in the right quantity, at the right time, at the right place, by the right man and in the right way or process. Each hospital is a distinct entity and as such each has to be tailored to the specific aims to be accomplished, the specific tasks to be performed, the volume of services to be rendered and the type of community to be served. The basic purpose of the hospital is "better patient care" and return the patient back to the community as a productive unit of that community. Hospital administration is an activity to secure better through optimum utilization of inputs.

The following steps could also be taken to improve matters:

- Effective coordination should be established between the medical services and the supportive services to ensure promptness and clarity.
- Effective coordination and cooperation must be ensured among the various departments of the hospital to help the patients in diagnosing their ailments. It is suggested that a medical board may meet once a week where all the specialities may be represented and the patients needing the attention of more than one speciality may be asked to attend the board.
- A receptionist well versed with the functioning of hospital-system may be appointed to guide the patients to approach the hospital properly.
- There is a need of play cards and signboards to guide the patients and their relatives.
- Provision of cheap and quality goods to be used by the patients or their relatives.
- Arrangement of stay of the relatives in Dharamsalas specially constructed for the purpose.
- Hospital beds may be given to patients according to the severity of the disease rather than other trifle consideration like obliging the VIPs.

In brief, the functioning of the hospital should be organized and re-organized to serve the patients most efficiently. All the personnel engaged in patient care must keep the following definitions of the "patient" in their minds.

The patient is the most important in the Hospital:

- The patient is not dependent upon us—we are dependent on him. The patient is not an interruption of our work—he is the purpose of it.
- The patient is not an outsider to our business—he is our business. The patient is a person and not a statistic. He has feelings, emotions, biases, and wants. It is our business to satisfy him.

At present there is no comprehensive legislation to guide the organization and management of hospitals. There is a need of a hospital legislation to ensure maintenance of standards, to define rights and duties of the hospital staff and to ensure the efficient functioning of hospitals. It is suggested that the Government of India may set-up a body Development Council for Hospitals with its branches in the States like the Medical Council of India, to lay down policies to ensure that the hospitals have requisite facilities and provide efficient services to the patients. It has become a common practice to set-up nursing homes in the private sector. These so called 'nursing homes' are often huge money making projects devised by the specialists in league with one another. All these nursing homes must be under the control of the proposed council. It should be the duty of the council to see that the specialities like the private industry do not fleece the people and provide medical care of right quality and at a reasonable price. Besides, the proposed council may attend to the complaints of the patients to ensure smooth relations between the hospital authorities and the beneficiaries and thus help in the building of a Welfare State, a cherished ideal in the constitutions of most of the states in the world.

We must attend to all these problems to ensure efficiency of the hospitals. These problems also emanate from a number of constraints on hospital authorities, e.g., shortage of staff at all levels, absence of proper accommodation to provide space to the ever increasing number of patients, shortages of funds, shortages of medicine, shortage of equipment, political and administrative interference, etc., which need to be attended to by the governments at the Union and State level to provide satisfactory hospital services. Besides, the patients and their relatives must cooperate with the hospital authorities to make the best use of the available resources. Thus, we shall have to have a three pronged attack increasing internal efficiency, mobilizing government support and enlisting people's cooperation to ensure the reputation, prestige, credibility and viability of the hospital services. We have divided all chapters in twelve volumes.

Authors would be rewarded if the recommendations made in various chapters are analysed and put to use to make hospitals efficient and effective in the twenty-first century.

Chandigarh

S.L. GOEL
R. KUMAR

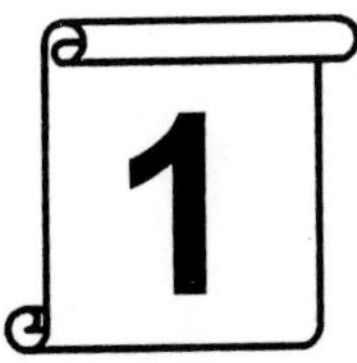

Health and Socio-Economic Development

MEANING AND GOALS OF DEVELOPMENT (See Chart 1.1)

The word 'development' is so often used in our daily life that we hardly care to think of its real meaning. The meaning of the term 'develop' is to unfold itself or to grow into a fuller or mature condition. And 'ment' stands for instrument of action, an act or process. So, in simple words development is to discover or unfold any hidden field. Development can be defined as a process of directed change towards some objectives which are accepted a.c; desirable goals. Development implies progressive improvements in the living conditions and quality of life enjoyed by society and shared by its members. It is a continuing process that takes place in all societies.

As stated in Dag Harnmarskjold Report, entitled What Now, Another Development Dialogue, 1975: 1/2, the goal of development is to ensure:

> "Development of every man and woman, and not just the growth of things, which are merely means 'for development geared to the satisfaction of needs beginning with the basic needs of the poor. ..'and for' development to ensure the humanisation of man by the satisfaction of his needs for expression, creativity, conviviality, and for deciding his own destiny." Development is a process of growth in the direction of modernity, especially towards nation-building and socio-economic progress. It has been stressed that "development is the rational process of organising and carrying out prudently conceived and staffed programmes or projects as one would organize and carry out military or engineering operations." Development has been defined in the same report, What Now Published by the Dag Hammarskjold Foundation, Uppasala, Sweden. It states,

Chart 1.1

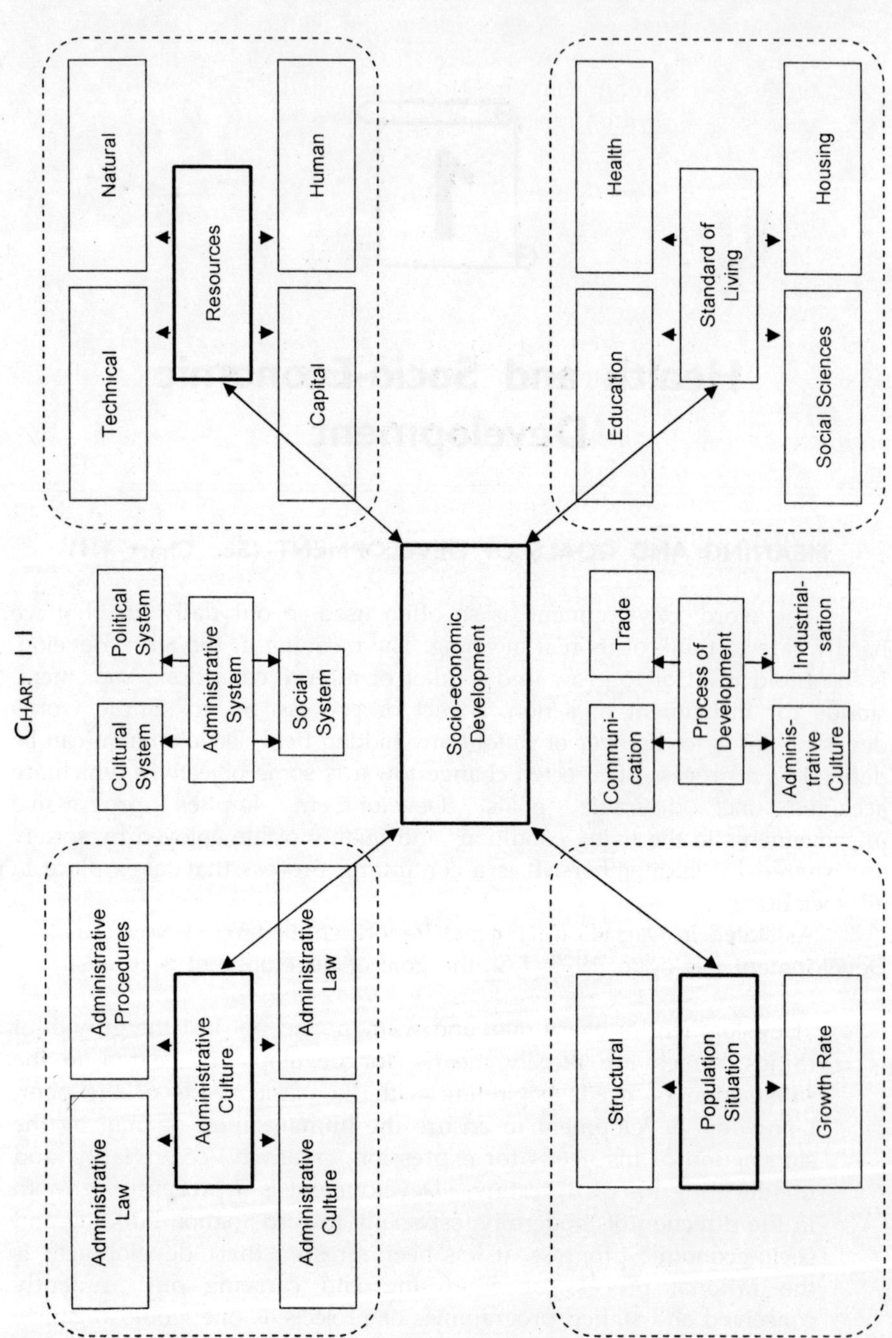
Socio-economic Development
Resources
Technical
Natural
Capital
Human
Standard of Living
Education
Health
Social Sciences
Housing
Administrative System
Cultural System
Political System
Social System
Process of Development
Communication
Trade
Administrative Culture
Industrialisation
Administrative Culture
Administrative Law
Administrative Procedures
Administrative Culture
Administrative Law
Population Situation
Structural
Growth Rate

> "Development is a whole; it is an integral, value loaded, cultural process; it encompasses the natural environment, social relations, education, production, consumption and well-being. Development is endogenous; it brings from the heart of each society, which relies first on its own strength and resources and defines in sovereignty the vision of its future, cooperating with societies sharing its problems and aspirations."[1]

We must be clear that the development is indeed a dynamic concept. Development implies growth plus social change. Nevertheless, development has often been conceived of primarily in economic terms, since sustained economic changes are necessary for the achievement of many social goals. This is not wholly correct. According to Dr. Candua, former Director-General of the WHO: "Among the objectives of the development are health and productivity. They are reciprocal and complementary. Without health, productivity can hardly flourish. On the other hand, productivity may increase means and opportunities for better health."[2]

Only a man who is healthy, enjoys working and is rewarded by a high degree of productivity. The hierarchy of goals of development may be shown in the form of a pyramid wherein at the base are basic minimum needs followed by economic and social necessities for bare subsistence. The fulfilment of these needs leads to a higher set of socio-political needs and ultimately to the goal of the full flowering of human personality or 'total development' and the release of the creative energies of every individual.[3]

4. Cultural	(4) full development of human potential and creativity,
3. Socio-political	(3) equity of distributive justice, social equality, redistribution of assets, democracy,
2. Economic-social	(2) higher growth with greater equity, mass consciousness, and
1. Basic minimum needs	(1) eradication of abject poverty and unemployment—access to minimum income and public services through employment with people participation.

According to Mr. K.S. Dadzie, United Nations Director-General for Development and International Economic Cooperation, "The final aim of development must be the constant increase of the well-being of the entire population on the basis of its full participation in the process of development and a fair distribution of benefits therefrom." Thus, the main aim of development should be to enrich the quality of life. Dr. T. Adeoya Lambo, Deputy Director-General, WHO, in his article, "Towards Justice in Health" in *World Health* (July, 1979) has rightly said:

> "What is happening around us shakes our complacency, challenges our faith in human progress and imbues us with an intense feeling of shame, doubt and guilt. In a world where the gigantic scientific

and phenomenal technological achievements command our admiration and almost fetish acceptance, we are witnessing an intolerable degradation of man. Our pride in belonging to a generation that for the first time since the genesis of man has set foot on another planet cannot, however, disguise the awful truth that it may be easier to travel to the moon than to erase from the surface of the earth, the image of inevitable poverty, human exploitation, injustice and the degradation of human welfare."

Our first concern is to redefine the whole purpose of development. Any process of growth that does not lead to human fulfilment or, even worse, that inhibits it is a travesty of the idea of development.

ASPECTS OF DEVELOPMENT

In fact, there the two aspects of development-economic and social, which cannot be isolated one from the other. P.C. Sikligar in his article, "Social Development: A Profile" in *IJPA*, April-June, 1998, rightly stresses the complimentary role of economic and social development. To quote him:

> "The term social development was separated from economic development in 1950s by the United Nations in their report on the World Social Situation, giving an impression that the human factors, like cultural dimension, value, social security, social justice, social welfare, social service, social policy, social work, political orientation, environmental issues, etc. were neglected since time immemorial in the framework of economic development. Earlier, social development was perceived as economic growth. Later on global economists also realised the importance of human factors which were neglected to economic development. Keeping in mind the human orientations, they accepted that the entire economic development could not become social development but it could only be a part of social development. In later stages, sociologists considered inclusion of needs of social values in the process of development. They emphasised that social development is more than economic development and the necessity to ensure development in all fields related to society's dimensions. In other words, it could be said that economic development could be helpful in the process of social development in a vital manner."

PERSPECTIVES OF ECONOMIC DEVELOPMENT: NEED OF SOCIAL DEVELOPMENT THRUST

Economic development—a high growth rate of the national product is a means to an end, i.e., it cannot in itself be the ultimate objective—the final goal of a dynamic society. Economic growth is never more than the method of obtaining the means through which a nation plans to achieve some form of social progress or social change. Developing nations have become increasingly conscious of the social aspects of economic planning. It is now generally realized that economic growth should be a means towards the eradication of hunger, illiteracy, disease, and reduction of existing social and economic inequalities. The consequences of growth without development are too painful to be ignored.[4] The correlation between economic growth and social development has tended to be low in the Asian, African and Latin American countries. In a recent study[5] this relationship has been critically examined. For this purpose, the authors devised a method of measuring development which combines social, economic and political factors. They, then studied the relationship between this measure and the per capita GNP—a usually accepted economic growth index among 74 developing countries. They found that per capita GNP is responsible only for about half of the variation in the indicators of meaningful development, bearing out the conclusion that economic growth has often failed to be really reflected in socio-economic development. The late Max Milikan had said: "There is a growing recognition that economic growth alone will not automatically bring with it all the virtues of modernization."[6] In other words, there is a realisation that development is a social as well as an economic process. Because of this intimate relationship, it is very difficult to isolate social development from the economic context.

> "If this inter-relationship is not taken into account material advances may be accompanied by loss of social cohesion, insecurity, delinquency, mental stress and other social ills. In fact, the trend is now for economic planning to give way to the socio-economic planning that involves planning for the social goals, with economic development as means rather than an end."[7]

Many writers have defined economic development in a broader sense. Myrdal has defined it as nothing less than the "upward movement of the entire social system,[8] or it may be interpreted as the attainment of ideals of modernisation "such as rise in productivity, industrialization, social and economic equalisation, development of modern knowledge, improved institution and attitudes, and a rationally coordinated system of policy measures that may on the one hand remove the host of undesirable conditions in the social system that have perpetuated a state of under development while on the other hand promote better nourishment, better health, better education, better living conditions, etc."[9] After over a quarter of a century's experience and experiments with economic growth models based on western models, we find that this model stands as the 'God that failed'. Nobel Laureate, Jan Tinbergen has rightly said: "The poor countries should reject the aim of initiating western patterns of life. Development is not linear process, and the aim of development is not to 'catch up' economically, socially, politically or culturally. Many aspects of western life have become wasteful and senseless and do not contribute to people's real happiness. For poor nations to attempt to imitate the rich may only mean that they trade one set of problems for another and in doing so discard or destroy much that is valuable in terms of their human resources and values."[10]

Thus began in the early seventies a search for another development (social development). To quote Mr. Mahbub Al Haq: "We are taught to take care of our GNP, since this would take care of poverty. Let us reverse this and take care first of poverty itself since GNP can take care of itself, for it is only a convenient summation, and not a motivation for human effort."[11]

PERSPECTIVES OF SOCIAL DEVELOPMENT (See Chart 1.2)

Social development is a broad concept encompassing improvement in the social status of the people enriching human capital. Social development lays stress on provision of health services—education, housing, cultural amenities, protection of children, a change in the status of women, regulation of labour and improved status for workers and reduction of disease, poverty and other social illness.

According to T.K.N. Unnithan,[12] "Social development may be seen as a process of ushering in a new order of existence. The quality of life and the quality of social relations which exist would indicate the level of the order of existence."

ECAFE meeting of the Working Party on Social Development held at Bangkok redefines the social development as: "The greater capacity of the social system, social structure, institutions and policy to utilize resources to generate favourable changes in levels of living interpreted in the broad sense as related to accepted social values, and a better distribution of income, wealth and opportunities."[13]

This is a comprehensive definition given by ECAFE (now ESCAP) in terms of the capacity of the social system to bring about favourable changes in the levels of living. The name of ECAFE has been changed to ESCAP to indicate the change in thrust to social development.

Social development is more concerned with the investment in human beings. A unit of investment in education, health, social welfare, etc., is, in the ultimate analysis, as productive as a unit of investment in agriculture, industry or trade. Research undertaken at the United Nations Research Institute for Social Development (UNRISD) in Geneva has indicated that developing countries, which have relatively high scores on social indicators, also tend to have high growth rates. Therefore, we must take a comprehensive view of development. Such a view of the development process would enable the planners to estimate realistically the social and economic changes and to accelerate those already taking place. Planning for 'people' must replace merely planning for aggregate production growth According to Dr. Salima Omer, Associate Professor, University or Nebraska, USA, social development is a "process that aims at the total development

CHART 1.2

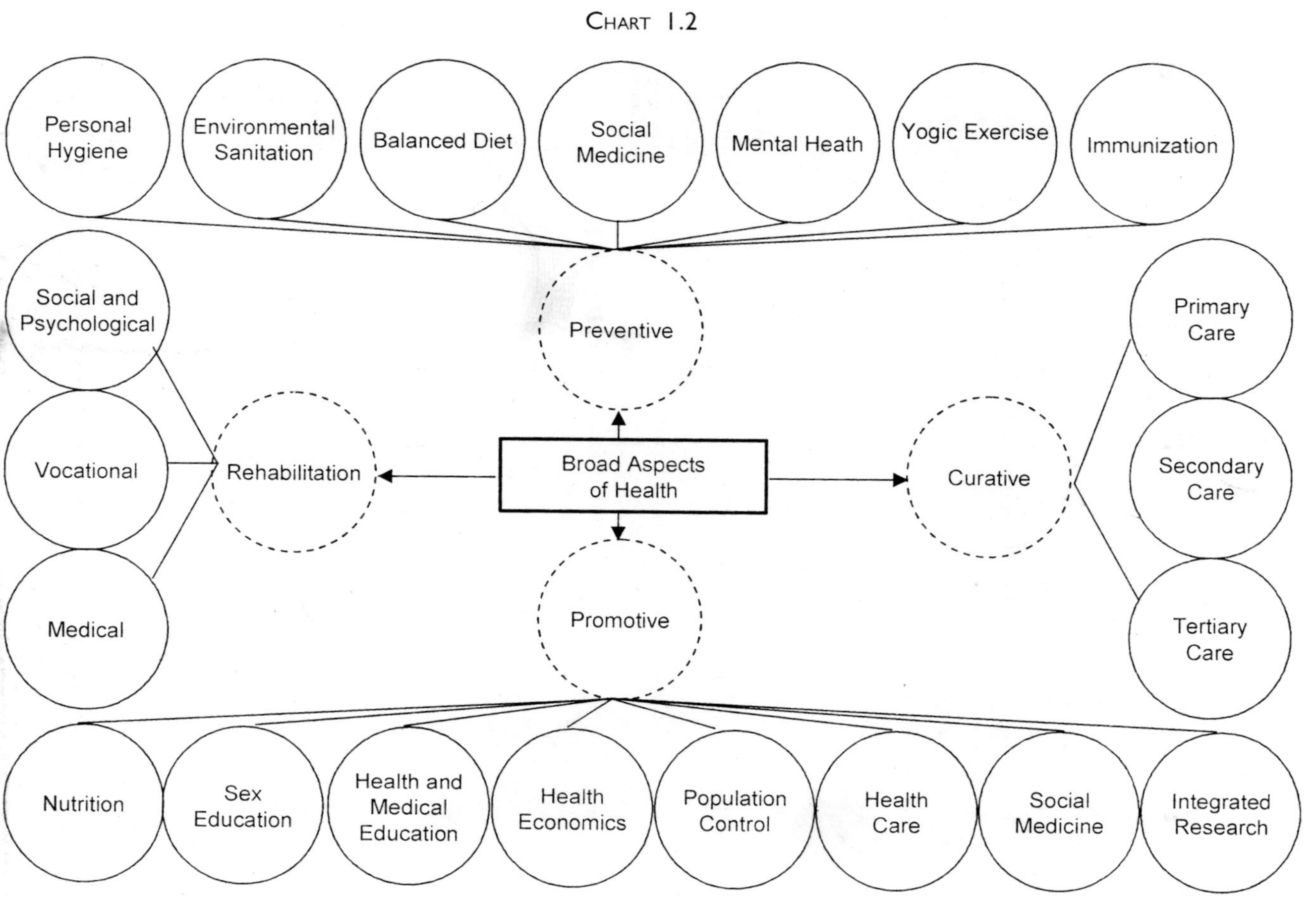
Personal Hygiene
Environmental Sanitation
Balanced Diet
Social Medicine
Mental Heath
Yogic Exercise
Immunization
Preventive
Social and Psychological
Vocational
Medical
Rehabilitation
Broad Aspects of Health
Curative
Primary Care
Secondary Care
Tertiary Care
Promotive
Nutrition
Sex Education
Health and Medical Education
Health Economics
Population Control
Health Care
Social Medicine
Integrated Research

of people. . . social development is inter-sectoral, inter-regional and inter-disciplinary and visualises institutional and structural reforms to provide greater social justice."[14]

It has been realised increasingly over the years that social development is necessary not only to provide opportunities to individuals for self-development but also as a vital contribution to economic development. The distinction between social and economic development is no longer tenable. Economic development is necessary to achieve most social goals and social development which is in turn is necessary to achieve most economic goals. The purpose of development is to permit people to lead economically productive and socially satisfying lives.

The emphasis of the strategy of UN Second Development Decade (1971-80) as well is on growth with social justice, removal of poverty and substantial rise in the level of employment. This strategy is fully based on the idea of total development, i.e., combining the social and economic development. To quote the strategy:

> "As the ultimate purpose of development is to provide increasing opportunities to all people for a better life, it is essential to bring about a more equitable distribution of income and wealth for promoting both social justice and efficiency of production, to raise substantially the level of employments, to achieve greater degree of income, security, to expand improved facilities for education, health, nutrition, housing and social welfare, and to safeguard the environment. Thus, qualitative and structural changes in the society must go hand in hand with rapid economic growth, and existing disparities—regional, sectoral and social should be substantially reduced."[15]

Dr. Mahler has very succinctly remarked in this connection:

> "Economic growth, without being specifically attuned to human needs and human realizations, is not worth very much. Once more you hear everywhere people speaking about nuclear energy, oil energy, solar energy, wind energy and everybody seems to be overlooking the fact that without human energy, there would be no kind of progress either socially or economically."[16]

Recently, four Asian scholars viewed development in terms of fundamental humanistic values rather than in narrow techno-economic terms. They mentioned five core principles, which stand inseparably together.

(1) Man as the end of development—which is therefore, to be judged by what it does to him.
(2) Delineation of man, in the sense that he feels at home with the

process of development in which he becomes the subject as well as the object.

(3) Development of collective personality of man in which he finds his richest experience.

(4) Participation as the true form of democracy.

(5) Self-reliance as the expression of man's faith in his own abilities.[17]

The three most vital players in the arena are the Elected Ruling Government, the appointment Administrative Machinery and the Demanding Public. While the ultimate responsibility and answerability/accountability rests with the first component, the actual job of delivering results rests on the administrative machinery. It is, in the ultimate analysis a joint team effort of the three but any weak link can jeopardize the outcomes and efforts of any other causing bad governance.

It may be useful to conclude with the remarks that the process of development is holistic in nature, encompassing political, social, economic and cultural aspects.

HEALTH CARE ADMINISTRATION AS A COMPONENT OF SOCIO-ECONOMIC DEVELOPMENT

In this work, we shall deal with one of the social services, i.e., health services. The health component and other components of the socio-economic system necessarily interact. Health not only affects the remainder of the socio-economic complex, but is also affected by it, sometimes favourably, sometimes unfavourably. K.S. Dodzie, United Nations Director-General for Development and International Economic Cooperation in his article, "The UN Answers the Challenge" in *World Health* (November, 1979) has rightly said: "The promotion and protection of the health of the people is essential to sustained economic and social development and contributes to a better quality of life and to world peace." The major areas in which health affects socio-economic development include problems arising out of the rate of population growth, rapid industrialisation and urbanisation, mental stress and social instability, environmental pollution and the growing disparity of living standards within and among nations. It needs to be reiterated here that social development not only continuously interacts with economic development but that the various aspects of social development keep on interacting with one another. 'A sound mind in a sound body' is an old proverb. Thus, changes in one sector of social activity produce changes in the other. We must see that these chain reactions are conducive to the attainment of overall objective of social development. Myrdal has summed up the position very succinctly as:

> "Standards of both health and education depend, in turn, on the whole social milieu, especially the prevailing attitudes and institutions."

In an overall and integrated concept of social and economic development of a country, health cannot be considered exclusively as an end itself. One must take into account also its role as one of the social sectors in overall development and try to establish measurable relationships between health and the microscopic variables, such as consumption, productivity and labour on which it depends or with which it is involved most directly. In other words, it is necessary to determine the investment in health required for development or the rate of development. The benefits accruing from health programmes are less difficult to measure. It is rarely, if ever, possible to identify all the consequences of a health programme, especially the long-term consequences. A health care is primarily a social service. Health programmes are mostly established because they contribute to the satisfaction of primary human needs, irrespective of economic considerations except in so far as they can be afforded and constitute an asset for the future. For this and other reasons, the cost and other data required to evaluate the contribution made by health programmes to development are rarely completely available, even when it would be feasible to obtain them.

To plan for health, that is, to meet the basic needs of the community and, at the same time, to satisfy the requirements of the overall pace for development is a complex process. It will be possible to achieve it fully when the economic benefits obtained with a specific health measure can be expressed in quantitative terms and when it is possible to measure precisely the degree of benefit to health from activities which are carried on outside this direct operational sphere. While health planners have always assumed that there is a good correlation between health and socio-economic development, doubts have been expressed by the general planners regarding such a correlation. Research is still in its infancy in this area. H. Leibenstein has rightly said that data on general relationship indicated that health and education were the most evident among the large 'residual' of factors that proved statistically more important than the usual economic indicators in explaining economic development.[18]

Prof. D. Banerji stresses the role of health as a contributor to economic growth and the need to integrate health activities into general economic activities so that the former do not interfere with the latter or vice versa. Dr. E.J. Thierry in his article, "Laying the Foundations", succinctly remarked that, "Health is man's most precious possession; it influences all his activities; it shapes the destinies of people. Without it, there can be no solid foundation for man's happiness. Nevertheless, all too often, social planners, forget this simple truth and leave health out of account: Integration of health schemes in overall development plans are of paramount importance."[19]

The tasks assigned to health economists in cooperation with planners include the development of instruments for measuring social phenomenon; the identification of the fields of health where the maximum results can be obtained with the available resources and the provision of and in improving the management of health services (e.g., in hospital establishment).[20]

Though progress has been made in the analysis and estimation of cost and benefits in public programmes, but cost-benefit analysis in public health area has lagged behind. The economics of health is a newer term than medical economics: it encompasses the medical care industry, extends into such fields as the analysis of the economic costs of diseases and the benefits of control programmes, return from investment in education and training, etc. Many have tried to evaluate man or, in other words, to put a price upon his economic worth. One of the earliest attempts was that of Sir William Petty (1623-87) who originated many ideas later used by the political economists. Adam Smith used in his Wealth of Nations and other works; Dublin Lotka and Spiegelman have attempted to translate the figures of life expectancy into terms of financial values to the community. It was observed that the period of infancy and early childhood represent a drain upon family and community resources. This investment made towards a productive age is therefore a loss to the community, not only in the investment made but also of future earnings of the individual. But, loss due to sickness, on the other hand, is limited to the duration of illness when the individual remains unproductive or underproductive from ill-health. Let us now mention the possible direct and positive effects of health on socio-economic development.

1. Many uninhabitable areas can be made fit for settlement and thus it can help in the exploitation of idle resources of that area, e.g., in Haryana, an area of Pehowa Block was made fit through the Malaria Eradication Programme. The area was infested with malarial parasites and was unfit for human settlement. Various studies have indicated the useful consequences of disease eradication programmes on agricultural development and ultimately economic growth.
2. It can help in the lowering of absenteeism rate resulting from poor health caused by diseases. Here, we must be cautious about its limitations in the developing countries where there is widespread unemployment or underemployment and where a sick person is readily replaceable without affecting the socio-economic conditions in these countries.[21]
3. Good health can promote good labour morale and productivity;, i.e., a healthy worker can work full-time and has a greater productivity potential. According to Benjamin, in these countries "where health conditions are worst and relatively simple, their low cost health programmes can produce dramatic lessening of the ability and disability of the labour force."[22]
4. Good health affects intelligence, improper nutrition and lack of mother-care can cause mental retardation and other mental problems. A study carried out by Correa and Cummins in

"Contribution of Nutrition to Economic Growth covering 18 countries for the period 1950-62, reveals that in 9 countries of Latin America, there was an increase in the national product, whereas the contribution was zero in the economically developed countries. The poorer the country, the greater the role of improved nutrition in its development.[23]

5. Good health is a basic right and produces civic consciousness. We should not look at health only as a means of economic development. What is more important is to view economic growth as contributing to the betterment of the health of the people, as it must be recognised that health is a basic human right, Thanis Kraivixien, the Prime Minister of Thailand, rightly said in his, inaugural address to the 30th WHO Regional Committee for South-East Asia, held at Bangkok, Thailand (28 August, 1977):

   "Any society should consider that a high quality of life, and the happiness of the people, which can only be obtained through a sufficient level of health, is not only a basic prerequisite to development but should be the basic objective of any development effort."[24]

6. Better health is generally associated with better capability and leadership. In a study by ILO on qualitative difference in the labour force, health was found to be the factor most clearly related to difference in economic growth.[25] According to Myrdal: The required personal qualities are certainly multiple and probably have a synergistic action. However, there can be no doubt that health plays an essential part."[26]

7. Better health induces positive attitudes conducive to economic growth and modernisation. The individuals become better citizens as they hope for future betterment and work hard to make the future more pleasant and enjoyable. Improved health may induce in the people to increase productivity and motivation to reduce family size.[27] The people with good health are generally enthusiastic and try to achieve higher and higher goals in life.

Let us now review some studies which have analysed the loss resulting from poor health or diseases. Sirton made an assessment of the financial loss due to malaria to the individual and the family alone at not less than Rs. 11,000 lakhs annually. In this conservative estimate of the annual financial loss to the country due to malaria; Sinton arrived at the figures of Rs. 1,000 crores. He stated:

"It constitutes one of the most important causes of economic misfortune engendering poverty, diminishing the quantity and quality of food supply, lowering the physical and intellectual standards of the nation and hampering increased prosperity and economic progress in every way."[28]

Tuberculosis is a widespread and contagious disease. A study was carried out by Dr. A.S. Sen and Dr. R.N. Basu, Consultant and Senior Research Officer, Planning Commission, Government of India, to measure the cost of tuberculosis in India.[29] They found that the total losses from mortality, morbidity and the direct cost[30] of the disease amounted to Rs. 420.4 crores, Rs. 288.58 crores and Rs. 29.68 crores respectively. The production loss due to mortality and morbidity from tuberculosis has been very large. As compared to these losses, the amount of direct expenditure which is being incurred on the control programme is very small. The annual direct cost for a population of about six million works out at Rs. 0:49 per person per annum. Hence, the eradication of tuberculosis is not only a social welfare activity but an ultimate economic gain.

Because of this inter-relationship, economic development cannot be isolated from the social context, health programmes cannot be related unilaterally to either the economic or the social spheres, as they influence both and are influenced by both. Thus, there is a need to promote, encourage and support research on the standardization of nomenclature, systems of health statistics, indices of health and socio-economic development, evaluation methods, and health economics theory and practice. The World Health Assembly Technical Discussion on the contribution of Health Programmes to socio-economic development (1972) arrived at the following general agreement:

> "It was recognised as a basic principle that health programmes are rarely ever justified solely on economic grounds, but rather as the means of, maintaining and improving health, which is perhaps the most important single factor in improving the quality of human life. It was accepted without question that health is an objective in its own right and represents one of the most important, manifestations of social progress."[31]

Thus, there is a clear indication of the need for knitting together social and economic components of development plans to attain intended objectives of development of the people, within a time schedule and resource schedule.[32]

All the countries of Asia, Africa and Latin America should apply development planning to accelerate socio-economic development, guided by social justice. Development planning relates to a teleologically-determined manipulation of policy measures and instruments devised so as to stimulate the authors of the socio-economic scene to act in the most conducive to the achievement of the national socio-economic development objectives and goals.[33] Thahane defines it as a "process of organizing national economic and social effort for the promotion or achievement of clearly defined national development goals."

The process of Development Planning can help us to get the benefits of modernisation which depends upon the "Systematic, sustained and purposeful application of human energies to the rational control of man's physical and social environment for various human purposes."[34]

The people inhabiting the developing world expect their governments to pull them out of the morass of distressing under development. This would be possible only provided the efforts of the Governments are comprehensive, selective, coordinated and sustained. Besides, timely action, backed by a strong will and determination at all decision-making and operational levels, can change the complexion of our socio-economic scene.

In the 21st century, development is going to pose a great challenge, because health of the people, which is a major component of development faces many challenges. We suggest here some ideas, which can promote health of the community and ultimately promote socio-economic development.

On the basis of our discussion and analysis, the following suggestions are given to revitalize the health care delivery system to meet the challenges and fulfil the basic health needs of the people:

(i) Will and determination on the part of the political elite, to accept innovative measures to meet the population's health needs and priorities.

(ii) Identification and implementation of a clear and comprehensive National Health Policy.

(iii) Decentralised planning, involving the participation of the target communities.

(iv) Mobilisation of existing and untapped resources—community, government (local and national), bilateral, multilateral and non-governmental—to provide adequate health care for all.

(v) Establishment of appropriate administrative structures with necessary competence and capability and devolution of authority and responsibility for the implementation and development of the programme in a team spirit and a well-designed information system to help in planning, implementation and evaluation.

(vi) Manpower development for national health needs.

(vii) Strengthening existing rural establishment and graded extension of national administrative structures to provide adequate and accessible referral, supervisory, logistical and other supporting services to ensure the judicious use of health services.

(viii) More allocation of financial resources based on the principles of equitable distribution and maximum utility.

(ix) Encouraging integration and coordination.

(x) Reorientation of Medical Education to suit the needs of the community.

(xi) Designing health technology to suit the environment and making the best use of existing technology of traditional system of medicine.

(xii) Improving research and development capacity to solve health problems.

(xiii) Devising measures to promote the use of simple, standardised equipment and drugs, placing reliance on available local resources whenever possible to foster self-reliance.

(xiv) The preventive health measures are crucial for sustained improvement and must be intensified to attain:

(a) Total coverage of the entire urban and rural population in the country with assured potable drinking water supply and sewerage;

(b) The disposal of urban wastes should also be given a high priority to ensure clean environment;

(c) For improving the environmental sanitation and hygiene, high priority must be given to town and country planning, provision of better working and living conditions, removal of congestion through the increased tempo of housing construction, slum clearance and prevention of water and air pollution;

(d) The nutritional status of the population must be raised and total prevention of food adulteration and drugs control should be achieved through rigorous controls; and

(e) Health education should be an integral part of all health programmes.

It is hoped that the implementation of these suggestions would ensure wider and more evenly distributed health care based on social justice, greater involvement and satisfaction of the beneficiaries and more efficient and more economical health services in new millennium.

O.P. Diwivedi[35] in his article, "Development Administration: an Over View" suggests challenges of sustainable development in the new millennium.

The challenge before the leaders and administrators of developing nations is then, how to achieve sustainable development and yet provide basic human needs (the provision of food, appropriate habitat, health and education), as well as social justice, removal of poverty and self-reliance with very limited resources.

They will have to be more self-reliant in the 21st Century, as they cannot expect the same level of development and as the attention of the West turns more towards helping Eastern Europe. So they must consider being self-reliant and using their own resources among and between themselves much more than they have done so far. For this they will require a cadre of professionally trained and dedicated administrators, as well as moral and just politicians who can stand against the forces of corrupt politics and unscrupulous commercial and business interests. Specially, development administrators have an obligation to serve the public in a manner which strengthens the integrity and process of governance. Such is the challenge and duty for the leaders and administrators of developing nations in the 21st Century.

Good Governance can provide all the inputs based on knowledge, creativity, innovation and motivation. People's participation, for development/productivity/efficiency and fulfil the dreams of millions of People enshrined in the constitution, budgetary, documents, five year Plans and often repeated promises of the executives. Good Governance can transform a developing country like India into a developed world where India can be counted among the few top countries of the world. It is expected that the executive machinery of the government of any political party should attend seriously politically intractable problems, avoid tendency to retain power by depriving citizens of basic human rights or manipulating ethnic conflict. The party should attend to all the problems affecting socio-economic development and for promoting the process of good governance leading to development modernization, dynamism. This will make resurgent of modern India contemplated by the leadership who got us Independence. The need of the hour is to develop dynamism, development, democracy through good governance based on innovation, creativity, talent, skill, etc. in order to usher an era where there is no poverty, no exploitation, no fear, as well as all follow the ethical values. The need of good Governance is of great significance in the new and emerging areas which have to take their roots.

Notes and References

1. Milton J. Esman, "The Politics of Development Administration," in Montgomery and Stimn, (eds.); Approaches to Development of Politics, Administration and Change, New York, McGraw Hill, 1965, p. 9.
2. Message from Dr. M.G. Candua, Director-General of the WHO, MI the *World Health*, March 1969, p. 5.
3. R.C. Malhotra, 'An Alternative Strategy for Self-sustained Development with focus on Participation by the Poor at the Local Lever, paper presented to Consultative Meeting on Alternate Strategy for Development with Focus on Local-level Planning Development (from 31st Oct. to 4th Nov. 1978)—UN Asian and Pacific Development Institute, Bangkok, April 1979, p. 5.
4. Salvatore Schiavo—Campo and Hans W. Sorger, Perspective of Economic Development (Houghton, Mifflin Co., Boston, 1970.)
5. Irma Adelman and Cyntila T. Morris, Society, Politics and Economic Development, John Hoptrus Press, 1967.
6. Max Milikan, "A Strategy for Development", Centre for Social and Economic Information, Executive Briefing Paper I, New York, 1970.
7. WHO, Public Health Paper, "Inter-relationship between Health Programmes and Socio-economic Development", 49, Geneva, 1973, p. 32.
8. Gunnar Myrdal, "Asian Drama", New York, 1968, p. 1869.
9. C.E. Black, The Dynamics of Modernization, New York, 1966, pp. 55-60.

10. Jan, Tinbergen, Reshaping the International Order: a Report to the Club of Rome, New York, E.P. Dutton and Co. Inc., 1976, Chapter 5, pp. 61-64.
11. Aly, Haq., Mahbub, The Poverty Curtain, p. 48.
12. T.K.N. Unnithan, "Development Processes in an Underdeveloped Country (India)" in Carle, C. Zimmerman and Richard E. Dumors (eds.); Sociology of Underdevelopment, Jaipur, Rawat, 1976 (Asian ed.), p. 402.
13. ECAFE, Seminar on Meeting of the Working Party on Social Development, (Bangkok, 8-15, December 1970).
14. UN, Asian and Pacific Development Institute, Proceedings of a Consultative Meeting, Bangkok, April 1979, p. II.
15. UN General Assembly Resolution, 24th October, 1973, para 83.
16. Text of Address of Dr. H. Mahler, Director General, WHO—WHO Regional Committee for South-East Asia, Thirteenth Session, Bangkok, Thailand, 28 Aug., 1977, Published in Final Report and Minutes of the Meeting of the Thirteenth Session, WHO, New Delhi, Sept., 1977, p. 64.
17. Haque Wahidul, Niranjan Mehta, Anjsur Rahman and Poona Wignaraja, "Towards A Theory of Rural Development,", Development dialogue, 1977; Dag Hammarskjold Foundation, Uppasala, Sweden in B.P. Desai, Planning in India (1951-78), Vikas Publishing House, Ghaziabad (UP), 1979, p. 158.
18. H. Leibenstein, Theories, Non-traditional Inputs and Interpretation of Economic History in P. Deprez (eds.) Population and Economic, Economic History Association, Winnipeg University of Manifolia, 1968.
19. Dr. F.J. Thierry, "Laying the Foundation" in *World Health*, March 1969, p.13.
20. D.C. Banerji, (1967), "Health Economics in Developing Countries", *Indian Medical Journal*, Ass. 49, pp. 417-21.
21. WHO, Public Health Papers, No. 64, p. 20.
22. B. Benjamin, Social and Economic Factors Affecting Mortality in Confluence, Surveys of Research in the Social Services, Vol. V. (Hague Mauton Co.), 1965.
23. H. Correa and G. Cummins (1970): "Contribution of Nutrition to Economic Growth," *American Journal Clin. Nutr*, 23, S60-63 in World Health Papers, 49, p. 47.
24. WHO, SEARO: SEA/RC. 30, p. 64.
25. Galenson and G. Pyatt, The Quality of Labour and Economic Development in Certain Countries, Geneva, ILO, 1964.
26. G. Myrdal, Asian Drama—An Inquiry into the Poverty of Nations, New York, Pantheon, 1968.
27. M. Perlman, "On Health. Population Change, and Economic Developments", in M. Perlman and other (eds.), Spatial, Regional and Population Economics, Essays in Honour of Edgar M. Hoover (New York and Breach, 1972), pp. 293-310.
28. J.A. Sinon, "What Molaria Costs in India Nationally, Socially and Economically", condensed and reprinted in Health Bulletin in 19S8, No. 26, Government of India Press, p. 125.
29. A.S. Sen and B.N. Basu, Economics of Health—The Cost of Tuberculosis Planning Commission, Government of India, Health Division, 1968, pp. 1-35.
30. Direct Cost means expenditure on hospitals, clinics, drugs, research, training, BCG vaccination, etc.
31. WHO: World Health Assembly, 1972, A/25, Technical Discussion, 66, p. 6.
32. UN: Proceedings of the Inter-regional Seminar on Organization and Administration of Development Planning Agencies, Vol. I, p. 113 (Sales No. E.74 II, H. 2).

33. T.T. Thahane, Planning for Development, in John Barratt und others, (eds.), Accelerated Development in Southern Africa, London, Macmillan, 1974, p. 451.
34. Quoted in Marrico B. Jansen, ed., Changing Japanese Àttitude Towards Modernisation, Princeton, 1965, pp. 23-24.
35. O.P. Dwivedi, "Development Administration.. An Overview" in *UPA*, July-Sept. 1997, pp. 321-22.

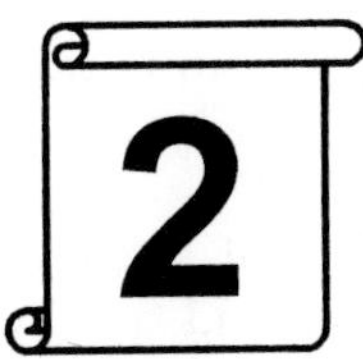

Functions and Role of Senior Chief Executives in Hospitals

(Director/Medical Supdt./Others)

In the health system, the top level positions are occupied by Director-General of health services at the Union Level, Director of health services at the state level and district health officers at district level. These top-level health functionaries are the chief executives in their respective jurisdiction. Since most of them occupy these higher offices on the basis of only seniority, they may not possess insight, vision, depth, and creative intelligence to tackle the health issues. It is very important that Government selects persons with right qualities of head and heart to occupy these positions to inject dynamism in health services. An organization is like a ladder. At the top of the ladder is the chief executive, who is responsible for hospital Administration and productivity.

In the sacred book, Bhagvad Geeta, Chapter III, Sloka 21, it has been rightly said that whatever a great man (chief executive) does, that very thing other men also do; whatever standard he sets, the generality of men follow the same.

The success of the organization depends, to a great extent, upon the personality, interest, ethos, perception and attitude of its chief executive. Therefore, there is a need for great care and forethought before appointing the chief executive of an organization.

As a member of the Hospital's senior management team, the Chief Executive Officer (CEO) will participate in planning and decision-making processes necessary for the successful attainment of the hospital's mission in addition to maintaining an awareness of changes in health care matters that could have an impact on the success of the hospital.

The responsibilities of the Medical superintendent/Chief Executive Officer include, but are not limited to:

1. Overall operations of the acute-care facility.
2. Working with system management to develop and implement policies and procedures, short- and long-range goals, objectives and plans.
3. Providing leadership to hospital managers, directors and officers that will enroll support, create ownership of goals, and encourage active participate in decisions that impact the hospital.
4. Ensuring the hospital meets necessary regulatory and compliance approvals and quality accreditations in conjunction with the hospital's Chief Nursing Officer.
5. Partnering with physicians who use, or will use, the hospital; taking a leadership role in the recruiting and retention of physicians.
6. Assisting in planning new services that generate additional sources of profitable revenue.
7. Creating an environment that will encourage the recruiting and retention of qualified hospital employees.
8. Managing costs by continually seeking data that will identify opportunities and take action to eliminate non-value costs in conjunction with the hospital's Chief Financial Officer and Chief Nursing Officer.
9. Developing and maintaining positive relations with community that the hospital is located as well as the community leaders.
10. Analyzing areas in planning, promoting and conducting organization-wide performance improvement activities.
11. Representing the hospital at meetings including medical staff, hospital board of director meetings as well as relevant community meetings; participates with leaders in designing and providing patient care and services. At each monthly meeting the committee of visitors he shall state the number of patients received and discharged, the number of deaths, the manner of employment, the number remaining in the hospital, distinguishing sexes, the weekly cost of maintenance with such matters as may appear as desirable.
12. Participating in the hospital's monthly operation reviews as well as participating in corporate office meetings as deemed necessary.
13. He shall have full control over all attendants and servants and shall regulate their duties and have authority to suspend them whenever he shall deem it expedient reporting the same of the first meeting of the Committee of Visitors.
14. He shall be responsible for the management and condition of the establishment and of the patients therein and shall have the direction of the medical, surgical and moral treatment of the patients and of all general arrangements within the hospital,

and in case of emergency shall have the power of calling on the assistance of any physician or surgeon. He shall also in all cases of fatal or dangerous accident or other emergency immediately communicate the fact in writing to one of the committee or to their clerk.

15. He shall ensure examination of every patient on admission and make proper entries thereof and take care that such medicines as he may think proper for their certain and speedy cure be duly administered. He shall see every patient once a day and oftener, if requested. He shall order and be responsible for the drugs, surgical instruments and books belonging to the asylum and he shall report the case of every patient fit for discharge to one or more of the Committee of Visitors.
16. He shall classify the patient of both sexes and shall regulate and determine at all times the diet of the sick and infirm patients. He shall also have the power from time to time to examine and report on the quality of all provisions furnished for the use of the patients.
17. He shall never be absent himself for one night or for any longer period without the previous written consent of the Managing Committee.
18. He shall sign all orders for the delivery of store or other articles for the use of the hospital such orders to be limited by the contract to be from time to time entered into by the Committee or if on an emergency he shall be given an extra order, it shall be reported to the next meeting of the Committee.
19. He shall be authorized to give directions for any requisite to buildings or works and shall report that same and other repairs needed to the Committee at their next meeting.

Public Relations Office (PRO): A case study of Lucknow Deemed University Hospital

The hospital has a Public Relations Office situated in the main building. It functions round the clock throughout the year to provide information and assistance to patients and their attendants. This was started in 1964. At present it is manned by 3 Public Relations Officers, 1 Enquiry Assistant and 2 other staff members of the hospital. The PRO has a unique functioning and is an important link between the hospital administration and the patient. Besides helping the patients, the office manages all the administrative matters of the hospital after working hours and on holidays. It has a close link with the police and press. A good number of security and other staff are attached to this office to maintain law and order and help in keeping the campus clean with regular supply of water and electricity. The ambulances are also under the control of this office. The present PRO's are: Smt. Homa Jafar, Mr. Rahul Singh and Mr. Manoj Srivastava.

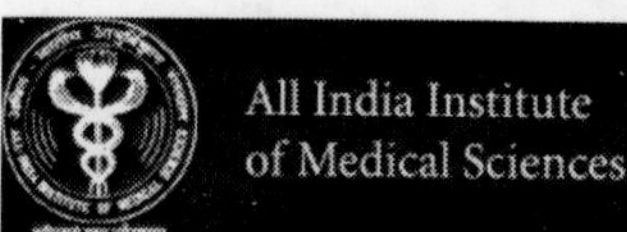

Administration

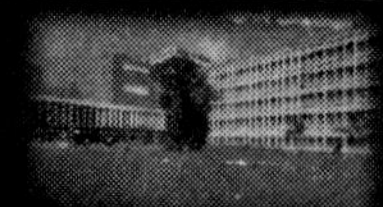

Organizational Structure
Constitution of various committees at AIIMS
Institute Body (IB)
Governing Body (GB)

Finance Committee	Academic Committee	Selection Committee	Estate Committee	Hospital Affairs Committee

President I.B.
Chairman G.B.
Director

Administration Deputy Director Administration	Academics Dean	Hospital Medical Superintendent	Centres Chiefs of Centres	Computer Facility Deputy Director Computer Facility

Administration
Deputy Director Administration

Sr. Financial Advisor	Sr. Administrative Officer	Estate Manager	Store Officer	Superintending Eng.	Security Officer	Public Relation Officer	Labour Officer

Gr. A, B, C & D Staff

Academics
Dean
Sub Dean

Registrar Academic Section	Examination Section	Head of Departments Faculty Asstt. Prof.	Assoc. Prof.	Addl. Prof	Professor

Hospital
Medical Superintendent
Additional Medical Superintendent
Deputy Medical Superintendent
Manager

Duty Officers for OPD and Casualty	All Clinical Laboratories	Hospital Records	Wards, Private Wards & Operation	Hospital Peripheral Services Laundry, Blood Bank etc.	Medical Stores	Nursing Staff

Centres
Chiefs of Various Centres

Chief of De-addiction Centre	Chief of CNC	Chief of RPC	Chief of IRCH

Head of Departments
Faculty
Officers & Other Staff
Under Graduate students
Post Graduate students
Senior Resident, Junior Resident
SRF, JRF

Computer Facility

Deputy Director & Head
System Analyst
Senior Programmer
Programmer

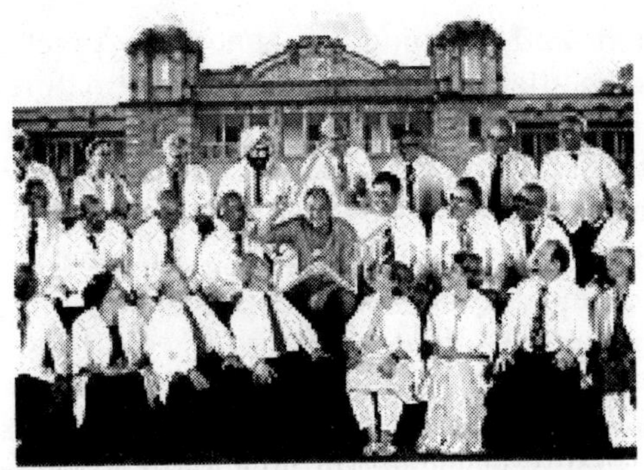

SOME OTHER SERVICES IN THE HOSPITAL ATTACHED TO THE UNIVERSITY

The medicines, drugs and gases, etc. are supplied in the hospital from the **Central Medical Store**, and surgical dressing material, spirit, tincture, stationery, case sheets, printed forms, cleansing material, etc. from the General Store. The stores are under supervision of Medical Officer (Stores). The hospital has its own **Dispensary** also where mixtures, ointments, etc. are prepared and distributed to OPD and indoor patients. This is under the supervision of Prabhari Adhikari Pharmacy, Sri Mumtaz Ahmed. He also monitors the supply of drugs, etc. to the wards. To assist him there are 3 Chief Pharmacists, Mr. J.K. Paliwal, Mr. R.C. Sinha and Mr. Ram Bharosey.

The **X-ray Department** of the hospital functions round the clock and is under the Head, Department of Radiodiagnosis, Prof. S. Bhadury.

The **Cobalt Therapy Unit** is under the Head, Department of Radiotherapy—Prof. Madhu Srivastava.

There are 2 whole body CT scan units obtained through wet lease—one for the Department of Radiotherapy and the other for the Department of Radiodiagnosis.

The hospital has a modern **Mortuary** where postmortem examinations of all medicolegal cases of Lucknow District are performed. This is under the control of the Superintendent of the hospital and Chief Medical Officer, Lucknow.

Lastly, the finances and accounts of the hospital and university are looked after by a **Finance, Accounts and Audit Office**, which has a staff of 50 officials under the administrative control of the Finance Officer, deputed by the State Government. The present Finance Officer is Sri Abdul Ghani.

CEOs of District (Community) Hospitals: A case study in South Africa

District hospitals play an important role in the delivery of health services at community level, especially in rural areas. These hospitals provide comprehensive level-one health services to their communities, and serve as a resource for the whole health district. Most district hospitals are situated in rural areas, with medical services in these hospitals being rendered by generalist medical practitioners.

The education and training of generalist practitioners for rural practice needs specific attention. Firstly, the unique nature of rural practice makes it necessary for doctors to undergo relevant and focused instruction. Rural family practice requires that doctors have the knowledge and skills to practice in settings where high technology and specialist resources are not available, while at the same time requiring that they be able to perform a wide range of advanced functions and procedures.

Secondly, it is argued that appropriate education and training for rural practice can positively influence the recruitment and retention of medical practitioners in rural areas. The teaching of the knowledge and skills required for rural practice should take place in an appropriate setting that promotes interest in rural practice and familiarizes the student with its particular challenges.

There is a paucity of data in South Africa on medical practitioners staffing district hospitals, especially in terms of their knowledge and skills levels. Such information is critical if rural hospitals are to deliver equitable and quality health services, and also for guiding appropriate undergraduate, postgraduate and continuing professional education for rural practice. With this as background, health service managers in the Western Cape requested a skills audit of medical officers in district hospitals to identify a possible gap in competencies that may impact on service delivery. The aim of this study was thus to identify the knowledge and skills of medical practitioners delivering these services in the Western Cape and to compare them with service needs in order to make recommendations for education and training.

This study reports on the results of the knowledge and skills gap analysis. The knowledge and skills gaps varied considerably according to the individuals' education, training and experience, as well as their circumstances and working conditions. The superior competencies of the older practitioners reinforce the importance of the recruitment and retention of more experienced practitioners. The uneven skill and knowledge base in aspects of HIV/AIDS management should be addressed urgently by initiatives such as the internet-based course on HIV/AIDS developed by the Family Medicine Education Consortium (FaMEC). Departments of Family Medicine should urgently re-orientate their curricula to meet the training needs for level-one hospital practice.

Qualities of Leadership

A Medical Superintendent/Director is the head of a hospital depending upon the size and complexity of a hospital. Secondary Health Care hospitals are manned by Senior Medical Officer (SMOs), medical Superintendents while tertiary health care has a higher-level post called Director. These posts require both technical as well as administrative knowledge to run the hospital efficiently. Since medical superintendents/ Directors are from medical background, they lack administrative skill resulting into poor performance.

The success or failure of the organization depends to a substantial extent upon the capacity, capability, motivation and perception of the chief executive and his team. The chief executive has to facilitate the accomplishment of desired objectives with the least friction and the most satisfaction to those for whom the task is done and those engaged in the enterprise. According to Edwin E. Chiselli (American Pshychologist, Vol. 18, No. 10), talented chief executives are well endowed intellectually, gifted with the capacity to direct the efforts of others, self-stimulated to action, confident in their abilities and striving for a position where they can most fully utilize them. Top executives are to provide leadership to the organization. According to Haimann, "Leadership is the process by which an executive or a manager imaginatively directs, guides and influences the work of others in choosing and attaining specified goals by mediating between the individual and the organization in such a manner that both will obtain the maximum statisfaction."[1]

To quote Keith Davis, "Leadership is the ability to persuade others to seek defined objectives enthusiastically. It is the human factor which binds a group together and motivates it towards its goals."[2] It is said that a critical part of health and medical reform to promote health executive development and the role that executives play in productivity. Effective management must start from the top and work downward. Standards and reasonable health and medical objectives should be developed from a high degree of involvement and inter-relationship at each level so that no instruction is given or goal set which is not shared and reasonable. In the final analysis, the work performed by an employee at the lowest level cannot be more effective than the work performed by the person setting the goals.[3]

Without the right hospital chief executives, administration will not merely retard the heading processes but may even retard the health and medical development effort. The quality of the men placed in top positions is more important than laying down of rules and methods of operation.

The hospital administrator is the key executive of the hospital. Success or failure of the hospital depends to a great extent upon the competence, capability, perception, ethos and dedication of hospital administrators. The most important qualification is technical knowledge and administrative knowledge. Either he should be a postgraduate in hospital administration or has attended courses in hospital administration.

Let us discuss the essential qualities required for medical Superintendent/Director in the field of Hospital Administration. So that they can be effective health and medical leaders.

The secret of right action in reality is not a secret. It does not lie in any formula that we repeat. There is no magic by means of which we can follow the path of idleness and yet make our life productive. No! The secret lies in our own motives, in our power of application. It is not the strong physical vehicle which makes the productive human being; it is skillfulness in action, knowing how to adjust ourselves quickly, how to perform a task with the least expenditure of energy. This is what gives immediate success.[4].

Robert M. Hutchines states, "Thus, all organizations can function and achieve excellence provided all its members strive to pursue the goals of the organization earnestly, sincerely, whole-heartedly and with dedication."[5]

Our thought is the seed, which determines the fruit of our action. If the seed is good, then the flowers and fruit, which come from the seed, must be good and must prove beneficial to ourselves and others. But if we plant in our hearts a poisonous seed, it will harm not only ourselves but all who come in contact with us. Human life is a great responsibility. Only a thoughtless man will say: I cannot help what happens, I am not responsible. We are constantly influencing ourselves and our fellow-beings by what we think, because our thought shapes our inner nature and we radiate consciously or unconsciously what we are. Let us be wakeful then. Let us be thoughtful in whatever we do. Let us be faithful to our true self; for all blessings must come to us, if we prove ourselves true to our higher nature.

Work Culture

Health and Medical Leaders must create work culture and not psycho-fancy. Work culture is at the lowest ebbs these days. Bata K. Dey in his Article, 'Work Culture in India-Achievements and Failure' rightly says that culture is not something, which can be imported or transplanted; it must grow from within; it grows, and it does, in fertile soil and congenial climate. Gap in capital equipment or technology can be filled by import. You can even buy management, but not dedication, commitment, culture. How to create that is a million dollar question. An inexpensive answer to such a costly question is that, work culture tends to be congruous with, and is an extension of, the societal, indeed national culture. And the latter, at the moment, is the elusive commodity, despite this country's ancient civilization and old culture. The search is on. And we shall succeed.[6]

Murtaza Mithani, Chairman and Managing Director of Wintech Group in his article, "The High Road", in *The Tribune*, dated June 28, 2000 expects his employees to be committed to their work. "As the head of an organization, I, expect my employees to be innovative, competitive and flexible. They should possess total commitment, be actively involved in every day work, and have no hastiness while interacting. He wants his team to be able to work in synergy with various departments. Failures and challenges should be treated as a stepping-stone to success. Think big, create your own space and help yourself." The health and medical leaders must create a work culture and among health and medical personnel to provide decent health care delivery.

Need of Commitment and Empathy

Quality needs teamwork and mutual understanding. Personnel in health and medical care must work in a team to achieve quality. S.J. Maricodoss mentions two ingredients of teamwork commitment and empathy. These can be developed by sound health and medical leadership. To quote him:

> Commitment is a deep and profound value of emotional intelligence. It means aligning oneself with the goals of a group or organization. It is applying oneself completely for a cause. People possessing this competence readily make sacrifice to meet larger organizational goals. Hence more than the individual interests, the group's mission or interest takes priority. It is very deep to the extent of sacrificing oneself. It also involves taking sides or taking stance.

Emotionally balanced people are generally empathetic and not sympathetic. Sympathy perpetuates oppression and makes people dependent. Sympathy is a form of judgment. We should therefore avoid being sympathetic towards others. Empathy means understanding the issue or concern that lie behind another's feeling. It is an ability to look at things from other's point of view or to read another's emotions or to put oneself into other's shoes and think from their angle. Avoiding pretension, it enables sensing and responding to a person's unspoken concern or feelings. It can be called the foundation skill for all the social competencies. Empathetic listening is a tremendous deposit in the Emotional Bank Account. Empathy includes understanding others, service orientation, developing others, leveraging diversity and political awareness.[7]

Azim Premji in his article, "Leader for the Knowledge Era" rightly suggests that leaders must build star performers and teams. They must not only attract the best of minds to join the organization but create a strong sense of ownership in them. Ownership is not just offering stock options. It has more to do with an emotional engagement and integration with the organization.

The most important quality on which actual role of medical and health leadership would depend is the integrity. In this context, Peter Drucker rightly observes that a person who does not have the integrity of character is unfit to be a manager and a gentleman. According to Ordway Tead, the Chief Executive, besides integrity, must possess the following qualities:[8]

(i) Physical and nervous energy;
(ii) Enthusiasm;
(iii) Sense of purpose and direction;
(iv) Technical mastery;
(v) Friendliness and affection;
(vi) Decisiveness;
(vii) Intelligence; and
(viii) Faith.

Chester Barnard mentions the following qualities:[9]

(i) Vitality and endurance;
(ii) Decisiveness;
(iii) Persuasiveness;
(iv) Stability in behaviour;
(v) Intellectual ability; and
(vi) Knowledge.

In spite of the awareness of the importance of the chief executive in an organization, the selection process of CEOs in public health sector leaves much to be desired and most of the CEOs are appointed purely on seniority or on political affiliations.

We must induct chief executives in health system from any source and as Paul H. Appleby has said, "The persons capable of serving well at high levels are rare birds, they must be sought wherever they may be found and developed by various methods." The need is to change the frame of mind of these chief executives, to make them more adventurous in style, more determined to change the way things are done, perhaps, braver.

There is a need to link the promotion of those personnel to position of the chief executives of health and medical organizations who are result-oriented. A chief executive who cannot take the right decision at the right time cannot aspire to be a successful executive. Therefore, seek those individuals in the organizations who have proved their worth in achieving productivity. To quote A.P. Saxena; Productivity will only be feasible if administration can provide a corpus of administrators, who are knowledgeable and skilful and have a sense of dedication to the goals of health and medical organizations. Such health and medical administrators will have to fulfil several roles. These will include:

(a) As experts who are capable of identifying problems and providing solutions, who will recognize priorities of productivity tasks and apply their expertise to these tasks;
(b) As change agents who know the conditions and directions of change, understand their roles and can direct efforts toward change, keeping the key focus on productivity; and
(c) As leaders who organize and mobilize people and resources, both physical and financial to fulfil the productivity tasks.[10]

There must be a regular appraisal system to screen the functioning of the chief executives. The appointing authorities must be prompt in taking quick decisions regarding the services of the chief executive on the basis of performance appraisal.

C. Rajagopalachari in his lecture delivered under 'Sardar Vallabhbhai Patel Lectures Series' on 14th August 1955 had said that character is by no means enough. But without it, let it be remembered, nothing else will be of any avail. It is like daylight, which we are apt to forget on account of its very importance. Therefore, there is a need to ensure that men of right character occupy high positions.

Let me quote a few words a thousand years old, they are as true toady. "The efficiency of the army consists partly in the order and partly in the general, but chiefly in the latter, because he does not depend upon the order, but the order depends upon him." Therefore, there is a great need to select and develop the right chief executives to produce social change and modernization in health system.

If the ideal of health administration is to provide better medical care to the people then we shall have to see that in a given situation we make the best possible use of our resources in terms of personnel and finances to achieve optimum results. For instance, in a developing country life India, the health administrator should normally be concerned with the following:

(a) that the patients are treated as close to their homes as possible in the smallest, cheapest and simply equipped unit such as a sub-centre which is capable of looking after them adequately;
(b) that the medical services should be organized and administrated in such a way that the quality of medical care improves gradually;
(c) that medical care services should be organized from the bottom-up and not from the top-down;
(d) that the services planned should meet the needs of the people;
(e) that the members of the health and medical personnel function as a well-knit team; and
(f) that new categories of health personnel such as multi-purpose health workers and community health workers should be given suitable training and support to provide simple medical care and preventive services to large sections of the community.

Generating Ethical and Moral Values

Chief Executives need to develop ethical and moral standards. Public services must also develop the normative linkages, i.e., they must develop professional standards which should help them in their best performances. Standards are contagious. They spread throughout an organization, a group, or a society. If an organization or group cherishes high standards, the behaviour of the individual who enters it is inevitably influenced. They should not develop an excessive sense of self-importance or arrogance. As has been said the Gita, "We should purse the path of excellence without fear or favour and work ceaselessly to achieve the objectives." Good organization building has to create around it a bracing atmosphere, a prideful tradition of integrity, excellence and fellowship. Human beings breathe an ethos around them almost unconsciously, these traditions make for that ethos."[11]

Functions of the Chief Executive of Health and Medical Organizations

The functions of the chief executive are increasing at a very fast rate in keeping with the complexity of the health and medical organization, like the evolution of man from a one-cell animal to a complex and specialized human being. With the growth in complexities, many tools, techniques and instruments have been developed, which can help the chief executive in attending to his modern and complex functions in an efficient manner.

Health system is becoming complex as new problems like non-communicable diseases, disease of modern life style, etc. are raising their head. So the health executives must be well equipped to tackle these problems before these become explosive. Let us enumerate some of the important functions of the health and medical executives.

I. *Allocating Work among Line, Staff and Auxiliary Agencies*

The chief executive carries out his work through line, staff and auxiliary agencies, as he cannot discharge his functions individually with speed and efficiency.

Line Agency

Line organization is the oldest and the simplest form of structure. The 'term' line has been borrowed from the military organization. Line agency is concerned with the carrying out of the primary objects of the organization and, thus, deals directly with the persons concerned. The citizens come directly in contract with line agencies. The following are the characteristics of a line agency:

(a) Authority flows from top level to the lower levels through delegation and decentralization to ensure the carrying out of activities at each level commensurate with responsibility.
(b) It consists of direct vertical relationships through various levels of the hierarchy of the organization.
(c) A superior exercises inherent authority to guide the operations of the persons at lower levels.
(d) All the persons engaged in line operations are directly involved in the fulfilment of the objectives of the organization.
(e) Lower levels report regularly to the upper hierarchy to keep the top persons duly informed.[12]

In health and medical organizations, the Chief Executive operates through medical and health personnel, as they constitute the key persons in providing medical and health care delivery system.

Staff Agency

The 'staff' idea also took birth in the army where it was observed that, with the growth of the army, the commander could not function only on the support of line agency. The 'line' was supplemented by the 'staff'. The staff refers to the officers who provide advice to line as to how to achieve results. The 'staff' became the think tank of the line agency. The larger the organization, the more is the need for the staff. Henri Fayol rightly stressed the need of staff, "Whatever their ability and their capacity for work, the heads of great enterprises cannot fulfil alone all their obligations. They are, thus, forced to have recourse to a group of men who have the strength, competence and time, which the head may lack. This group of men constitutes the staff of the management. It is a help, or reinforcement; a sort of extension of the manager's personality to assist him in carrying out his duties. The staff appears as a separate body only in large undertakings and its importance increases with the importance of the undertakings."[13]

Pfiffner and Presthus, mention the following as staff functions:

1. Advising, teaching, consultation.
2. Coordination, not merely through plans but also through human contacts, trouble-shooting and winning over opposition at all levels of organization.
3. Fact-finding and research.
4. Planning.
5. Contact with other organizations and individuals to know what is going on.
6. Assisting the line without infringing its authority.
7. Sometimes exercising delegated authority from the line commander.[14]

The information technology has made the staff agency indispensable as these agencies through the analysis of information help the line agency in policy-making, planning, decision-making, co-coordinating, control, etc.[15] For example, the Planning Commission in India helps the Union and State Governments in optimizing their resources through planning. Similarly, University Grants Commission helps the Union and State Governments in controlling standards of the university education. Science and technology is providing great opportunities to Governments to provide good services to the people and raise their standard of living. Staff agency can help the line agency in making use of science and technology. L.D. White mentions the following advantages, which can accrue to top line personnel through staff help:

(1) To ensure that the chief executive is adequately and currently informed;
(2) To assist him in foreseeing problems and planning future programmes;
(3) To ensure that matters for his decision reach his desk promptly, in condition to be settled intelligently and without delay, and to protect him against hasty or ill-considered judgments;
(4) To protect his time;
(5) To exclude every matter that can be settled elsewhere in the system; and

(6) To ensure means of ensuring compliances by the subordinate with establishment policy and execution direction.[16]

In tertiary hospitals, medical superintendent, Deputy Director Finance, Deans, etc. help the health and medical Chief Executive.

Auxiliary agencies also help the line agency in the performance of its duties. These are institutionalized services to the line agency. Besides, the auxiliary agency provides expert services in its area of operations economically. Some of the experts make no distinction between staff and auxiliary agencies. Others make the following distinctions: (i) Auxiliary agencies are operating services while staff agencies are engaged in thinking, planning, research, etc. (ii) Auxiliary agencies are not directly involved with the major policies of the organization while the staff is engaged in policy formulation and other advice regarding functioning of the organization. Such services make the cost of the product cheaper because of large scale operation and expertise developed.[17] Such organizations in a hospital or health organizations are drug stores, sterilization units, dietary arrangements, etc.

2. *Ensuring Authority and Responsibility Through Active Involvement of all Health and Medical Functionaries*

Authority is the right or power of a person to command other people to do things and to get work done from them. Responsibility means a charge for which one is responsible or accountable. Since it would not do just to hold a person responsible for performing a task without first giving him/her the authority necessary to get the job done, responsibility should always be coupled with commensurate authority. This parity is not mathematical but rather co-extensive both related to the same assignments. According to Ernest Dale, "Authority should be equal to responsibility. That is, if a man is responsible for results of a given operation, he should be given enough authority to take the action necessary to ensure success."[18] The trend today is to make use of authority in collaboration with colleagues-developing team work. Teamwork is a plan of health care to provide optimum care. Every health functionary should be a team member. The team leader must ensure effective communication to ensure effective participation.

Thus, the fuller staff participation is important both as a means of tapping the practical and intellectual resources of all the health personnel for the benefit of the health organization and as a way of making work in the organization more meaningful for everyone.

Such participation though theoretically available in one form or the other is practically non-existent. Most of the health functionaries interviewed revealed that the leaders allow superficial participation, indicating the presence of distrust in the minds of the health personnel.

The following advantages would result from the participative management:

- Participation yields personal commitment and involvement toward organizational goals;
- Participation produces the free flow of communications for an informal work force and atmosphere;
- Control systems are primarily of self-monitoring and guidance and not needed for external control;
- Through participation a leader is likely to obtain stronger motivation towards an objective. Even those who disagree will feel compelled to show loyalty by the sheer weight of the group opinion; and
- A high degree of confidence is shown in subordinates which facilitates interpersonal processes.

These qualities—interest, intelligence, and energy—are fundamental to strength of personality. But they must also be in balance. Unless the individual's traits are so combined that they enable one to win and hold the devotion of other colleagues, one will have little chance of meeting the demands made on him or her. The personnel must be able to feel that they know their leader and can trust because he is the leader of their team. More specially, an executive must have that quality about his or her personality, which enables him or her, without sacrificing integrity of purpose, to lubricate human relationships.

3. *Effective use of Delegation and Decentralization to Promote Efficiency of Health Systems*

The decentralization and delegation can lighten the burden of the health executives and enable them to devote attention to important aspects of planning, policy-making and coordination. They should clearly make use of delegation and decentralization through staff to achieve the objective of best patient care. According to Fayol, "Everything that goes to increase the importance of subordinate's role is decentralization. Everything which goes to reduce it is centralization."[19]

Besides, proper delegation of authority promotes effective control over operations, due to a clear definition of responsibility and action at each level. When decisions are no longer to be referred up the line, the delay in execution is minimized.[20]

The importance of delegation was also stressed by Goddard: "Delegation of responsibility and authority is an important aspect of successful administration, to place the responsibility for decision at the lowest possible organizational level in order to attain decision as speedily as possible. No administrator can do in detail all the work he is administering, for by definition an administrator manages the work of others. Therefore, the principle of delegation of responsibility should be followed to the utmost extent consistent with efficiency and coordination of policy. The responsibility and authority of individuals should be clearly defined in writing, and the authority placed in each position must correspond to the responsibility which the position carries."[21]

4. *Administrative Functions and Responsibilities*

Administrative functions constitute the major activities of the chief executive. This involves the management of men, money and material. His administrative functions are summed up by Gullick in the word 'POSDCORB'. These elementary functions have become highly complex and developed. The chief executives must understand this complexity with the help of advanced techniques and use them to discharge administrative functions. In health and medical organizations, the Chief Executive lack in performing these functions. There is a need of intensive training to make them efficient. Let us mention these briefly as given by Gullick:

(a) Planning, that is, working out in outline the things that need to be done and the methods for doing them to accomplish the purpose set for the enterprises.

(b) Organizing, that is, the establishment of the formal structure of authority through which work sub-divisions are arranged, defined and coordinated for the defined objective.

(c) Staffing, that is, the whole personnel function of bringing in and training the staff and maintaining favourable conditions of work.

(d) Directing, that is, the continuous task of making decisions and embodying them in specific and general orders and instructions, and serving as the leader of the enterprise.

(e) Coordinating, that is, the all-important duty of interrelating the various parts of the work.

(f) Reporting, that is, keeping those to whom the executive is responsible informed as to what is going, on which, thus, includes keeping himself and his subordinates informed through records, research and inspection.

(g) Budgeting with all that goes with budgeting in the form of planning, accounting and control.[22]

5. *Administrative Improvements and Reforms to keep the Health System Efficient*

The Chief Executive needs to keep his organization well designed through improvements and reforms to ensure maximum output.

The chief executive may check the organization intermittently in the context of the essentials of a good organization.

Proper appreciation and application of principles of organization can help in the evolution of a framework required for this purpose, and in ensuring that the organizational structure continue to meet the changing overall needs of the enterprise.

6. *Control over Internal Management*

Internal functioning of health and medical work is deteriorating day by day even in institutions of International importance like AIIMS, PGI,

Destnet Hospital, etc. One of the very important tasks of the chief executive is to supervise, direct and control the performance of the organization within the scope of law, policy and regulations already established to ensure decent delivery of health services. He can achieve effective supervision through a number of methods, viz., setting of service standards, budgetary control, reporting system, inspections, etc. In order to be effective as a supervisor, he must possess three qualities, i.e. job competence, the ability to guide the subordinates and the personal traits like ability to cooperate and motivate others.

7. *Public Relations*

People talk of high inefficiency in health and medical institutions. There is no body to listen this inspite of the operation of Right to Information Act, 2005. The Chief Executive is to ensure participation of people in the formulation and implementation of plans and programmes. Imaginative measures are needed on the part of the chief executive to promote and sustain the interests of the citizens in the administration, to give them a sense of participation in the decisions that immediately affect them and to enable them to contribute to better administration.

8. *Implementation of Health and Medical Programmes*

Words, written or spoken, are of no use unless they are put into action. The emphasis should be more on performance rather than paper planning. Khalil Gibran has rightly said, that "believing is a fine thing, but placing those beliefs into execution is a test of strength. Many are those who talk like the roar of sea, but their lives are shallow and stagnant, like the rotting marshes. Many are those who lift their heads above the mountain top, but their sprit remains dormant to the obscurity of the caverns."[23]

Swami Vivekananda has also mentioned that we must act decisively to regenerate the potentialities of our country. "Let us all work hard, my brethren; this is no time for sleep. On our work depends the coming of the India of the future. She is there ready waiting. She is only sleeping. Arise and awake, and see her seated here, on her eternal throne, rejuvenated more glorious than she ever was, this Motherland of ours." The Union and State Governments are announcing health and medical schemes for the poor frequently but what is the result? Their half-hearted implementations lead the criticism of Government and loss of already short finances.

9. *Creating Commitment to the Ideals of the Health and Medical Organization*

No organization can develop until and unless the top persons working in the organization are committed to achieve its ideals. An attitude of dedication to the goals of an organization should be an indispensable trait of the top leaders. This is their primary requisite to operate and function effectively and efficiently to build self-confidence in themselves and, in turn, in the public.

Administrative functions constitute the major activities of the chief executive. This involves the management of men, money and material for which most of health and medical executives are not well grounded. They instead of giving directions are rather dependent upon their junior staff. This needs to be improved.

10. Generating Ethical and Moral Values in Health and Medical Organizations

Chief executives especially in the foiled of health and medical organizations need to develop ethical and moral standards. Health and medical services must also develop the normative linkages, i.e. they must develop professional standards, which should help them in their best performances. Standards are contagious. They spread throughout an organization, a group, or a society. If an organization or group cherishes high standards, the behaviour of the individuals who enters it is inevitably influenced. They should not develop an excessive sense of self-importance or arrogance. As has been said in the Gita, "we should pursue the path of excellence without fear or favour and work ceaselessly to achieve the objective." Good organization building has to create around it a bracing atmosphere, a prideful tradition of integrity, excellence and fellowship. Human beings breathe an ethos around them almost unconsciously, and these traditions make for the ethos."[24] The health and medical leaders must promote it.

Let me quote Josiah Gilbert Holland, who, through this couplet, mentions the required moral ingredients of the top men, especially health and medical personnel.

> God, Give us Men!
> God, give us men! A time like this demands; Strong minds, great hearts, true faith and ready hands; Men whom the lust of office does not kill;
> Men whom the spoils of office cannot buy;
> Men who possess opinions and a will;
> Men who have honour; men who will not lie.

A chief executive like Director of a AIIMS is not supposed to carry out by himself all the functions entrusted to his care. The actual day-to-day administration is carried out by the permanent heads of the departments like Cardiology, Urology, Orthopaedies, etc. His actual role is that of "a trouble shooter, a supervisor and promoter of the future programme." The chief executive is a leader to motivate and coordinate the work of others. He has staff and line organization working under him. His great virtue lies not in himself administrating the work but in making others administer. As Prof. Dimock says, "First, he must keep the enterprise on an even keel. Second, he must delegate everything he can. Third, if the programme is going on satisfactorily, he then has the time and nervous energy with which to chart that lies ahead."

The Chief Executive must infuse such a sense of responsibility among his colleagues so that they work whole heartedly to ensure high quality of life through the provision of preventive, promotive, curative and rehabilitative health services. In this way reputation and prestige of health system would shine.

11. Direct access to the people

A health and medical leader has to be accessible to the people he leads. He cannot afford to run his organization from behind the closed doors of his office. He has to be on the shop floor, working with the rest of his team and leading from the front.

Robert H. Rosen has stressed that a new way of leading is emerging-one, that is lowly, quietly and decisively transforming our organizations. Never before have our challenges been so great and the need for responsible leaders so profound. Successful enterprises know how to excel and compete. They make the most of their resources—their financial, marketing, and technological capabilities-but it is their people who make the deciding difference they are the engine for growth and productivity. Mature-wise leaders make it happen. He should promote the culture of "I AM OK", YOU ARE OK."

12. Creativity to see work as a potential for creating joy and to experience the happiness of creating something totally new

It is immensely satisfying to do work, which contributes to the lives of others and creates radical transformation in the quality of life of those around us. Creative work, which creates a new form, which is original, is very satisfying. Work which is without an effect, or which can be done equally well by anyone else, never inspires us. We all like to give our special touch to whatever we do. This creates an interesting paradox; whether our responses influence the quality of work or does work influence the quality of our responses? The answer is to go beyond the dichotomy?[25]

13. Leadership

Leadership—Medical Superintendent/Directors must provide leadership to technical and non-technical workers working under him. Leadership is the process to direct and co-ordinate the activities of members of an organization towards the achievement of goals, honestly and efficiently.

A leader is a person who plans, organizes, makes decisions and influences people. Leaders have a positive attitude towards people and towards their work. Leaders are always hopeful; they expect their efforts to lead to success. A number of factors are involved in the ability to lead, including the following:

(a) Insight into human behaviour;
(b) Ability to plan, organize and direct efforts of others;

(c) Decision-making ability on a practical and realistic basis;
(d) Ability to co-ordinate the efforts of others; and
(e) Keep the environment of work place stimulating.[26]

Hospital Administrator can function effectively provided he gets all the facilities like adequate and qualified manpower, adequate building (space), adequate equipment and drugs and sufficient resources to run the hospital. The hospital administrator must also optimize the use of resources and discourage wastages. Hospital Administrator must keep in mind that hospital administration is an art and science, which can make the maximum use of resources for the welfare of the patient. The hospital administration is to achieve results at a given point of time with whatever resources are available to him. That is why it has been said that put a good man in a bad setup he will make things go through; put a bad man in a good setup, he will create a mess of the whole situation. Therefore, right selection of the hospital administrator is the *sine-quo-non* for the success of hospital administration

Let us support with the help of an Article by Attar Singh Rajindra Hospital Chronically ill" in *The Tribute* dated September 2007.

The Government Rajindra Hospital, Patiala, once a premier health care institution of Punjab that attracted patients from all over the region, is now in a state of neglect. Lack of funds, government apathy and shortage of specialists are some of the factors that have contributed to the slump in its reputation.

Several specialty departments, including cardiology, urogology, and nephrology, are running only for academic purposes. These departments are woefully short of staff, particularly senior faculty, which has resulted in a sharp fall in the number of patients visiting the hospital. Masters courses in paediatrics surgery and plastic surgery have been dropped for the want of senior faculty to teach students. The fate of another course in the department of urology, which had been planned to be introduced, hangs in the balance.

Several senior faculty members of the hospital have left the hospital in the past one decade and started their own practice. The patients that were once treated at the hospital by the doctors are now spotted at the latter's private nursing homes.

The government has done precious little to stem this and there has been no concerted effort to check the exodus of doctors from the hospital.

The facilities at the hospital have also been at the receiving end of the government apathy. This 1,000-bed hospital is faced with a fiscal crisis due to lack of funds. The emergency wing has virtually no medicines at its disposal. The hospital, which is attached to the Government Medical College, is the oldest referral hospital in the State. However, the situation has come to such a pass the doctors struggle to rune even emergency procedures without outside support. The emergency department does not get any funds separately and has limited medicines at its disposal. These medicines too are used in extreme emergency situations. The incinerator at the hospital has been out of order ever since its installation over 10 years ago. Hazardous biomedical waste is dumped outside in a corner near the main building of the hospital. The waste, which is carted off by the municipal corporation, has been a constant source of infection at the hospital.

Also, the incinerator, which was purchased in 1991, has never been in operation. Initially, the incinerator could not be used due to a dispute between the private firm that supplied it and the public works department.

Later, the high cost of operation went against it's use.

The incinerator room, which is situated near the doctors' hostel, is a picture of neglect with wild overgrowth all around it. The health administrators should possess the following qualities:

Intelligence, Alertness, Verbal, Facility, Originality, Judgment, Dependability, Initiative, Persistence, Aggressiveness, Self-confidence, Desire to excel, Activity, Sociability, Cooperation, Adaptability, Humour, Mental Level, Status, Skill needs and Interest of followers, objectives to be achieved, etc.

If the ideal of health administration is to provide better medical care to the people then we shall have to see that in a given situation we make the best possible use of our resources in terms of personnel and finance to achieve optimum results.

Administrative Functions

I. Administrative Functions constitute one of the major activities of the Chief Executives

This involves management of men, money and material. His administrative functions are summed up by Gullick in the word 'POSDCORB'. Let us mention these briefly:

(a) Planning, that is, working out an outline of the things that need to be done and the methods for doing them to accomplish the purpose set for the enterprise.

(b) Organizing, that is, the establishment of the formal structure of authority through which work sub-divisions are arranged, defined and coordinated for the defined objective.

(c) Staffing, that is the whole personnel function of bringing in and training the staff and maintaining favourable conditions of work.

(d) Directing, that is, the continuous task of making decisions and embodying them in specific and general orders and instructions, and serving as the leader of the enterprise.

(e) Coordinating, that is, the all-important duty of interrelating various parts of the work.

(f) Reporting, that is, keeping those to whom the executive is responsible, informed as to what is going on, which, thus, includes keeping himself and his subordinates informed through records, research and inspection.

(g) Budgeting with all that goes with budgeting in the form of planning, accounting and control.[27]

These elementary functions have become highly complex and developed. The Medical Superintendent/Doctor must understand this complexity with the help of advanced techniques and use them to discharge administrative functions.

2. *Understanding and Directing Change*

New millennium is going to be different and the new millennium needs leaders who can understand and redirect this change into fruitful changes. Leadership and change are closely linked. An awareness of the changing atmosphere at the workplace calls for leaders who can understand and deal with the changing paradigms of corporate culture. No longer is it enough for a manager to limit his job to doing things on time, within budget and the way they were done yesterday, only five percent better. Leaders are today treading on completely unfamiliar territory where yesterday's rules no longer apply. Uncertainty is now an inescapable fact and things no longer happen in a predictable manner. Innovation is the new mantra for the leaders of today. They make new rules almost as fast as the old ones become redundant. Under these circumstances, it is imperative for a leader to have a clear vision of where his organization is headed. In the absence of such vision, it is all too easy for organization, both old and new, to flounder and fail.

3. *Emotional Intelligence (EI)*

Emotional intelligence is concerned with achieving one's goals through the ability to manage one's own feelings and emotions, to be sensitive to, and influence other key people, and to balance one's motives and drives with conscientious and ethical behaviours. The following are the characteristics of EI:

(a) Inter-personal sensitivity covering competencies like listening and sensitivity.

(b) Motivating, including impact and energy.

(c) Emotional Resilience.

(d) Influence and Adaptability covering both influencing and negotiating ability and being adaptable in various types of situations and cultures.

(e) Decisiveness and assertiveness.

(f) Leadership including motivating other people.

4. Code of Ethics for the Medial Personnel in India

The document prepared by Department of Administrative Reforms and Public Grievances has chalked out a Code of Ethics, which need implementation. The objective of Code is to prescribe standards of integrity and conduct that are to apply in the medical and health services. The principles stated below underlie and supplement the rules and laws to regulate the public and private conduct of various health and medical services.

Selflessness: Holders of public office should take decisions solely in terms of the public interest. They should not do so in order to gain financial or other material benefits for themselves, their family, or their friends.

Integrity: Holders of public office should not place themselves under any financial or other obligation to outside individuals or organizations that might influence them in the performance of their official duties.

Objective: In carrying out public business, including making public appointments, awarding contracts, or recommending individuals for rewards and benefits, holders of public office should make choice on merit.

Accountability: Holders of public office are accountable for their decisions and actions to the public and must submit themselves to whatever scrutiny is appropriate to their office.

Openness: Holders of public office should be as open as possible about all the decisions and action that they take. They should give reasons for their decisions and restrict information only when the wider public interest clearly demands.

Honesty: Holders of public office have a duty to declare any private interest relating to their public duties and to take steps to resolve any conflicts arising in a way that protects the public interest.

Leadership: Holders of public office should promote and support these principles by leadership and example.

These principles apply to all aspects of public life. The Committee has set them out here for the benefits of all who serve the public in any way. Medical Profession needs to follow the following:

- Health and Medical Professionals must maintain highest standards of behaviour so that their actions and decisions result in the benefits for industry, employees, customers, shareholders and society.
- Health and service must conform to the commitment promised to patients.
- Patients must be given best possible service and treated with respect and fairness.
- Best way of promoting high standards of medical practices is through self-regulation. The Code has been designed as an instrument of self-regulation to serve as voluntary guideline towards better quality of life and higher standards of medical practices.

Health Leaders have to work hard to remove callousness, negligence, non-punctuality among doctors working in hospitals under their charge. The doctors are deteriorating in their efficiency, as they remain busy in their private practice. The Hospital Leaders must act decisively to solve existing and emerging problems.

The CEO of a hospital has numerous and varied functions like ensuring perfect MIS system, Material finances, human development, medico-legal aspects, etc. It will be difficult to give a comprehensive list.

Top executives in hospital administration must be the persons with vision, initiative and desire to achieve the operational goals with dedication and perseverance. In the words of Jawaharlal Nehru, "No administrator, I suppose, or anyone else for the matter of that, can really do first class work without a sense of function, without some measures of a crusading spirit. I am doing this, I have to achieve this, as a part of great movement in a big cause. That gives a sense of function, not the sense of individual's narrow approach of doing a job in an office for a salary or wage, something connected with your life's outlook or anything, perhaps being interested, as people inevitably are, one's personal preferment in that particular work."[28]

Notes and References

1. Haiman, Professional Management, Eurasia Publishing House, New Delhi, 1966, p. 440.
2. Keith Davis, Human Relations at Work, McGraw-Hill, New York, 1967, pp. 96-97.
3. Remarks by Richard A. Shelling, Governor of Vermont, Conference Report, Recapturing Confidence in Government, Public Personnel Management Reform, February 1979.
4. Management Techniques: Principles and Practices, "Ecology of Management Techniques, 2001, p. 29
5. M.R. Pinto, Values in Public Services, *IJPA*, January-March, 1989.
6. Bata K. Dey, *IJPA*, April-June 1989, p. 175.
7. Robert H. Rosen, Learning to lead, in Frances Hassellein *et al*. "the Peter Drucker Foundation," 1997, p. 302.
8. Tead Ordway, The Art of Leadership, McGraw Hill, New York, 1935, p. 83
9. Cheser Barnard, The Functions of Executive, Harvard University Press, Cambridge, 1938, p. 260.
10. Dilip Thakor, "Successive Planning in Indian Industry, in *Business World*, August 31-Sept. 13, 1981.
11. Moddie, A.D., The Brahmanical Culture and Modernity, Asia Publishing House, New York, pp. 106-14.
12. S.L. Goel, Advanced Public Administration, New Delhi, Sterling, 1994, p. 88.
13. Henri Fayol, in Gullik and Urwick (eds.) Papers in the Science of Administration, p. 86.
14. Pfiffner and Presthus, *op. cit.*, p. 86.
15. S.L. Goel, *op. cit.*, p. 88.
16. S.D. Mooney, Principles of Organization, p. 41.
17. S.L. Goel, *op. cit.*, p. 91.
18. Ernest Dale, Management—Theory and Practice, 1973, Tokyo, McGraw-Hill, p. 149.

19. Henri Foyal, General and International Management, London, Pitman, 1956, p. 26.
20. L.D. White, Encyclopaedia of the Social Science, The Macmillian, 1951, Vol. V, p. 43.
21. H.A. Goddard, Principles of Administration Applied to Nursing Services, WHO, Geneva, 1958, p. 85.
22. Gulick, Luther, 'Notes on the Theory of Organization', in Luther Gulick and L. Urwick, Papers on the Science of Administration, New York, Institute of Public Administration, 1937, p. 13.
23. Gibran Khalid, Between Night and Morn, The Philosophical Library, New York, 1971, pp. 8-9.
24. Moddie, A.D., The Brahmanical Culture and Modernity, Asia Publishing House, New York, pp. 106-14.
25. S.L. Goel, Management Techniques: Principles and Practices, Leadership, p. 265.
26. *Ibid., op. cit.*, p. 256.
27. Gullick, Luther, 'Notes on the Theory of Organization in Luther Gullick and L. Urwick, Papers on the Science of Administration, New York, Institute of Public Administration, 1937, p. 13.
28. Jawaharlal Nehru and Public Administration, *IJPA*, New Delhi, 1975, p. 88.

3

Qualities and Essentials for Medical Personnel in a Hospital

The profession of medicine is highly respected in the society and that is why doctor is considered as the image of God. Doctors are angels to the suffering humanity. Doctors whether they are only Graduates or postgraduates or possess other high qualifications need some basic human qualities to serve the humanity as well as get job satisfaction. It is difficult to mention all the qualities. We mention here some of the important qualities which are basis for the efficient functioning of doctors.

Human development and improving the quality of life of people are the ultimate goals of all activities of any government. Quality of life and development can be achieved only with healthy mind and body. Health is the vital ingredient of all development activities.[1]

That poor socio-economic conditions worsen the health of the people is well known and accepted by all. Neither wealth nor technological progress will ensure the health of any nation unless they are equitably distributed among its entire population. The United States, arguably the wealthiest, the most powerful and the most technologically advanced among the nations of the world ranks 46th in the human index—behind even economically weaker countries such as Cuba—precisely because the bonanzas of progress have not reached as many as 45 million (more than 15%) of her citizens who do not have health insurance. No country can shine if it is blinded by the glare of glittering wealth and media hype to take notice of the poor and deprived masses existing beyond the arc lights of rightist elitism.

Social inequalities similarly have a profound adverse effect on health and health care delivery. Perhaps the most neglected and least understood among them, and one that is prevalent universally, is the differential impact of gender on disease and health care seeking behaviour. Admittedly the impact is more on women; but men are also not immune to it. Unfortunately little or no attention is paid to the gender dimensions of health by teaching institutions and medical curricula anywhere in the world.[2]

Health care has long ceased to be the exclusive preserve of the doctors. We, as doctors, know that effective and efficient health care can only be delivered if all members of the team work in a concerted fashion. No matter who we are or what is our particular field of specialization, no matter whether we are physicians, surgeons, anesthesiologists, dental specialists, nurses, physiotherapists, laboratory technologists or any of the several allied health scientists, our common goal is to help heal the sick through our areas of expertise.[3]

"There should be an attitude of care and compassion while dealing with a patient or his attendants, since he/she is already in pain, distress or depression. In big public hospitals, where the load of work is generally excessive, the outlook of various personnel, especially the Class III and IV category employees has become highly bureaucratic and impersonal, if not in human—be it stretcher bearer, sweeper, lift operator, O.T. or ward boy or even nurses and junior doctors. Many senior doctors tend to forget the Hippocratic oath and neglect the patients with impurity to satisfy their ego or whims. Many of them become unhelpful, since they consider certain simple jobs/interventions below dignity—in the process patients further suffers.

PGI's Nehru Hospital is one example of good infrastructure but without the attitude of 'Care'. While a stream of hapless patients from far and wide throng the premises of this large hospital, with the belief that it offers ultimate in diagnosis and treatment—he and his relatives are treated with apathy/antipathy by all concerned, as and when he makes an attempt to enter the hospital. The approach of the staff lacks the content of service, sensitivity, responsiveness, urgency, helpfulness and even humaneness. Except the senior members of the faculty, who are dedicated, devoted, accessible, knowledgeable and caring, rest of the staff needs intensive training and supervision in 'How to approach a patient and his distressed relatives' and further the provisions have to be enforced, the erring and arrogant have to be purged, the systems of management which have collapsed have to be restored and a semblance of administration to address the grievances of ailing public, set-up. These feelings are evoked in all, who have attempted to seek service in this hospital for himself or ones relative.

While we watch in the movies/media that in the event of an emergency just one phone call is enough to access the best of service, in the civilised societies, in Nehru hospital one may not get allotment of even a room/bed for several days due to procedures which are neither easy to understand nor transparent nor a helpful person around to guide the persons in pain and misery. While the city is proud to possess maximum number of ambulances, one may not be available get it, if you don't have links when an ambulance approaches the giant building of this hospital, it is refused entry to that gate, which may be convenient to the patient several cane bearers will shoo it away from one gate to another, even before the patient is unloaded. These are the experiences of a senior doctor-patient, who had to get admitted to this hospital recently. While the patient is struggling to come out of ambulance, her lone attendant, her aging husband is fishing for a wheel chair in the vast campus, without success when a patient descends from above in a trolley, he runs like an athlete to grab the same. The onlookers, the staff members including ward attendants find the scene amusing, but do not get moved to lend a helping hand. This was not the end of woes—just a beginning.

While in the ward, the nurses are big bosses and are not available to assist or nurse the patient. Their duty ends by customary recording of blood pressure/temperature, sometimes after cursory examination and often with guess work examination. The ward boys and sweepers are there in large numbers, but wait for their palm to be greased, to come forward. Getting an appointment for major investigations is a difficult task in the first instance. Even after getting one, it is meaningless—either the equipment is out of order—more often than not or endless wait on the wheelchair in the corridor, even for a severely disabled case, with nobody to listen around. The patient may remain admitted for days on end, waiting to be investigated by the elusive machine, for which the engineer/part will come from abroad.

The patient is handed over a slip to buy medicines/dressings/ syringes, etc. every few minutes. The junior doctors/nurses/ward attendants all boss over the patient's relatives or the patient herself. Similarly, he is shuttled from one floor to another every few hours for investigations or his blood is to be distributed to several blocks situated at far off and unknown destinations. All this is to be done by the attendants of the patient and not the hospital attendants. First of all it would be difficult to arrange and afford so many attendants by the patient, secondly, they are detained by the security or pushed out by the ward attendants. Collection of reports from different departments and making payments at counters, which are difficult to discover is no less an ordeal.

At the end when the patient is to be discharged getting a discharge slip or getting no dues certificate, requires waiting and running around which involves testing the fitness of the patients' attendants. If you have to get certificate for medical leave/reimbursement, etc. another round of arduous exercise starts. The men in the medical superintendent's office are always less than co-operative and generally sullen faced and arrogant.

Those at the helm of affairs of Nehru hospital can at least provide an easy access to ambulance, wheelchair and stretcher-bearers to serious/ disabled patients. They can provide helpful people bearing badges can I help you to give guidance/help to the needy. Those patients who require extra care may be provided a nurse on the pattern of Escorts hospital. Above all each staff member has to realise and act in the manner that he is for the good of the patients and not to cause any harassment to him or his attendant—who are in distress anyway.

The following are some of the qualities and essentials for doctors and other staff in a hospital for better care.

I. Competence

The education and training to medical personnel must be thorough so that they can face the challenges of health faced by patients and society. The Doctor who is competent in his field can help the patients with confidence and faith. Competence of a doctor is lifting of his performance to higher standard, the building of he is personality beyond to normal limitations. However, competence acquired in a medical college is not sufficient as science and technology is developing fast, therefore there is a need to keep in time with the latest developments in his area. This would muster a lot of strength to him and he would be motivated to move in medical field higher and higher. This is called getting continuous medical education. Medical knowledge is not static but dynamic. If we wish to safeguard the future, it is high that all those who are engaged in medical profession should get concerned with creativity and change that is take a second look at their work system and style as well as contour of advanced medical technology to promote creativity and total change if not a revolution.

You are poised on the threshold of a world of opportunities. Some of you will choose to be scientists, discoverers and inventors; some will opt for teaching; but most of you, I am sure, will prosper in professional practice. Whichever fields you may choose, or find yourself in, I wish you a glorious future. But please do remember always that our fellow human being-their health, happiness and meaningful life—are the ultimate reason for our existence. Treat them with care, compassion and empathy. Treat them, as we would like to be treated. Nothing more is required; nothing less is acceptable. Go out and conquer the world by winning the hearts and minds of the people through professional competence, dedicated service and humane treatment.[4]

Unquestionably a physician (and by the word 'physician', I include a doctor practicing any specialty he or she chooses), must need be competent. It is the university and its teachers, which provide and equip you with this competence. However, the acquisition of a degree in my opinion is merely a license to practice medicine is your chosen specialty, your consummation as a physician can only come after you have gone out into the world of sickness and suffering and grappled long with death and disease. Unless the unfortunate values of present-day living have poisoned your mind, dulled your sensibilities and blunted your sympathies, you will learn that there is more to a true physician than the mere knowledge of the science of medicine. It is only when the art and philosophy of medicine have encrusted science, and have permeated into its very core that you will have blossomed into a true physician. Bear in mind that competence needs to be perpetually reinforced and renewed. A physician is first and foremost a student for life. Young and old, we are all undergraduates in the school of experience.

I will not detail what constitutes competence. But I would urge you in this machine-age not to forget the use of your eyes, ears and hands. None are so blind as those who have eyes and yet not see, or so deaf as those who have ears and yet not hear, or so unfeeling as those who can touch and yet not feel. The art and science of medicine is not taught by books; it is acquired only if you have lived with disease and made your home at the bedside of patients.

Competence however is not enough. Competence must be associated in even greater measure with what is best termed 'humanity'. Humanity is the sensibility, which enables a physician to feel for the distress and suffering of a patient, prompting him to provide relief. Humanity embraces both care and compassion; it forms the core of a doctor-patient relationship, a relationship which has been increasingly eroded in our present age.[5]

Medical sciences is becoming more knowledge-oriented, integrating inputs from many allied fields, and advances are taking place in all these fields. The common saying that 'education is a lifelong process' is more true in the case of medical experts. Keeping track of the advances elsewhere in the world and fetching those advances to the teeming millions in the rural areas in the country using a cost effective, timely delivery system calls for updated knowledge and continuing efforts. Yet another challenge, the doctors must be cognizant is that the society is increasingly becoming educated and demanding, and thus, have rising expectations. The future knowledge society needs constant updating of skills and extraordinary teamwork across multi-disciplinary fields. I always remind the youngsters that being best in the country is not just enough; one has to be best in the world.

Let me leave with you a word of advice given more than 100 years back by Sir William Osier, the first physician-in-chief of John Hopkins Hospital, and the author of many books including the one titled "The Principles and Practice of Medicine":

> ". . . Learn to see, learn to hear, learn to feel, learn to smell, and know that by practice alone can you become experts."[6]

Medical and Health Education must equip the medical personnel to pay more attentions to preventive care.

It is also necessary to appreciate that the effective delivery of health care services would depend very largely on the nature of education, training and appropriate orientation towards community health of all categories of medical and health personnel and their capacity to function as an integrated team, each of its members performing given tasks within a coordinated action programme. It is, therefore, of crucial importance that the entire basis and approach towards medical and health education, at all levels, is reviewed in terms of national needs and priorities and the curricular programmes restructured to produce personnel of various grades of skill and competence, who are professionally equipped and socially motivated to effectively deal with day-to-day problems, within the existing constraints. Towards this end, it is necessary to formulate, separately, a National Medical and Health Education Policy which (i) sets out the changes required to be brought about in the curricular contents and training programme of medical and health personnel, at various levels of functioning; (ii) takes into account the need for establishing the extremely essential inter-relations between functionaries of various grades; (iii) provides guidelines for the production of health personnel on the basis of realistically assessed manpower requirements; (iv) seeks to resolve the existing sharp regional imbalances in their availability; and (v) ensures that personnel at all levels are socially towards the rendering of community health services.

2. Dedication and Commitment to Promote Individual and Community Health Care

In the patient care scenario you dedicate your life to the care of the individual patient. I recall not long ago in middle of the night a patient who was transferred to our hospital, had a complication during a delivery of her third child. She had severe lung disease following abruptio placenta, 10 year ago she would have died, but for the combination of the dedication of the staff with physicians, nurses, pharmacists and respiratory therapist who stayed at this woman's bedside throughout the night.

Within a weeks' time she left the hospital to go back to care for her other children. So, these children now have a mother because of the efforts of this team that individual care could not have saved a decade ago. Someone's life is being saved because of your efforts. Unfortunately, there are many diseases such as diabetes, chronic lung disease, and some forms of cancer that we can't cure. There you work with your patients to help with the illness, you understand how the illness has influenced their life. You do what you can, to make it easier for them. This may be your life calling. In this patient care approached medicine you take care of one patient at a time. You do the best you can for that patient and for the records of the lifetime you will make a difference in thousands, if not hundreds, of thousand of lives.[7]

- I qualified as a doctor a little over 25 years ago and was sworn into medical practice by a modernized version of the Hippocratic oath, devised by the Dean of Medicine at Tufts University in the USA. It may be pertinent to recount that to you now.
- I swear to fulfil, to the best of my ability and judgment, this covenant.
- I will respect the hard-won scientific gains of those physicians/ health care workers in whose steps I walk, and gladly share such knowledge as is mine with those who are to follow.
- I will apply, for the benefit of the sick, all measures, which are

required, avoiding those twin traps of over treatment and therapeutic nihilism.

- I will remember that there is art to medicine as well as science, and that warmth, sympathy, and understanding may outweigh the surgeon's knife or the chemist's drug.
- I will not be ashamed to say "I know not," nor will fail to call in my colleagues when the skills of another are needed for a patient's recovery.
- I will respect the privacy of my patients, for their problems are not disclosed to me that the world may know. Most especially must I tread with care in matters of life and death. If it is given me to save a life, all thanks. But it may also be within my power to take a life; this awesome responsibility must be faced with great humbleness and awareness of my own frailty. Above all, I must not play at God.
- I will remember that I do not treat a fever chart, a cancerous growth, but a sick human being, whose illness may affect the person's family and economic stability. My responsibility includes these related problems, if I am to care adequately for the sick.
- I will prevent disease whenever I can, for prevention is preferable to cure.
- I will remember that I remain a member of society, with special obligation to all my fellow human beings, those sound of mind and body as well as the infirm.

If I do not violate this oath, may I enjoy life and art, respected while I live and remembered with affection thereafter. May I always act so as to preserve the finest traditions of my calling and may I long experience the joy of healing those who seek my help. Adapted from that written in 1964 by Louis Lasagna, Academic Dean of the School of Medicine at Tufts University, and used in many medical schools today.

There is a sentence in the oath there that is very poignant—that you will remain a member of society. So when you are at work, don't forget that patient in front of you is someone's mother, father, brother, sister, or child and how would you want that relative of yours treated. Take pride in what you have achieved so far in graduating and what you will do now.[8]

The late Bertrand Russell also expressed the view that mere knowledge does not have any motivation within it; that comes from a different source, namely, the field of emotions and sentiments in man. Something must stimulate knowledge; otherwise, it remains static and unable to influence human action. Our knowledge, said Russell, that any two sides of a triangle together are greater than the third side, does not motivate us, while walking, that we should go by the short side and not by the long sides. That motivation comes from some other inner source in man. Mere knowledge that obtains in our schools and colleges and universities, even at its best—and it is rarely that it rises to that level—contains no energy of emotion and sentiment relating to ideals of human excellence or to patriotism and national dedication, which alone can stimulate relating to ideals of human excellence or to patriotism and national dedication, which alone can stimulate that knowledge to develop into character-excellence and to make it dynamic, make it into a 'man-making education' leading to a 'nation-building' resolve, in the luminous words of Swami Vivekananda.[9]

A spirit of service and dedication must pervade among the providers of the health care as they are considered second God on earth by the receivers of health care. In the new millennium, we must empower the patients by the looking after them carefully and making them feel important.

The progress and achievements of the past 50 years are solid foundations for a healthier and better world. It is already time to build on them. Life in the 21st century could and should be better for all. We can pass no greater gift to the next generation than a healthier future. That is our vision. Together, the people of the world can make it a reality.

3. Ethical Values

On graduation, the doctor took the oath of honesty, purity, etc., which stressed all the ethical values. Later, with Western medicine becoming popular in the country, the medical students were asked to take the Hippocratic oath, which originated in Greece. The Hindu version of such an oath has been in existence long before the Hippocratic oath. But most Indians have not heard about it or have forgotten it. Since independence, this practice of Oath-taking has been given up in most places.

The training of the medical students and the oath that they took on graduation fully reflected the great ethical values that were instilled into all medical students and doctors. Thus medical ethics became the bedrock of medical practice and dharmic ideals prevailed. As regards remuneration for services rendered, this always took a secondary place. The medical students and the medical profession were indoctrinated with the principle that medical treatment is based on compassion towards all beings and it is not primarily meant for earning money or for fulfiling other desires.

In Vedic India and even later for many centuries, physicians were told that medical practice was never fruitless; it always gave some benefit or other for the doctor, not necessarily material or monetary. A Sanskrit-verse described this idea as follows:

> Sometimes punya, sometimes friendship,
> Somewhere money, somewhere else fame,
> Often knowledge and experience,
> Never is treatment without its fruit.[10]

Ethical or dharmic values are essential for the existence and for the progress of any Society and have to be preserved and practiced if human civilization has to progress. Of these values, ethics in medicine is of the greatest importance, as medicine deals with problems of life and death. To argue that the practice of values in medicine will depend on the condition of society is untenable, as the members of the medical profession belong to the elite in society and must shoulder greater responsibilities. They must have much greater concern about values than any other section of society. The doctor and the teacher—the Vaidya and the Upadhyaya—have to set a noble example to others in any civilized society.[11]

Doctors should not be influenced by pharmacy. They must see that pharmacy suits their requirement and is affordable. Doctors can play a great role in bettering services.

A well informed society expects for accountability, transparency and sound professional services from the health care providers. This requirement is fulfiled by professionalism and ethical practice of profession. The core element of profession is a specialized body of knowledge and commitment to service. Integrity of knowledge base and its expansion through research and ensuring the highest ethical standards in its use in the best advantage of the patient is a professional commitment of a pharmacist. Any failure in his duty is an indicator of falling standards of the profession. Licensing bodies and professional associations have the responsibility and social obligation to discipline unprofessional and incompetent pharmacists. Society believes the profession places the welfare of society above that of the profession. The education institutions have an important obligation to inculcate these values in their graduates.[12]

4. Modern Knowledge of Informatics

All hospital personnel directly involved in looking after patients are obliged to process a large amount of information, so as to provide good care. Physicians, for instance, must obtain each patient's demographic data and a history of the illness, note the signs and symptoms manifested, and compile a past treatment history and associated diagnosis for treatment. Nurses, in turn, need much of this information to formulate a proper care plan, after which they must note the patient's daily progress. Laboratory technicians require details as well, to conduct tests that the doctor has ordered, the results of which are sent back to physicians. Pharmacists too need certain data, to supply the necessary medication. All these examples show that a large part of the daily work of doctors, nurses, laboratory technicians, and pharmacists consists of information handling, perhaps up to 40 per cent of their hospital working day.

5. Time-savers

Fortunately, new technologists are now emerging which help to process this information far more accurately and efficiently. To the computer are now added allied machines that can undertake, for instance, imaging in the audio-visual field and rapid data transmission. Gradually, all these time-servers have been brought into hospitals to solve the problems created by the information explosion. Such technologies have been melded into a uniform system which is designed to meet hospital needs and is generally called a hospital information system.

The basic concept of such a system is to create a cumulative file of each patient's data, which can be quickly updated on a continuing basis. This type of data file in computer terminology is called a database.

Once each patient's database is created and regularly updated, data handling at the hospital improves tremendously, enabling a section requiring specific information on a patient to obtain it rapidly from the database. The information is delivered by a printout from a computer terminal in a standardized form. Or the physician may type an order into the computer database, which the computer then transmits to the laboratory as an instruction to perform clinical tests for a certain patient, the laboratory also receiving pertinent data that is stored in the patient's database. Similarly, when a physician uses his or her computer terminal to write a prescription into the patient's database, the computer transmits the prescription immediately to the pharmacy, while the prescription information is kept and accumulated in the database, which provides this information to the administrator in the form of hospital supply statistics.

However, technological progress will make it possible to transmit the data contained in hospital information systems through a telephone line to the clinics. Once this computer networking is established, the health care provided to the patient at either the clinic or the hospital will be more accurate. And while the privacy of each patient must always be protected, the accumulation of accurate data concerning matters of health that can be achieved through computer linkage with other health care facilities within a district and, ultimately, throughout the country will contribute to better health research and planning for the benefit of all.[13]

6. Data files

Health professionals are increasingly interested in the use of computers and especially micro-computers, for health statistics and epidemiology, not least because the price of today's microcomputer hardware now makes these machines affordable to them and, in some cases, to students. Microcomputers can now be found on the office desks of doctors and in the research laboratories of health scientists. These individuals have been asking about microcomputer-based statistical software that they could use with their desk-top machines to carry out data handling and management functions.[14]

7. Effective Communication

A basic doctor, to effectively deliver health care to the country must be an astute clinician, a good communicator, and a sound administrator, so as to effectively lead an ever-expanding health team for a positive health action. Work and action domain of the doctor has crossed the boundaries to drugs and dispensaries and presently extends to a large extent to the families and to the communities—hence the need for the basic doctor to be a community physician. Thus, has emerged the need for developing a well-designed and structured programme of education for basic doctors with general applicability, departing from the present MBBS curriculum, and with emphasis on the primary health needs of the country. In addition, human values and medical ethics need to be incorporated as a part of the curriculum. In essence, the National Education Policy in Health Sciences aims at, and strives towards, the production of basic doctors equipped with adequate knowledge, requisite skills and appropriate behavioural attributes to meet the health needs of the country.[15]

All the health experts from top to both including auxiliary health services need be taught as to how preventive health services through health education can be developed to avoid opening of more and more hospitals and assuring an effective and efficient health services.

Essential of Communication

The essentials of communication are:

(a) Clarity of Thought

The first *sine qua non* of good health communication is that the idea to be transmitted must be absolutely clear in the mind of the communicator. It must spring out form a 'clear' head. It should be understood by the personnel so that it may be fully appreciated and acted upon.

(b) Importance of Action Rather than Words

In all communication, actions are more significant than words. Example is better than precept. A health officer who is not punctual cannot succeed in enforcing the time-rules on the subordinates.

(c) Participation

In this connection it is essential that both the parties (the communicator and the recipient) should participate in the communication. It is the only way to make the communication effective and made health programmes successful.

(d) Transmission

The communicator must plan carefully what to communicate, with whom to communicate and how to communicate. How can the top personnel communicate with the workers when they themselves do not know or cannot understand all the facts about the new plans? Further, delegation of authority without responsibility breaks down the spirit of communication.

(e) Keep the System Always Alive

The system of communication should be kept open and alive all the year round. It is only by honest attempts that good communicative relations can be developed.

(f) Cordial Employer-employee Relations

Effective communication requires good employer-employee relations, which enable mutual appreciation of different viewpoints.

According to Terry, eight factors are essential in making communication effective:

(a) Inform yourself fully;
(b) Establish a mutual trust in others;
(c) Find a common ground of experience;
(d) Use mutually known words;
(e) Have regard for context;
(f) Secure and hold the receiver's attention;
(g) Employ examples and visual aids; and
(h) Practice delaying relations.

According to Millet, seven factors make communication effective it should be clear, consistent with the expectation of the recipient, adequate, timely, uniform, flexible and acceptable.

8. Need of Effective and Efficient: Good Public Relations to Promote Health Education

The creation of awareness is integral to social and economic development. The possibility for the power of communication to liberate the minds and essential qualities for health professionals, potential of people to critical awareness is real in every field linked to human development, and the generation of public will hinges on effective communication of information and ideas that relate to people's needs, aspirations and capacities for progress in thought the action. In this sense, getting and development process started is largely the task of information, education and communication through public relations. Health Education through public relations is of cardinal importance.

Public relations is the establishment of a climate of understanding. It means interpreting the programme of an organization to the public and *vice-versa*. "Public relations in health is the composite of all the primary and secondary contacts between the health education and the citizens and all the interaction of influences and attitudes established in these contacts."

According to Harwood: "Public relations may be defined as those aspects of our personal and corporate behaviour which have a social rather than private and personal significance."

The purpose of public relations is not only to supply information, but also to encourage an understanding and cooperation between to citizens and the health professionals. The objectives of public relations should be to increase prestige and goodwill and to protect the life of the health organization by safeguarding it against unwarranted attacks as well as to remove the genuine complaints and grievances of the people.[16]

9. Relationship with Patients and Relatives

The hospital today is more than the combination of medical and therapeutic treatment by specialists, greater and refined medical and surgical knowledge and even better and more effective facilities and equipment. It includes these factors as the core of its efficient operation but an additional dimension—one, which is too often ignored or at least minimized—is the human and social element in the structure of the organization.[17]

The ideal of service must be encouraged among the personnel responsible for health care. It is the responsibility of the Health authorities to set the pattern for the philosophy of patient care. It was rightly mentioned by Gardner that:

No society can reach heights of greatness unless in all fields critical to its growth and creativity there is an ample supply of dedicated men and women.[18]

CHART 3.1

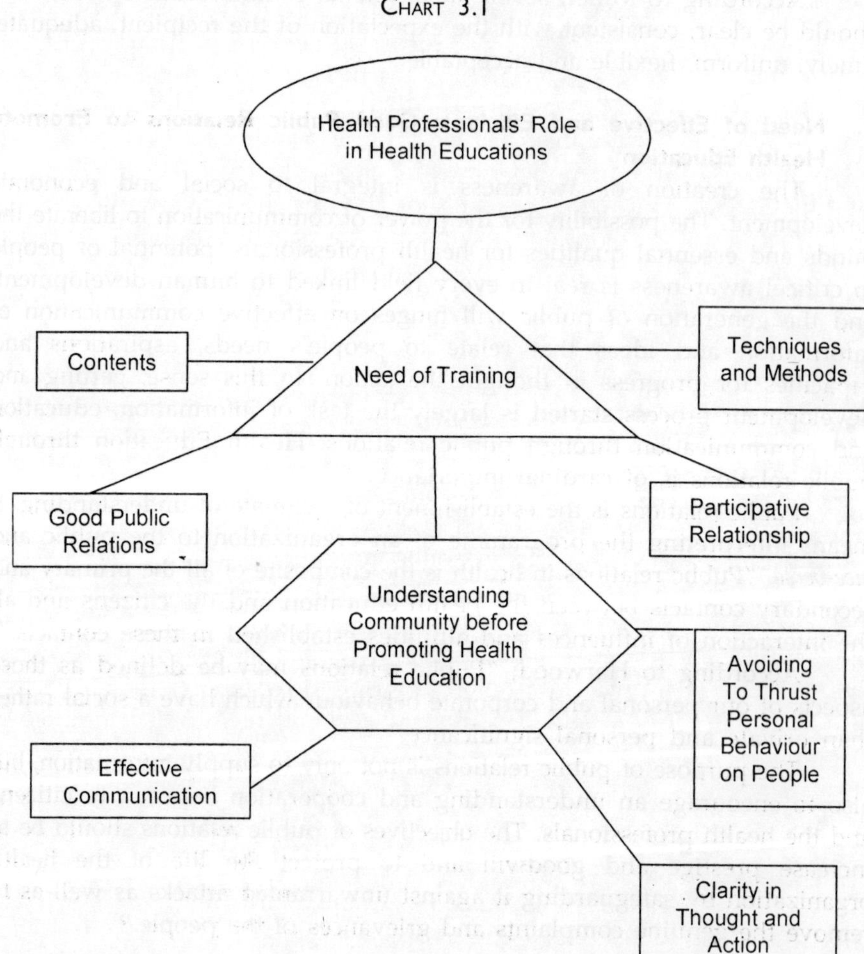

All the personnel engaged in patient care must keep the following definitions of the "patient" in their minds.[19]

- The patient is the most important in the Hospital.
- The patient is not dependant upon us—we are dependent on him.
- The patient is an interruption of our work—he is the purpose of it.
- The patient is not an outsider to our business-he is our business.
- The patient is a person and not a statistic. He has feelings, emotions, biases, and wants.
- It is our business to satisfy him.

10. Holistic Medicine

Medicine for very long time unfortunately differentiated the body-mind binomial. Traditionally, it also separated the disease from the afflicted person, making doctors "specialists in the disease" and "not in the cure as a whole." This attitude was also reflected in medical institutions and in their relationship with their patients. Most institutions have tended to adopt the same attitude in their structure and in their sense of the problems that they faced. You will agree with me that the dissociation of mind and body that permeates the relationship with the patient, rules the institution. However, time has come for all of us to try and help today's medicine to become more humane and complete. This goal-expression effectively informs several professional practices in the treatment of people in hospitals and institutions to adopt "Quality" as a never-ending process.

The modern physician must also be a soul, which strives to attain a moral ideal and to establish equanimity with fellow souls. He should have intense urge to search for a light in the ignorance and the darkness of this world. While treating patients our action must blend with their physiological processes. We should learn to respect their personal rhythm, unique composition and socio-economic individuality.

The distrust, which the public feels towards medicine, the inefficiency, and sometimes the ridicule, of therapeutics are perhaps due to the fact the patients are seen as diseases described in medicine. Obviously, the remaking of a physician should be inspired by the precise knowledge of his body and of his soul. This remaking would require development of institutions wherein body and mind can be shaped according to the natural laws. One would have to learn to control the mind rather than be controlled by it.[20]

11. Equanimity

Last but not the least we come to an important attribute of every good physician or surgeon, Equanimity or Aequanimitas as Sir William Osler termed it. Equanimity means imperturbability, the ability to be unruffled, to be cool, calm amid stress and storm, to be clear in thinking and judgment, during an emergency, or during grave crisis or peril. It is the ability not to betray the emotions of worry, anxiety and above all of fear when treating critically ill patients. Some physicians are born with the gift of aequanimitas, some cultivate it with practice and experience. To be possessed of true equanimity within the without is a divine gift. But even if you cannot help the storm that rages within you, train yourself to hide this, so that you present a picture of fortitude and calm from which your patient imbibes sustenance and strength.[21]

Peaceful Mind

From anger arises infatuation; from infatuation confusion of memory; from confusion of memory, loss of reason; and from loss of reason one goes to complete ruin.

When anger is aroused in the heart of man, it deprives him of his power of discrimination. He is unable to weigh the pros and cons of a question. He will not heed the consequences of whatever he does in a fit of anger. Such is the nature of infatuation caused by anger.

Emotional intelligence is concerned with achieving one's goals through the ability to manage one's own feelings and emotions, to be sensitive to, and influence other key people, and to balance one's motives and drives with conscientious and ethical behaviours. The following are the characteristics of Emotional Intelligence:

(a) Inter personal sensitivity covering competencies like listening and sensitivity.
(b) Motivating, including impact and energy.
(c) Emotional Resilience.
(d) Influence and Adaptability covering both influencing and negotiating ability and being adaptable in various types of situations and cultures.
(e) Decisiveness and assertiveness.
(f) Integrity.
(g) Leadership including motivating other people.[22]

For medical profession, peaceful mind is of utmost significance as a minor wrong decision taken during a disturbed mind can ruin the life of patients. Doctor is dealing with patients and not some statistical data.

12. Action Oriented

Don't wait for your ideas to happen, make them happen. As Adman Carl Ally puts it, "Either you let your life slip away by not doing the things you want to do or you get up and do them." Passion for doing something should be matched with your core capability. It starts with you. You have to be in control to create control. If you can't control yourself you can't control the situation. Once you have control inside you will have control outside. Control doesn't mean suppression. It means regulation. It means channelization. Control adds tempo to performance, daring to vision, and brilliance in performance.[23] The more a doctor would work with patients, the more he would enjoy life. A doctor can be rusted by not acting.

Love and Affection towards all these who are seeking the help of medical personnel—Administration is manned by and meant for people. We must attend to their problems with love and affection, which would in return give strength and bliss.

Happiness on earth and bliss above are certainly the fruits of living the life of love. The changeless abode of the soul is reached by the path of love. Those that are devoid of love are just the skeleton covered with skin.

The journey of this world is delightful to one, who after the removal of his errors and dispersion of the cloud of his ignorance, has come to the knowledge of truth.[24]

13. Honesty and Integrity

"Some say Knowledge is Powers,
Others say the above is not True,
Character is Power and Wealth,"

—*Sri Satya Sai Baba*

Integrity is one of the essentials for Character-building and personality development. Integrity means to be pure in thought and action. Integrity is very easy to accept but very difficult to put in practice. A man or woman of integrity is never influenced by temptations and pressures from outside as he or she would only respond to one's conscience. In today's world, it is very difficult to adhere to integrity as every one is in material race.

Honesty and integrity are other attributes integral to a physician. The need for honesty and integrity in all matters pertaining to patients and to the outside world is obvious enough. I however, refer specially to intellectual honesty. Self-delusion comes easy to one and all in medicine and I too admit to the crime of Procrustes was a robber who had become an innkeeper. When a traveler stopped for the night at his inn, Procerustes would show him to his bed. When the guest was asleep the robber would determine how the guest fitted the bed. If he was short, he would bind him and stretch him so as to fit the bed; if he was too long he would chop off his legs so that he fitted the bed. In medicine it is common to jump to a preformed diagnosis and then delude yourself by making the clinical features fit this diagnosis. You add to what is not or subtract from what is, in order to justify a hasty preformed conclusion.

To err is human, and there is no physician on earth who has not made mistakes. The best-trained faculties may falter in observation, and even in the most experienced, errors in judgment must inevitably occur in an art and science, which often consists in the balancing of probabilities. Cultivate an honesty of mind, which recognizes, regrets and proclaims these mistakes. Only then will you learn from them and perhaps not repeat them. Do not hide your mistakes under a bushel or pretend that they never existed. It you do so, you will be increasingly unable to recognize truth; you will tread the unfortunate path of self-deception and delusion and your mistakes will multiply.

Can there be a true doctor who does not practice, charity? Unquestionably not. Never refuse a patient who seeks your help but cannot afford your fees. You will be twice blessed—both by the patient and by the Lord who values the poor more than the rich. You have the right to live in reasonable comfort but let me quote you a pertinent saying—"No one should approach the temple of science with the soul of a money-changer."[25]

14. Humility and Selfless Services

Humility is the hall-mark of a true physician. The grace of humility is a precious gift. "Knowledge is proud that he knows so much, Wisdom is humble that he knows no more." Extend you charity, humility and consideration not only to your patients, but also to you colleagues, so that you do unto them as you would have them do unto you.

In my opinion, what distinguishes a great physician from an ordinary one is the power of judgment. Hippocrates said, "Judgment is difficult, and indeed medicine has been defined as the art of coming to a conclusion on insufficient evidence." We can increase our power of observation by constant practice. We can become more knowing and more wise through study and experience, but can we improve on our judgment? To an extent judgment is an inborn faculty; "the result of a union of mind and character, which a man either has or has not, and it is almost a difficult for him to increase it as to add a cubit to his stature."

Perhaps the only way to help improve judgment is to improve our mind, not by scientific training alone, but by an exposure to art, culture, literature, history, philosophy—the other great fields of human endeavour. A broader study of the humanities will enable you to understand Man and his afflictions far better than the detailed study of medicine alone. Dip therefore into the treasures of the world around you. Medicine is the study of Man. Study mankind and you will have enhanced your study of Man.[26]

The essence of the spirit of service is contained in the following words of Vivekananda: "This is the gist of all worship—to be pure and to do good to others. He who sees Shiva in the poor, in the weak, and in the diseased, really worships Shiva; and if he sees Shiva only in the image, his worship is but preliminary. He who has served and helped one poor man seeing Shiva in him, without thinking of his caste, or creed, or race, or anything, with him Shiva is more pleased than with the man who sees Him only in the temples. He who wants to serve the father must serve the children first. He who wants to serve Shiva must serve His children and all creatures in the world first."[27]

Swami Chinmayananda rightly observes that in order to live and to bring out the maximum happiness from ourselves, to work out the best for ourselves, everyone of us must have a goal in life, a mission, an inspiring ideal; looking up to that ideal and hitching our eyes to it, we must work on in the world outside. Thereby, the work becomes chastened; the work itself become its own reward for the individual and a great joy wells up in his mind, not in terms of what he gets on the first of the month, but what he gives to the society as best as he can, from the place where he is.[28]

Let us explain the role of serving others with the help of medical profession.

Dr. H. Mahler is very critical about the inability of health workers in contemporary society to influence those social and environmental factors which truly determine public health. He states:

> "There persist widespread negative attitudes among health professionals towards the health care of the poorest strata in the rural and urban population in the developing countries. Most of these attitudes imply-with a repetitiveness of an old gramophones records caught in a narrow, arrogant, condescending and indifferent groove—that these poor people are too apathetic, too superstitious, too illiterate to benefit from the health care potentially availability to them. Health professionals and those who train them should be much more radicals in accepting a social responsibility for the health needs of the people in these poor rural-urban communities so that they can act as agents for change."[29]

In the words of Swami Ranganathananda, "The subject of the philosophy of service, therefore, is not meant for academic discussion in the dull philosophy course of our universities; it should stir the minds and hearts of every section of the population. It is thus, that the nation will get the necessary strength to meet the recurring challenges that this age of revolutionary transition will throw at it. If India succeeds in responding to these challenges adequately, she will become a beacon of hope not only to herself but also to the whole of humanity. We have responded successfully to many a challenge to our national existence and integrity in our long history. And we shall face and overcome this challenge as well. With this faith in ourselves and in our national destiny, let us, from this day onwards, enter our respective fields of life and activity with hope and courage."[30]

To the mechanization of medicine is added the sin of commercialization. This is an age of consumerism where the lure of money—which brings with it power, luxury, comfort and enjoyment of life in all its varied physical forms is paramount. Dreadful as it may sound, medicine is fast becoming a business rather than a profession, and that too, not uncommonly a nefarious, corrupt business. What could be more nefarious than charging exorbitant fees from those who cannot afford them? What could be more corrupt than the practice of doctors who on purpose refer unsuspecting vulnerable patients from one specialist to another for no reason other than profit? What could be more corrupt than the unethical practice of commissions demanded by general practitioners from a specialist to whom a patient is referred?

Another major drawback of contemporary medicine is the crippling expense an ill patient often incurs-an expense that is often ruinous to the family. This is partly due to the fact that the physician of today has forgotten the art of medicine and remains solely pre-occupied with its science. His rapport is with machines and not with patients; it is technology that dictates his course of action and not his clinical judgment. History taking is a neglected art; he forgets to use his sense—his eyes, ears and hands, but remembers numbers, equations and formulae. Expensive investigations and expensive modes of treatment result, when simple tests and simpler measures would have sufficed.

Institutionalized medicine has also led to malpractice. Expensive glittering machines and foyers resembling five star hotels are the landmarks of modern institutions. To meet the cost, and, hopefully, make profit, machines have to be fed, and patients become the fodder for these machines. If an audit were to be carried out on the cost-effectiveness of modern day investigations, the result would indeed be shocking.

Why has there been such a decline in the ethics of contemporary medicine? It is almost certainly related to the decline in the sense of values in our present-day world. This decline is observed in all professions and in the whole of society, perhaps even to a greater extent than that observed in medicine. A burning desire for material gain and wealth dominates life today. It is indeed difficult for a profession to remain an island of virtue when surrounded by a sea of filth and corruption. The island is first eroded and then gradually swamped. But please remember what we have an ancient heritage to cherish and maintain. We must therefore combine and rise to root out the canker eating into the heart of medicine.[31]

Mahatma Gandhi nicely observed, "Living the Gandhian life is supremely hard, for it means stripping oneself of all wants. The people at Sewagram and Sabarmati have made their own uneasy compromises with modernity, but what gives their lives meaning and purpose is that they continue along the Gandhian path. In doing so they remind us that there are higher goals than earning a livelihood, and that in serving our fellowmen, we may best serve ourselves."

15. Keeping Abreast with Latest Knowledge and Changes

Rapid advances in our understanding of the structure and function of the human body, the aetiopathology of diseases and their path physiological consequences have enabled us to help our fellow human beings to overcome disease and disability to a considerable extent. Concomitant technological developments have furthered our ability to devise more precise management strategies to successfully deal with an ever-expanding spectrum of congenital and acquired anomalies. The frontiers of medicine are in fact advancing at an accelerating pace and are destined to continue so in the coming years. Mapping of the human genome, the steady unraveling of the genetic basis of health and ill health and the resultant progress in gene therapy and gene modification are opening up new vistas of diagnosis and therapy. The merging fields of stem cells, tissue engineering and Nan technology hold forth fascinating possibilities in the not too distant future. And the prospective marriage between molecular biology and powerful computational technology could transform the process of the designing and delivery of drugs. These and several other avenues of research have the potential to bring about a major paradigm shift in our understanding and approach to human health during your professional lifetime. And this possibility of medicine moving from the species level to the level of the individual—that is, moving from the current assumption that drugs and diseases work the same way in all human beings to the realization that there are subtle but significant individual variations—may become a reality as you progress in your practice of medicine.[32]

The human body is undoubtedly the most wonderful, the most intricately designed and the most functionally efficient machine—a machine that was perfected through billions of years of experiment and evolution of life by Nature. It has withstood the ravages of disease, famine and other hostile environmental conditions—and survived. A true gift of Nature. Preservation and promotion of health of the Nature's gift, I believe, is the *Raison d'etre* of our profession. While we do have to treat the sick, it should always be our endeavour to prevent sickness in the first place. For, despite all the scientific and technological advances—past, present and future—the old adage, 'prevention is better than cure,' I believe, will always hold true.

16. Team Work

Health care has long ceased to be the exclusive preserve of the doctors. We, as doctors, know that effective and efficient health care can only be delivered if all members of the team work in a concerted fashion. No matter who we are or what is our particular field of specialization, no matter whether we are physicians, surgeons, anaesthesiologists, dental socialists, nurses, physiotherapists, laboratory technologists or any of the several allied health scientists, our common goal is to help heal the sick through our areas of expertise.[33]

17. Treat the Patients with Dedication

Ever increasing population and lack of adequate, affordable health care facilities, particularly for the rural masses, is a matter of serious concern for India. A large proportion of our population has no access to even safe drinking water. The continued practice of open drainage system, indiscriminate disposal of waste and industrial effluents into water bodies, and added to this, increased migration from rural areas to cities resulting in uncontrolled growth of large slums in the urban centers without any sanitation facilities, etc., have created an environment unsuitable for healthy living. It has aggravated the spread of water-borne diseases like cholera, typhoid, tuberculosis, dysentery, and gastroenteritis. Yet another area of concern to the country is the spread of vector-borne diseases such as malaria, filariasis, Japanese encephalitis, and dengue to newer areas with mosquitoes, the vectors carrying these diseases, breeding in stagnated water bodies. It is said that in India alone, over two million cases of malaria are reported every year. Vector Borne Diseases are spreading to newer areas due to increased risk of transmission fuelled by developmental activities, demographic changes and introduction of new chemicals, to name a few possible causes.

Healthcare for our rural populace has become a nightmare with no facilities nearby, and forcing the rural poor to travel long distances for medical help. While specialist medical practitioners are particularly scarce in rural areas, those few who chose to serve in rural areas suffer from lack of infrastructure facilities and technological advances including missing the essential professional interactions found in larger medical centers in the cities. Hardly 2% of the doctors go to villages to practice and more than 70% of our population lives in those villages, and they do not have access to better facilities compared to their privileged urban brethren. Of the 650 million people dwelling in the rural areas in our country, 360 million people are illiterate and almost 70% of them are below poverty line. For these disadvantaged people, health services are distant dreams. It is one of the major issues, the country is facing today. Even as India is hailed as an upcoming developing country with consistent economic growth wherewithal's in the 'knowledge society, we have a long way to go in health care and you have a major role to play in that'.[34]

18. Health Education

Education must create a true health mentality, so that the application of rules for a healthy life becomes part and parcel of the daily round.

For thousands of years, disease and death have been accepted with resignation as normal ingredients of daily life—aspects of a tragic destiny, which strikes some and spares others without rhyme or reason. Today this resignation is unacceptable. We are aware that the dangers that threaten our health are often caused by imperfections in our social structures or in our own behaviour. We can afford to scoff at some of these threats, now that a correct application of new discoveries in medicine enables us to reduce them to reasonable proportions.

The task of education is to apprise people of their responsibilities, since diseases and accidents are so often linked with ignorance, carelessness, and inadequate precautions on the part of national authorities.

Studies made in different countries of the world have shown that fluctuations in the toll of disease and death depend even more on the level of education than on the social and economic conditions in which people live. Ignorance can be just as much a killer as poverty, and these two often go hand in hand.

Informing people is not enough; they have to be motivated. Education must create a true health mentality, so that the application of rules for a healthy life becomes part and parcel of the daily round; it must not limit itself to the domain of ideas. So in the filed of education, we have to draw a distinction between real needs and felt needs. Providing water in a desert area is a powerful felt need. But pure water that is not contaminated by microbes or parasites is a real need rather than a felt need, and one which only education can make apparent.[35]

19. Personal-relationship

It is the fallacy of modernity that we believe we communicate better through machines. Human beings communicate through bonds of mutual confidence. It is the prime task of the health communicator to facilitate a state of communal trust. Unfortunately, the staff of the public health services belongs to the educated elite. Therefore, typical bourgeois values permeate the hierarchy from the top to the level of the field-worker. Reality is seen through the reports of the latter, who knows that his superiors only welcome "facts" which are consistent with their social values and views. Large amounts of pseudo-information are concentrated around the false fact that poverty and ill-health are caused by ignorance. This allows the establishment to launch masses of educational programmes, the purpose and result of which only distract attention from the need for a structural change in society and a redistribution of wealth. In the process, the livelihood of the health education establishment is sustained.

Health and nutrition messages processed by the system have been devised and meted out according to the measure stick of the middle-class bureaucrat behind a desk. With their frequent characterizations of rural or village people's actions as mistakes, habits as bad and attitudes as wrong, they reflect a feudalistic lack of trust in the ability of common people to cope with their lives. There is little doubt that the pattern of working life in an organizational bureaucracy of which health services are a part tends to retard emerging moves towards change.[36]

20. Need of Vision among Medical Professionals to Inject Quality

Medical profession through, Indian Council of Medical Research, Medical Council of India and other organizations should define the role of the medical profession in the new millennium in the context of social development and improvement of the quality of life of the people.

A nation without a 'Vision' perishes. It is the vision that drives the progress of the nation. More than 500 experts drawn from various fields have prepared the "Technology Vision 2020" document for the country, which was released by the Prime Minister in August 1996. This vision document consists of 17 major technology packages. It deals with agricultural infrastructure and production, food-processing, health care, electric power, water-ways, life sciences and bio-technology, inland transportation, civil aviation, engineering industries, electronics, information and communication technology, material technologies and strategic industries, etc.

The Technology Vision Report aims to develop variety of indigenous technologies to transform India into a developed nation by the year 2020. With effective use of indigenously developed technologies in the next quarter century some of the visible results by the year 2020 will be, enhanced wealth of the nation, abundant production in various areas, well being of the people and national security.[37]

21. Human Resource Development: Star Performers—Need of the Hour

For a service industry like health care, human resource is a critical asset and an important differentiator between a good and a great hospital. Therefore, it is essential not only to recruit the right people for the right job, but also to keep them engaged and delighted, provide them an environment to excel and ensure that they stay motivated.

Needless to say, employees who bring direct revenue for the hospital are most valued employees. But apart from them, employees who perform their duty with ease and aplomb, demonstrate traits like initiative, creativity, incisive mind, quick decision-making, ability to guide others, high-level of commitment and sense of responsibility are described as Star Performers (SP). According to Dr. NC Borah, Chairman, Guwahati Neurological Research Centre, Guwahati, "SPs add value to the brand image of the hospital and are very crucial, especially during the initial growth period of any new project." They also display keenness to contribute towards the goal and growth of the organization. What would ultimately differentiate them is the style of working. Super performers should be judged not just by mere outcome. The differentiating factor should be the method of working, which should be systematic.

As per Pareto's Law, 20 per cent employees in any organisation drive the other 80 per cent. But these 20 per cent employees need not be in leadership positions. "Any employee in any position can usher in positive changes in the way a particular process is executed or help device methodologies to enhance throughput and increase efficiency of the department," says Ankush Gupta, Manager, HR, PD Hinduja Hospital, Mumbai. In a hospital set-up where teamwork is crucial, interdepartmental productivity becomes an even more decisive factor for a SP.

Scientific methods of recruitment, performance management system, feedback from colleagues and department heads are some tools that help identify SPs. Moving a step ahead from conventional tools, CMRI and BM Birla Heart Research Centre, Kolkata recently introduced the concept of 'balance score card' to evaluate an individual's performance.

This concept, used for measuring a company's activities in terms of its vision and strategies, forces managers to focus on the important performance metrics that drive success. It balances a financial perspective with the customer, internal process and learning and growth perspectives.

"Through balance score card, parameters are set prior to a person joining any department. Targets are maintained on a daily basis and performance is measured", explains Rupak Barua, Director, Growth and Development, BM Birla Heart Research Centre. The Hospital has also introduced a 'Talent Search' programme whereby management trainees are put on particular projects and monitored for six months to analyse their performance. (see box on how hospitals identify SPs) How hospitals identify star performers?

Hinduja Hospital

Relies on the concept of 'best employee of the month' to identify SPs. Based on parameters like discipline, sense of responsibility, decision-making ability and others, the Hospital assesses the social behaviour and performance of an individual. Every month, the HR department sends out a best employee nomination form to the heads of various departments, who rate their employees and send it back. A committee consisting of senior professionals screens the nominations to determine the best employee of the month.

Apollo Hospitals Group

Employs a scientific outlook to the idea of identifying and defining the targets for their employees. Their performance management system takes into cognisance two Ps—Performance and Potential of their employees. To analyse the performance of an employee, the hospital works on their key result areas (KRAs). At the beginning of the financial year, based on the annual operating plan of the unit, the heads of the units prepare KRAs which are cascaded down to the department heads and then the executives. The exercise is to align the organisational KRAs to individual KRAs. The job performance is evaluated in four major components like financial, customer perspective (as it is a service industry), employee perspective (because it is team effort) and process-related issues.

The test examines capabilities like whether an employee possesses the potential to get into higher responsibilities and has acquired the personality traits required to deal with his/her own work area. At the end of every year, the hospital tracks the individual's performance by incorporating results through performance management system.

Wockhardt Hospitals Group

It relies on performance appraisal system, the kind of business result that employees bring in and customer feedback to spot SPs.

Indian Spinal Injuries Centre (ISIC)

The SP is rewarded as the 'best employee of the year' award and honoured by placing his name on the department 'honour board'. He also gets the privilege to have a meal with the top management apart from a token of appreciation.

Detecting talent also aids in examining whether the employee is apt for the work assigned to him. If a person from one department has a personality trait which can be best leveraged in another area, he or she can be shifted to that domain. This is done with an eye to enhancing the productivity of the employee.

"Once the super performer is identified, a detailed growth pattern should be chalked out for him/her. We give them higher responsibilities based on three factors—targets achieved on time, the potential to assume higher responsibilities and level of excellence with the customers," explains T. Karunakar, GM-HR, Apollo Hospitals, Hyderabad.

Roping in Stars

Any new induction obviously is based on the job specifications and the job description for the specific vacancy. It also depends on the level of hierarchy at which the person is to be inducted. If the position is that of a decision-maker and the person will impact the way a particular function is run, analysing the traits of a SP in him becomes *sine qua non*.

In Apollo Hospitals Group, psychometric tools like Thomas Profiling are used for candidates during selection, to identify their behavioural traits. The test maps the behaviour of the applicant to his promised work profile, helping the company identify the right profile for the job. This in the long-term helps in choosing more SPs in the organisation.

"Though the test is not completely foolproof, it gives some insight into the person's ability to match the job profile. Since some jobs need less creativity while some require more creativity and problem-solving skill, one should be able to match skill set requirements with competencies and competencies with personalities," states Sangita Reddy, Executive Director-Operations, Apollo Hospitals Group. Initial right selection can obviously lead to harvesting potential star performers in the organisation.

Directing star power

The problems with managing creative employees are myriad. Often they leave the organisation if they feel they are stagnating or their efforts have not been acknowledged.

"The biggest hurdle with managing SPs is meeting their expectations in terms of rewards, better salaries, better flexibilities, more authority and faster climb in the organisation," states Kumar S. Krishnaswamy, Group Head, HRD, Wockhardt Hospitals Group, Bangalore.

And, there can be ego issues. Tensions can also occur in work environment when senior people have to work under a young and dynamic performer.

When the SP gets restless and more lucrative job offers come in his way, he threatens to leave. This leads to organisations grappling with retention of their best talent. Organisations have realised that it is easy to lose a SP, but difficult to retain one and still more arduous to replace one. However, organisations are not always in a position to fulfil the demands and expectations of SPs in the process of retaining them. There are other employees in the organisation who are vital, and always heeding the demands of the SP might crush the growth of other employees.

Thus, the approach for retaining should not be a last-minute one, when the person is calling it quits. Instead, the organisation should take a proactive approach. The three-tier strategy that most hospitals adopt is: appreciate them, train them and chalk a clear career path. "Good appreciation of their efforts, involvement in challenging assignments, slightly non-routine job responsibilities, and clear growth in the organisation are the time-tested ways to manage and retain high performers," opines Gupta.

Nurturing the Star

Motivating and training star employees to deliver continuously is another issue. Talent needs to be nurtured and the right skill set has to be imbibed.

According to Dr. Ravindra Karanjekar, GM, Wockhardt Hospitals, Mumbai, "The best method to hone the super performer is to continuously give him challenging situations and empower him to take decisions."

Recently, in Wockhardt Hospital, Mumbai, a group from the administrative department was given a Herculean task of creating a liver transplant unit in just seven days. There was a time constraint as well as sterile conditions to be complied with in the whole operational process.

"I told them to plan the project, study the intricacies and gave them complete freedom. By the the end of the project, all persons involved automatically evolved as SPs," reveals Dr. Karanjekar.

Besides challenging tasks, it is mandatory that continuous training on behavioural as well as technical skills be imparted. "Continuous training would ensure consistency of performance," explains Dr. Karanjekar.

Confidence building is a constant process and SPs need to be taken into confidence through constant monitoring. Experts underscore the procedure of sensitisation, through which SPs are given the realisation that they are not indispensable and can make mistakes.

The Star in Spotlight

More than monetary benefits, it is essential to acknowledge them publicly. Thus, in the Star Programme at Apollo Hospitals, the employees are rewarded in front of everybody. Similarly, 'compliment a colleague' concept tracks the appreciation of one colleague's better performance by another. These strategies have helped Apollo Hospitals build the concept of oneness among all. "Give them importance, recognise their contribution and at the same time tactfully make them understand that the contribution of other members of the team is equally important for his/her success," states Dr. Borah.

Motivation is the key for better performance and more enthusiastic employees, opines Dr. R.K. Anand, Medical Director, Jaslok Hospital, Mumbai.

He cites a recent example to prove his point. "The charity commissioner visited our hospital recently and the medical social worker (MSW) who was taking the commissioner around did exceptionally well in the task assigned to her. She not just knew every patient, but could also cite the medical diagnosis of that patient.

"After this incident, in the presence of the charity commissioner, we acknowledged her work," explains Dr. Anand. The result is a motivated employee, who is now working on many more projects.

"Money is not always a motivator. If someone is skilful, he will never really feel the dearth of money. Highlighting them in public gatherings as potential leaders and trainers will motivate them like nothing else," says Dr. Bidhan Das, Former Director, Operations, Rockland Hospital, New Delhi and now a consultant, Quality Council of India at Bhopal.

They say that equipment and technology do not make a hospital. The employees do. And being able to make super performers of their employees will differentiate a good organisation from a great one.

As one expert puts it, not having SPs is the failure of organization and not of employees.

ICMR should prepare a document for the new millennium to ensure quality health care which should not be second to developed countries so that our people do not rush to the health institutions of advanced countries and waste financial resources and bring discredit to the country. We should develop our own health system which should possess all quality standards.

CONCLUSION

The success of medical profession that is delivery of health services to the people depends upon the sincerity, dignity, honesty, integrity, perfection, etc. of medical professionals. The medical professionals can create confidence and credibility among patients and usher an era of best health services.

Medical professional can promote health and make India healthy and strong. India has its own well developed indigenous systems of health care like ayurveda, yoga, siddha, unani, etc. along with diverse ecosystem specific, local health traditions. These systems could be used to complement the allopathic system, as they could be more useful in certain areas of curative/preventive health care. This would enhance the quality and outreach of public health services, which are currently unable to meet the health needs of our people. However, care would have to be taken to ensure that we do not substitute the allopathic system of health care in areas like immunization, etc. where it has not alternative.

At present, our health care system suffers from a severe shortage of trained personnel. Across states, 6.30% posts of doctors remain vacant and random checks show that 29-67% doctors are absent. One way of overcoming the difficulty in recruiting qualified doctors to serve in rural areas is to make greater use of trained paramedical personnel. There is a strong case for reintroducing the 2-year licentiate course in medicine, which existed earlier but was abolished. We also need to devise ways of training and accrediting the rural health providers (popularly called RMPs) and permitting them to provide select services under the supervision of a licensed medical practitioner.[38]

Health is of great significance for the overall development of the country. Until and unless people of a country are not healthy, they cannot contribute their potential energy to socio-economic development, nation-building and modernization.

Dr. E.J. Thierry in his article, "Laying the Foundations", succinctly remarked that,

> "Health is man's most precious possession; it influences all his activities; it shapes the destinies of people. Without it, there can be no solid foundation for man's happiness. Nevertheless, all too often, social planners forget this simple truth and leave health out of account. Integration of health schemes in overall development plans are of paramount importance."

Health is fundamental to the national progress in any sphere. In terms of resources for economic development, nothing can be considered of higher importance than the health of the people which is a measure of their energy and capacity as well as of the potential man-hours for productive work in relation to the total number of persons maintained by the nation. For the efficiency of industry and of agriculture, the health of the worker is an essential consideration.

To improve understanding between the citizens and the hospital personnel, public relations need to be developed in an effective manner to create favourable community opinion towards the hospital services. This would create confidence in the minds of the people towards the competence, fairness, honesty, impartiality and sincerity of the hospital personnel. The following do's and don't may always be kept in mind for better public relations:

1. The patient is never interruption to work: the patient is our work. Everything else can wait!
2. Greet every patient with a friendly smile. Patients are people and they like friendly contact. They usually return it.
3. Call patients by name. Make a game of learning patients' names, and see how many you can remember.
4. Teach your staff members that for patients, all staff members are as important as the doctor.
5. Never argue with a patient. The patient is always right (in his or her own eyes). Be a good listener, agree with them where you can, and do what you can to make them happy.
6. Never say, "I don't know." If you don't know the answer to a

patient's question, say, "That is a good question. Let me see it can find out for you."

7. Remember that the patient pays your salary: treat him like your boss!
8. Choose positive words when speaking to a patient. This is a valuable habit that will help you become an effective communicator.
9. Brighten every patient's day, and you'll soon discover that your own life is happier and brighter.
10. Always go the extra mile, do just a little more than the patient expects you to do. For example, make it a habit to phone the patient after discharge from the hospital, to ensure he is doing well. Exceeding patient expectations is the best way to keep your patients happy and keep them as your patients for life.

WHO in its Report of WHO Inter-country meeting on quality assurance in health care from 16-20 December 1996 at Indonesia suggested the following for South-East Asian countries:

(1) Ensure that quality of health care is an integral part of health services delivery at all levels of health care covering public and private sectors;
(2) Organize advocacy/awareness workshops on quality assurance for policy-makers administrators and the leadership of health care to get their commitment for quality assurance;
(3) Establish a coordinating mechanism for quality assurance activities at national level through the nomination of focal point(s) and constitute a multi-disciplinary task force of national experts to provide advice on technical aspects of quality assurance;
(4) Initiate quality assurance of health care in selected hospitals and in primary health care through the district health system approach, document the experiences and expand gradually to more health care facilities;
(5) Organize national strategic planning workshops with technical assistance from WHO;
(6) Formulate guidelines to set standards and select national key indicators on quality assurance to monitor compliance and measure performance;
(7) Invest on building local capacity in health care quality through the creation of a critical mass of expertise with in the country;
(8) Mobilize potential resources from within the country including support from international agencies; and
(9) Ensure that orientation on quality assurance be integrated in both basic and in-service training programmes of all health care professionals.

Implementation of TQM in health institution calls for a total change in culture in terms of customs, practices and improvement by creating increased sense of caring brought about by improved communication, involvement and training. It involves the integration of all functions, processes and personnel with an organization in order to achieve continuous improvement in the quality of health care delivery systems.

By following TQM principles we can bring about harmony and quality working style in all the facets of the health institution and help it gain the top position and maintain it.

Finally, TQM consists in doing for the institution what should be done as a matter of course. The fruits of implementation of TQM may not be available instantly, lie magic tree, but it is sure to show improvements in health standards over a period of time.

Notes and References

1. Y.S. Rajasekhram, A Holistic Approach to Achieve the Health Targed, *University News*, 44 (16), April 17-23, 2006, p. 15.
2. K. Mohandas, 'Presentation and Promotion of Health', *University News*, 44 (33), August 14-20, 2006, p. 20.
3. K. Mohandas, 'Presentation and Promotion of Health', *University News*, 44 (33), August 14-20, 2006, p. 20.
4. *Ibid.*, p. 20.
5. *University News*, 42 (34), August 23-29, 2004, pp. 13-14.
6. *University News*, 43 (15), April 11-17, 2005, p. 20.
7. Jeffrey on Dragen, Care of the individual patient, *University News*, 42 (36), September 06-12, 2004, p. 15.
8. Steven Hla Myint, Training For Global Health Care Market, *University News*, 44 (21), May 22-28, 2006, p. 21.
9. Swami Ranganathananda, "Democratic Administration in the light of Practical Vedanta," p. 47.
10. Dr. B. Ramamurthi, Values in the Medical Field, in values, p. 171.
11. *Ibid.*, p. 178.
12. Y.C. Simadhri, Societal Relevance of Pharmacy Education, *University News*, 42 (26), June 28-July 04, 2004, p. 23.
13. Shigekoto Kailhara, "Information explosion", *World Health*, August/September 1989, pp. 6-7 and 8.
14. *Ibid.*, p. 11.
15. Prof. K.J. Nath, Public Health in India Five Decades, Vol. 1, pp. 6-7.
16. Harwood, Childs L., An Introduction to Public Opinions, *op. cit.*, p. 2.
17. Mary D. Shanks and Dorothy A. Kennedy. The Theory and Practice of Nursing Service Administration, McGraw-Hill, London, 1965, p. 95.
18. John W. Gardner, Excellence, New York, 1961, Harper and Brothers, p. 154.
19. Edythe Alexander *et. al.*, Nursing Service Administration (ed.), New York, C.V. Mosby Co., 1962, p. 63.
20. Mahendra Bhandari, Holistic Medicine and a Complete Human Physcians, *University News*, 44 (08), February 20-26, 2006, pp. 18-19.
21. *University News*, 42 (34), August 23-29, 2004, p. 14.
22. Aruna Goel, "Good Governance and Ancient Sanskrit Literature," New Delhi, Deep & Deep, 2003, pp. 59-60.

23. *Ibid.*, p. 60.
24. *Ibid.*, p. 108.
25. *University News*, 42 (34), August 23-29, 2004, p. 14.
26. *Ibid*.
27. The Complete Works of Swami Vivekananda, Vol. IV, p. 324.
28. Swami Chinmayananda, Kindle Life, *op. cit.*, p. 192.
29. Text of Address by Dr. H. Mahler, to the Thirteenth Session of Regional Committee of South East Asia.
30. Swami Ranganathanand, *op. cit.*, p. 251.
31. *University News*, 42 (34), August 23-29, 2004, pp. 15-16.
32. R. Mohandas, Preservation and Promotion of Health, *University News*, 44 (33), August 14-20, 2006, pp. 19-20.
33. *Ibid.*, p. 20.
34. *University News*, 43 (15), April 11-17, 2005, p. 17.
35. Etienne Berthet, A New role for teachers, *World Health*, May 1979, pp. 23-24.
36. Andreas Fuglesang, "Folk-wisdom and pseudo-information," *World Health*, January-February, 1989, p. 7.
37. *University News*, March 2, 1998, p. 12.
38. Government of India, Planning Commission, New Delhi, December 2006, Towards Faster and More Inclusive Growth, An Approach to the 11th Five Year Plan (2007-12), p. 68.

APPENDIX

Teaching Managerial Skills to Medical Students Undergoing Health Services Programme: An Experience from Eastern Nepal

NILAMBAR JHA, K.C. PREMARAJAN, S. NAGESH, SANJAY KUMAR, SURYA RAJ NIRAULA, SAILESH BHATTARAI, DEEPAK, K.C.

Abstract

When young medical graduates take up responsible positions in government hospitals, private hospitals, health centres and in national health programmes, they are given a lot of managerial responsibilities in addition to their technical role. Due to lack of training and exposure in health management they feel incompetent and insecure in their jobs, leading to frustration and low productivity. Management skills become more crucial at the peripheral health care institutions where a doctor is the team leader and has to implement a number of health programmes with the help of other health staff. So, skills like planning, leadership, supervision, monitoring and communication are a must for any doctor in order to make an impact on the health scenario of the country. It was against this background that the Department of Community Medicine at the BP Koirala Institute of Health Sciences (BPKIHS), Dharan, Nepal started a two-week residential programme on managerial skills development for the Eighth Semester MBBS students in March 2004. This article discusses the students' feedback about the programme and their own achievements during various postings.

Introduction

The weakest link in the health care delivery system in most developing countries like Nepal is the poor planning and management at different levels of health care services. This is mainly due to the lack of manpower trained in hospital and health management and also due to outdated policies and procedures. Hospital services are becoming more and more complex and sophisticated on the one hand, and health programmes on the other hand need to be more community- and result-oriented. A well-trained workforce in health and hospital management is required for optimum utilization of scarce health care resources in the country, for improving public health.

When the young medical graduates take up responsible positions in government hospitals, private hospitals, health centres and in national health programmes, they are given a lot of managerial responsibilities in addition to their technical role. Due to lack of training and exposure in health management they feel incompetent and insecure in their jobs, leading to frustration and low productivity. Management skills become more crucial at the peripheral health care institutions where a doctor is the team leader and has to implement a number of health programmes with the help of other health staff. So, skills like planning, leadership, supervision, monitoring and communication are a must for any doctor in order to make an impact on the health scenario of the country. It was against this background that the Department of Community Medicine at the BP Koirala Institute of Health Sciences (BPKIHS), Dharan, Nepal started a two-week residential programme on managerial skills development for the Eighth Semester MBBS students in March 2004.

The BPKIHS is an autonomous health science university with a tertiary care hospital situated in eastern Nepal:

1. The MBBS curriculum of BPKIHS is thoroughly integrated and community-oriented. It is partially problem-based, and incorporates the organ system and a need-based approach.
2. Teaching of community medicine throughout the MBBS course is the unique feature of this programme. The emphasis on early clinical and community exposure and self-directed learning is another innovative feature.
3. The MBBS students have to undertake six weeks of residential field posting in the community organized by the Department of Community Medicine. This posting is conducted in three blocks of two weeks each. This article discusses one of the residential field postings, to teach managerial skills under the health service programme (Health-Man) in zonal hospitals and district public health offices (DPHOs). The objectives of the programme are as follows:

At the end of the posting, the student will be able to:

- Recognize the importance of managerial skills in health care delivery services at different levels;
- Observe all activities of the Zonal Hospital and the district public health system;
- Familiarize oneself with activities at all levels of the health care system in Nepal, including national health programmes;
- Familiarize oneself with the mechanism of monitoring and supervision;
- Describe the Health Management Information System (HMIS) in Nepal; and
- Develop the skill to work as a group leader.

The health care delivery system in Nepal has a three-tier system starting from sub-health post (SHP) as a basic unit in each village development committee. One health post is situated among five to six village development committees and primary health centre in each Parliamentary constituency. These are the primary levels of health care delivery institutions. The District Health Office (DHO) is the secondary level of health care delivery system, present in the district. It provides promotive, curative and preventative services. The DHO is also responsible for implementation of all national health programmes.

The Zonal Hospital in Nepal provides tertiary care and is generally a 200-300- bedded hospital with specialist services like medicine, surgery, obstetrics and gynecology, paediatrics, ophthalmology, dermatology, psychiatry and orthopaedics, etc. The District Public Health Office is present as a separate office in the district headquarters, and looks after all national health programmes and public health activities in that district. For this posting, students are not posted at district hospitals because the students from the Fifth semester of MBBS start visiting the district hospital once in a week till the ninth semester with their supervisors from all clinical and community medicine departments under a separate programme called "Learning in Field" (LIF). It is felt that this exposure is not adequate to impart the skills of health management to students. Hence a two-weeks intensive exposure is planned every year in March.

Materials and Methods

The eighth semester MBBS students were divided into three groups on a random basis (52 in 2004 and 59 in 2005) and each group had 18 to 20 students. Each group of students, alongwith the faculty supervisors were posted at the Zonal Hospital and the District Public Health Office (DPHO) at one of the following three zones in the eastern development region of Nepal, such as Mechi, Koshi and Sagarmatha. The first two days were allotted for theoretical orientation on health and hospital management topics, including the need for management training for medical students and for briefing them on the learning objectives of the posting.

This was followed by the field posting at zonal hospitals and DPHOs at Bhadrapur, Biratnagar and Rajbiraj. From the DPHO they were posted for a day each to the primary health Centre, health post and sub-health post in that area. In addition, one day was allotted to study the functioning of a key non-governmental organization (NGO) working in the health care field in the region.

The process of learning involved observations during health facility visits, interaction with key service providers at the facility, study of the records and interviews with the patients and other beneficiaries in the community. Every evening, the students discussed their observations and management issues identified during the visit, with their resource persons to complete their learning experience. After the field posting, each group prepared a comprehensive report on its observations and comments. On the last day each group made a power point presentation to the whole class and the institute's faculty.

Prior to the posting, a series of departmental meetings were held to finalize the schedule. The Programme Coordinator and the faculty from the Department of Community Medicine visited each place of posting. They briefed the Medical Superintendents of zonal hospitals and district public health officers about the objectives of the posting and sought their support and cooperation in organizing the various learning activities during the posting.

On the first day of the posting, students were briefed about their role and responsibility. They were told that the purpose of the posting was to make them good health managers for the future with the possibility of their being posted to such places and to work with these limited resources and in such environments after obtaining their degrees. The total duration of the posting was two weeks. The students participated in all activities of the Zonal Hospital and the DPHO. Student evaluation and feedback were recorded at the end of the posting.

Results

These two residential field postings in health management were conducted in March 2004 and March 2005, respectively. Students received good support and cooperation from the local health authorities in zonal hospitals and DPHOs.

Students were posted for two days in the Zonal Hospital during which they visited the various patient care facilities such as the Outpatient Department (OPD), laboratory services, wards and the Operation Theatre. During the visit they studied the staffing, functions, organization, services, patient flow, work load, facility layout, and policies and procedures, as well as management problems. They also looked at resources utilization like bed occupancy rate, and average OPD load, etc. Following this, they studied supportive services such as housekeeping, sterilization, hospital waste management and laundry. They were also briefed on the administrative aspects, such as *Regional Health Forum, Volume 10, Number 1, 2006,* personnel management, and budgeting and expenditure pattern. The interaction of students with the Medical Superintendent and Nursing In-charge helped them to get an overview of the hospital administration and managerial problems like shortage of medical and nursing staff, limited resources, and delay in receiving funds, etc.

During posting at the DPHO, students got to know its various functions, especially its role in implementing various national health programmes and in managing the peripheral health institutions. Students interacted with the staff responsible for various public health programmes in the district to get an understanding of how programmes were implemented at the field level. They also learned how training programmes were organized by the DPHO to update the knowledge and skills of health workers.

Following this, they spent a day each at a primary health centre, health post and sub-health post. Here they got an opportunity to directly observe the functions, facilities and staff availability. In some places students were able to appreciate the gross underutilization of available facilities. They also studied the information flow from the periphery to the district level as part of the Health Management Information System (HMIS) by going through the monthly and quarterly reports. At the PHC and Health Post, students got an opportunity to directly observe the implementation of DOTS, as well as Leprosy and diarrhoea control programmes, etc.

Visits to NGOs working in health and development sector and NGO-supported hospitals enabled the students to understand the functioning and role of NGOs in supplementing the health care services provided by the government. They could appreciate the efficiency and dedication of NGOs compared to the government sector. All students (both batches 111) felt the objectives of the programme were clear to them. Table 1 shows the visits of students to different levels of the health care system of Nepal. Many students felt that the visits had been useful for them to learn the problems and possible solutions in the field of management. They also learnt supervisory skills during these visits. The students prioritized the managerial skills learnt during these visits.

Discussion

Primary health care is a complex concept requiring the most efficient use of resources, which are almost always scarce, and implying choice and the setting up of priorities. It involves communities in making decisions about their own health care and in accepting responsibility for protecting their own health. Generally, it requires the best use to be made of various categories of health workers, many of whom may be inadequately trained for the work they are expected to do, unused to working in teams, or dissatisfied with their working conditions. Health care is often a matter of persuading or educating people to change certain kinds of behaviour that affects their health.

In the students' opinion, visits to international nongovernmental organizations (INGOs)/NGOs working in the field of health were the most useful (100%), followed by DPHO (98.2%), Health Post (93.2%) and Sub-health Post (89.2%). The reasons could be that they visited INGO/NGOs for the first time, and also because these offices work efficiently and effectively as compared to government offices.

The DPHO visit was ranked second in terms of usefulness to students. The reason for this may be that students learnt hands-on about national health programmes and their implementation in the community. Another reason could be that there was maximum possibility for them to work at the district-level health care system after completion of their course.. During posting, students learnt various managerial skills from the team concept to multiple approaches to solving a problems.

Motivation and mobilization, however, depend not only on management, but also on leadership: hence the need to develop leadership skills among personnel with supervisory responsibilities. Supervision is one of the functions of both management and leadership and has been defined as the overall range of measures to ensure that personnel carry out their activities effectively and become more competent at their work. A supervisor thus appears as the interface between management techniques and the qualities of leadership, which all primary health workers in positions of responsibility should, in theory, possess and in practice display at all levels of the health system.

Another benefit of this posting is that it improves the supervisory skills. Health care services are a human resource intensive field. A good human relation is a must for any manager to get maximum productivity from the health team. During this field posting, students got the opportunity to interact with peripheral-level health workers, and to study their job responsibilities, working conditions, resource constraints, and field logistic problems, etc. This experience will be very useful for them to become good supervisors who can support and guide other team members. A study from the East Caroline University School of Medicine, USA.

Has reported on the training of medical students about leadership skills with community leaders through seminars. These leadership skills are useful for students to participate in community activities. A study conducted after the introduction of training in primary health care programme management into the curriculum in Gezira Medical School showed positive results for students' achievement and acceptance. The experience proved the feasibility of integrating health care programme management into the undergraduate curriculum. A similar training of medical students in primary health care in Nigeria showed favourable response from students and the faculty. These skills are really important to make a good health manager. These managerial and leadership skills are also the components of a "Five Star Doctor."

Other components are being a good communicator, team leader and care-giver. Management is a systematic way of eliciting cooperation from all possible sectors. Its principles and methods are the same whether resources are plentiful or scarce, or whether conditions are favourable or unfavourable. When resources are scarce and conditions difficult the necessary management effort can also be difficult. Good managers perseveres, however, and never loses sight of basic principles. Management principles are applied at all levels of a health care system at the central or national level, in zonal, district and primary level. It is a common mistake to regard management as a function of those at the top of the pyramid only, and to give little attention to intermediate and district levels. The effect is that well conceived programmes fail because of confusion at the lower levels of the pyramid.

Through this posting, students were able to understand the need for managerial skills at the primary level also. Good management is to organization what health is to the body—for the smooth functioning of all its parts. It highlights priorities, adapts services to needs and changing situations, makes the most of limited resources, improves the standard and quality of services, and maintains high staff morale. Early exposure to management process and problems in health care field helps in not only sensitizing oneself to management issues but also in making them letter equipped to take up managerial responsibility in future. Therefore, as a result of the positive feedback received from students of the Health-Man programme, there is hope that they will become good managers of their respective organizations.

Acknowledgement

The authors are grateful to the faculty and staff of the Department of Community Medicine, as well as to the students involved in the programme.

References

Agrawal, C.S. and Karki, P. Evolution of the second medical school in Nepal: A case study. *Medical Teacher*. 1999; 21(2):204-206.

BPKIHS, Dharan, Nepal. The first version of MBBS curriculum 1996.

Naga Rani, M.A., Koirala, S., Das, B.P. and Rauniyar, G.P. A brief review of the pre-clinical curriculum of the BP Koirala Institute of Health Sciences, Dharan, Nepal. *Medical Education*, 2002;36: 393:394.

McMoham, R., Barton, E. and Piot, M. *et al.*, On being in change. World Health Organization, Geneva, 1992.

Flahault, D. and Roemer, M.I. Leadership for Primary Health Care. Public Health Paper No. 82. World Health Organization, Geneva, 1986.

Job Ac, Coale M.M., Kolasa, K., Willis, L., Irons, T.G. Leadership development for medical students beyond the prescription pad. *Fam Med*. 1993; 25(3): 179-81.

Abdel Rahim, I.M., Abdeen, A.Z., Faki, B.A., Mustfa, A.E., Nalder, S. Introducing training in Primary Health Care program management into the curriculum. *Med. Educ.*, 1987; 21(4): 288-92.

Akpala, Co., Medical education and primary health care in Nigeria: The Sokoto University experience. *Cent Afr J Med*, 1991; 37(11): 347-8.

Boelen, C., Medical education reforms: the need for global action. *Academic Medicine*, 1992; 67(11): 745-49.

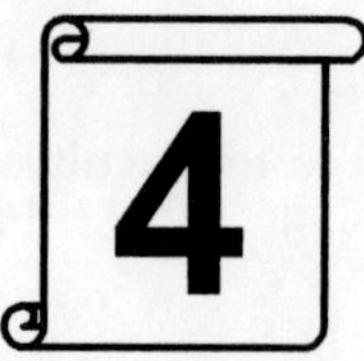

Doctor-Patient Relationship

Doctor-patient relationship is of utmost significance in medical science. In this context the first and foremost requirement is that the doctor need to develop a good rapport with the patients, which would enable him to know about him. There are large number of questions in the mind of the patient, which are creating problems and bad health. Doctor can remove many of his doubts through discussion. It is of great significance for the doctor to take the patient in confidence. Doctors and patients are intimately connected as the existence of one without the other is not possible.

In Ancient Universities in India, convocation address to the medical personnel . . . said:

> "..........Everyday you should continuously and whole-heartedly try to promote the health of the patients. Even if your own life is in danger, you should not desert your patients. You should not entertain an evil thought about the wealth or wives of others. Your dress should be modest, not foppish. Avoid drinking; do not commit a sin, nor help one who is committing it. Your speech should be smooth, polished, truthful and to the point. Taking all facts into consideration, you should make a deliberate endeavour to increase the stock of your knowledge and instruments...When you enter a patient's room, all your attention should be centered on the patients, his expression, movements and medicines, to the exclusion of anything else..."
>
> "Though well grounded in your line you should not praise your knowledge much; for some people get disgusted even with their friends and relatives if they are given to boasting. One can never get a mastery of the entire medical science...One should therefore pass one's time in making a constant effort to learn something more. A wise man will indeed gather something from every quarter; a fool

only thinks otherwise, and shows jealously. Taking all things into consideration, a wise physician should listen to and derive benefit from the discoveries or observations even of an enemy, if they are calculated to promote one's fame and prosperity in this world."[1]

The harmonious relationship depends upon the sincerity, earnestness and co-operation between the Doctor and the Patient. The achievement of good relations between the Doctor and the patient is a matter that does not depend by any means solely on the conduct of Doctors. It equally depends on the attitude of patients and thus their relations. People must behave well towards Doctors. If loose and unsubstantiated allegations are made about their incompetence, dishonesty, laziness and indifference to the public interests, it is unlikely that doctors will develop or display qualities of integrity, industry and public spirit. Both the doctors and the public must exhibit harmonious relationship between them. This would promote good rapport between the two, which would promote good relationship. Doctor-Patient relationship means the development of cordial, equitable and therefore mutually profitable relations between the two. Let us now discuss the essential features of their relationship.

Patients are demanding a more substantive, collaborative role in their own health care decision-making. Collaborative healthware is the application of information and communication technologies designed to enhance decision-making and communication between providers, patients, and their families. The emergence of collaborative healthware will play an important role in supporting the relationship between patient and provider and will assist patients in better understanding their illness experience and how their own values affect decision-making. Collaborative healthware is defined as "software for health care, tightly integrated with people systems"[2] and its creative and successful implementation will improve patient care and care management.

Collaborative healthware supports the relationship between health care provider and patient by engaging patients and their families as full partners in the health care process. In a collaborative partnership, patients expect that their clinicians will provide information's and guidance. Patients expect that their clinicians will educate them and their families on illnesses, available therapies, potential outcomes, and complications, so that decisions can be made based on the patient's individual preferences.[3]

More often patients are presented with opportunities to actively participate in decisions that affect their lives and well-being.[4] While patient preferences for participation in clinical decisions vary greatly,[5] the desire for information about their health and health care is high.[6] Patients want information that addresses their individual concerns and conditions as well as interactive tools to manage their health and disease.[7] Providing patients with enhanced health-related information favorably affects their trust in, relationship with, and confidence in their health care providers.[8]

1. INTRODUCTION

The study of doctor-patient relationship is of paramount importance, in the context of good patient care. It is to be realised that in this set-up both the participants are under a degree of stress. The doctor has to use his professional knowledge and skill, observing a degree of discipline and ethics to improve the patient's lot, who in turn looks upon him as a man of knowledge and science and who is pictured as kind, friendly, thoughtful and warm person, committed to do everything possible for patient's welfare. In this task he may be constrained by his ability, time, communication, money, attitude of the referral hospital, hospital systems, hospital environment, etc.

In India, medical attention is claimed as a Fundamental Right and in turn a good deal of sympathy and human approach is shown in most of the clinics/hospitals (unlike in advanced countries like U.S.A, where monetary considerations rule supreme). It would be desirable to keep the Doctor free from hunger, wants, exploitation and extraneous stresses, if the health care delivery is to be saved from complete commercialisation. This entails giving him the conditions of confidence and comfort, so that he is neither affected by ego, nor enters into unhealthy competition to muster more and more money.

2. PHYSICAL AND SOCIAL FACTORS

Man's social and physical environment determines his exposure and susceptibility to disease-conditions. His pattern of life, the work which he does, the place in which he lives, recreation which he pursues, may all increase or decrease the likelihood of his contracting a particular disease and may encourage or impede their development. Some diseases maybe found among the poor, others among the rich, some among women others among men, some among young others among old, some in married others among single, some among a particular occupation, some among those living in a particular locality and so on. Despite the spectacular advances in medical science, there is much that remains unknown about chronic degenerative and incurable diseases. Since the cause may be the product of the interaction of several factors, it is necessary to explore the patient's environment.

Illness is something that happens between the patient and the doctor—the first contributing the mystery of his symptoms and the second proposing an explanation. Behind the patient is the whole weight of collective representative which he, his friends and relatives have of illness, and behind the doctor are the systems which he learnt in books and during training. The therapeutic dialogue is therefore an exchange between two elements of society rather than two individuals. So, illness is not something absolute or isolated condition, it should be understood by evaluating the meaning of the situation for the participants, in terms of their perception of the benefits and drawbacks of particular courses of action.

When people seek medical care, there are two inter-related set of demands, action-values and social interactions: between one, the everyday life of the patient and the other professional therapeutic system of organised medicine, both may have conflicting interests and priorities. The patient may be more concerned with primary symptoms of pain than the underlying disease, the doctor may be more concerned about the diagnosis and treatment of illness (and its cause), than to produce an immediate comfort. This may lead to conflict. Why?

Similarly, a well read layman's effort at self-diagnosis and self-treatment are as much damaging to the doctor's dignity, as they are dangerous to the patients' health and welfare.

3. WHAT BRINGS A PATIENT TO THE DOCTOR?

It is not the disease always. It could be morbid episode of life, illness conditions, disabilities, disorders, psychological stress, symptoms, non-diseases as well as their attempted cures. Whatever may be the complaint, it indicates disturbance in smooth pattern of existence or a change in his/her external or internal environment. Hence, while diagnosing and treating diseases, if is often important to study illness behaviour, i.e., the way in which given symptoms may be differentially perceived, evaluated and acted (or not acted) upon by different kinds of persons. Their full understanding requires paying attention to the underlying social and psychological context, as the cause of disturbance or studying the reasons for reduced tolerance of symptoms and his capacity to cope with the stress.

It may be related to the growth and development (as at puberty or menopause) or social events, e.g., marriage, getting or loosing job, first love, first child, bereavement, illness, etc. For instance, a neglected child may present as a case of abdominal pain, a divorcee with indigestion, elderly widow with painful knees, etc. the real cause being the underlying stress.

Else a young mother may bring her first child suffering from cold for fear of pneumonia, the newly wed arrives with vaginal discharge or urinary infection and 40 years old worrying about his chest pain. If the value of these symptoms is wrongly assessed, a patient may be sent away with an issue dangerously unresolved or physical symptoms due to psychological stress, distressingly and expensively investigated.

After a death in the family or that of a friend, the survivors UI! more at risk to present to the doctor with varying complaints, especially like the ones which the deceased had suffered. A woman who loses her mother early in life, may be more vulnerable to depression in her later life. Even events like marriage or birth of a child may imply some loss, reduced independence or privacy leading to depressive episodes.

The confrontation of a doctor and patient can be turned into a positive, congenial and curative relationship, with mutual support and co-operation. Patients do not always find it easy to reveal their worst, anxieties or betray their real notions without encouragement and certainly not outside the framework of relationship based on mutual confidence and respect. Understanding the patients symptoms will require a peep into in his work environment, his relation with employer and the associates at work, his sexual life, his social inter-relations and his friends.

Whether the patient's basic complaint is physical or emotional the doctor's work starts with imaginative listening so that the patient feels that his condition is being taken seriously. It should be possible to strike a happy mean between a cold impersonal attitude adopted for the sake of objectivity and an over-identification with the patient, resulting in personal emotional involvement, with an unnecessary impairment clinical skill.

4. THE RELATIONSHIPS

It is the Doctor-Patient relationship where the lay and professional perspectives and priorities most intimately meet, accommodate each other and clash. Besides patients, doctors too very widely in their responses to illness situations. However, the doctor being member of a particular professional group, his actions are defined and confined by the law, ethics, time, space, inter-professional relations and organisation of medical practice. Any contact between a patient and his doctor is usually a result of conscious choice on the part of the patient. Such a contact on the part of the patient may represent a desire as much for emotional support as for physical diagnosis or medication. The patient's assessment of the professional's performance will be based upon his view of such things as the doctor's interest in him, the amount of information given to him, the willingness of the doctor to show concern, to take an interest, and his commitment to the welfare of the patient. This relationship has been analysed by a legal luminary, in great detail, elsewhere in this book.

4.1 The Interaction

The doctor-patient relationship is that of expert-layman and it is the physician's expertise which is ultimate resource in his interaction with others. This relationship varies from complete passivity on the part of the patient, to the patient's consent to accept the advice and follow it. The interaction is expected to follow the model of guidance-cooperation; the physician initiating more of the interaction than the patient. A patient is expected to do what he is told by the expert. It may extend to mutual participation where patients are able or are required to take care of themselves, e.g., in diabetes. Two other models of interaction are possible: (i) the patient guides and the doctor cooperates, (ii) the patient is active and the doctor passive. In a fee-for-service situation, it may be certainly a case that the patient guides and the doctor co-operates.

What model would you choose as a doctor or as a patient?

4.2 Privileged Access

The doctor often deals with human beings in a manner, which

outside the context of the patient-doctor relationship would be criminal, immoral, scandalous or ridiculous. As part of the doctor's basic task, it is frequently necessary that the patient's body be exposed and touched, that it should be mutilated in some way or that it's bio-chemical functioning should be interfered with. While such activities become part of the professional's take for granted perspective, it is clearly a source of conflict, tension and upset for patients, who must readjust their usual conception of appropriate behaviour in relation to their body. To see a person naked when this is not usual and to touch and manipulate their body is a privileged access. Some of the doctors' contacts such as vaginal or rectal examination, may not be permitted to any other person; even a sexual partner. The patient's usual concept of the inviolability of his body play have to be temporarily shelved when procedural, antibiotic drugs can be harmful, they involve a certain element of risk for the patients. Thus, good medical strategy is to use antibiotics for prophylactic purposes only, when the risk of infection is high. Some take the position that the gains from antibiotics justify their use, even when the risks of infection are only moderate.

4.3 The Prescription

It is not surprising that practitioners frequently choose to treat rather than to wait, when they think that the patient expects to be treated. Prescriptions are seen as rewards at the end of nearly all consultations. Often the time honoured methods to send the patient away after consultation, e.g., sliding one's chair back, rising to one's feet, holding the door open, fail to work, only a prescription succeeds. Since a primary expectation from the doctor is that he should do everything he can for his patients, it can easily be the case in a situation of uncertainty that the doctor may be under great pressure to do something. But the doctor must weight the risk of doing some things against the risk of delaying or deciding not to do anything. The doctor may develop a vested interest in the perpetuation of this system of doing something, since he will earn after each prescription or medicines dispenses. This will reduce the chances of real patients getting due attention. Should the reward for declaring a person perfectly fit or free of disease be also not available?

4.4 Non-Diseases and Non-Medical Problems

A bias toward illness in situations or uncertainty has been identified, i.e., a professional's typical assumption is that it is better to impute disease than to deny it or risk overlooking or missing it. Non-disease is defined as a diagnostic label which is established after person has been incorrectly diagnosed as ill or suspected of having disease and than after subsequent examination and tests is ruled not to have it. Such false positives are non-diseases. The cause may be mimickery, normal variation or a laboratory error. It would seem that having a non-disease is hardly serious and involves nothing more than a certain amount of worry and time wasted on one or more visits to clinic.

The medical decisions rule argues that it is more serious to mills the diagnosis by carelessness, ignorance or accident than to make a false positive diagnosis. The non-diseases highlight the importance of a variety of emotional and psycho-social problems and the tendency on the part of some doctors to define them out of the sphere of medic competence as non-medical problems. But the doctor is too close to his patients and the community to shirk in this manner. It is natural that such problems be presented to the doctor, whether he sees them as a part of his task or not. If not a doctor, then who else would deal with such problem.

4.5 Informed Consent

The controversy about the informed consent has been there in connection with clinical research or with non-therapeutic research, such as drug trials where the benefit is not for that particular patient (or volunteers), but for patients in general at sometimes in the future. In such cases the medical personnel has to seek consent of the subjects after giving an adequate information about the facts and outcome of the drug trial, etc.

5. MEDICAL ETHICS

The hippocratic oath which represents the ethical considerations prevailing in the practice of medicine, has its early reference in the first century A.D. The oath was seen in those days as an ideal to be attained rather than a norm to be observed and it was not until 14th century that it was an obligatory requirement to take the oath before starting the practice of medicine. Since then several declarations have been made, while the oath reflects a high standard of morality, many of its provisions have become obsolete. Still it is an inspiring document towards the total welfare of the patients.

Till recently, the concept of medical ethics was simple one, since it did not have to deal with knotty problems like enthanasia, abortion forensic medicine, introgenic diseases, etc. Medical ethics, in the context of drug industry, public service, registration, hospital services, nursing home as a business venture, specialisation to promote professionalism, an association of medical-men safeguarding their own interests in the community, which was irrelevant in the practice of medicine in the earlier times is now a practical necessity. Indian Medical Association has drawn a code of medical ethics which is comprehensive and a model one with its core content laying down the ethical obligation to one's patients, colleagues and society and those for issuing certificates, notification, reports, etc. Various declarations made from time to time carry moral authority with them. These can be used whenever it is appropriate to refer to the ethical dimensions of human rights. Ethics is a self-imposed regulation and an exercise in nobility of the profession. But can nobility alone fulfil the various materialistic needs of the medical personnel ?

6. PRACTISING DOCTOR

A practising doctor in India is responsible for good deal of primary medical care, notwithstanding the stiff competition offered to him by quacks of different hues. But with due planning and trust by the government and the community he can be made more responsible to cover all aspects of primary and preventive health care as well. This would entail treating the private doctor as a member of continuing health care team rather than as an outsider or an adversary. This would further require change in the training programme of medical education, to make it more realistic to the needs of the society through agile imagination and capacity to speak and act in vernacular.

As today, when a doctor starts practice he finds 9/10th of his patients tend to present such symptoms which he was never taught to cure. He tends to find physical cause for every symptom overlooking the emotional and psychological reasons. But a large number of patients who consult their doctors have nothing demonstrably wrong with their bodies, but still they feel unwell. Why?

6.1 Minor Ailments

Once the doctor and the patient is aware of the vast field of untreated minor emotional or psychiatric illness, it will be possible to offer considerable help by listening patients. Ventilation of problem in this way may be much more helpful than a vast armamentarium of apparently more sophisticated investigations and explorations. When a patient of common cold presents to the doctor, it is necessary to ask what is the reason of his visit, rather than ridiculing the patient. May be the patient has something more to unburden, if sympathetically treated, which he needs to settle by discussion and advice.

6.2 Why a Patient Attends for Common Cold

A patient may have different notions about the outcome of his visit to the doctor:

(1) in the hope that the doctor has some magic cure for cold,
(2) for getting medical certificate for getting sick leave sanctioned, which may also imply his dislike for his job,
(3) fear of underlying tuberculosis or polio which may have started as a common cold,
(4) to prevent complications like bronchitis, sinusitis, pneumonia, etc., and
(5) low threshold due to anxiety or depression.

6.3 The Neurotic

A patient with minor psychiatric problem cannot be willing to visit a psychiatrist even if referred. Also the psychiatric services will be overburdened if patients start coming for psychiatric help in all neurotic problems. More so, a psychiatrist is not the best person to treat minor aberrations in behaviour and inner experience. Best to treat such a case is one's own doctor, who knows the person and his environment. It would be prudent that there is none in this world who does not have any neurotic trait.

It will be useful to attach psychiatric social workers/medical social workers as assistants to doctors in practice as well as the working in hospitals, to reduce their workload and to provide psychotherapy based on present situation and difficulties alone. Such a social worker can attempt to manipulate the patient's environment after studying his social difficulties and assets, as well as his organic and emotional problems. It will take several visits for the patient, before he accepts the ailment to be of emotional origin. This arrangement will provide an effective assessment of the patient's non-medical problems and would prove less expensive, time-saving and acceptable.

6.4 First Line of Defence

A family doctor in the first line of defence for a patient of minor ailment and similarly minor ailment is the bread and butter of a practitioner. So the two participants have a mutual co-existence. A patient with a wart who thinks to be cancerous needs as much reassurance as the patient with pneumonia is in need of treatment. Similarly, practitioner cannot thrive on the income from serious patients alone.

One important function of a practising doctor is to refer a seriously ill patient to a hospital. But, it is in the interest of the patient, to first contact their own doctor to avoid getting dangerous and expensive hospital investigations, say in case of anxiety neurosis. Obviously, specialists are not good in the diagnosis and treatment of anxiety neurosis. The practitioner will have continued responsibility and would be able to co-ordinate the activities of various specialists if required at a later stage. The danger of over-diagnosis and self-treatment (e.g., referral to specialists) is specially there, if two disorders co-exist, one of which may easily be missed, particularly if it is of psychiatric origin. It is no good to consult a surgeon to get the gall bladder out, where underlying depression is overlooked, since the symptoms will persist even after the surgery.

Another function of a practising doctor is to be available for emergencies or to make arrangement for attendance at odd hours. A practitioner is your personal doctor who fulfils the role of an adviser, a confident and a friend. Such doctor has to maintain a degree of impersonal objectivity. Too personalized doctoring may encourage ill-health, by encouraging an infantile dependency, but too impersonal doctoring may lead to lack of faith in the treatment.

Yet another function of a practitioner is to know the patient's environment, his family background, his liabilities, stress susceptibilities, etc.

Further, the practising doctor has the responsibility of imparting health education by explaining various aspects of illness and dispelling misconceptions. In this process, the doctor has to be careful not to weigh heavily on the pocket of the patient and the community has to see that the doctor is not harassed or exploited in the name of his noble profession.

7. THE GOVERNMENT DOCTOR

In our set-up, most of the hospitals, dispensaries, and the so-called health centres are managed and financed by the Central Government/State Government/Municipalities, etc. The salary of the staff, including that of the doctors is paid from the public funds. The patients have generally not to pay any fee to get consultation and other services.

7.1 Impersonal Attitude

Since it is not a fee for service situation, the doctors and others tend to be impersonal to the extent of being apathetic. The human beings in distress are treated more like subjects or even objects. With the result, the ailing citizens tend to get a feeling of non-attendance, neglect and indifference, even if the treatment administered is timely, correct and adequate. Though, it is the citizen, who is the master of all—since he votes the Government in/out—it is he who is neglected the most. He is not given any information. No one treats him as a person, since his social, personal and emotional needs are overlooked.

7.2 Indifference to Job

The Government doctor often refuses to develop any relationship with the OPD/Ward patients and tends to just mark his time. Some them attend to only VIPs, who can bestow favours in one way or other, others do it for a consideration. Some of them report only on the day of 'visit of the boss' other tend to limit it to the salary day. Many of them continue to run their business outside, even during stipulated hours of the hospitals. A minority of them who earnestly and with devotion, are called worldly unwise, eccentric, even foolish.

In this process, the patient care is wholly or partially sacrificed. When the reluctance to even look after the seriously ill is visible, where is the scope for preventive health, community education or to look into the promotions or rehabilitation aspects?

7.3 Private Doctors are Step-Sons

Private doctors, who work to earn their livelihood (some of them to amass wealth on a commercial scale) have always been looked upon as step-sons (or daughters) by the Government or the doctors war in Government hospitals. While the Government has not taken any steps, may not, even given a thought to treat the large number of practising doctors as a vast resource (for the curative and preventive health of the community) the hospital colleagues view them some who are foreigners, inferior, rival and even cheats—who are foreigners, inferior, rival and even cheats—who are engaged in minting money hook or crook.

Little do they realise that it is the practising doctor, who can undertake to provide the care medical and health care. Since their thriving depends upon the fee, directly collected from the members of the community, they have to build and maintain their reputation—which can rest on result-oriented service and not on cheating or misleading anyone.

If a practising doctor visits a hospital to help one of his patients in distress, who was taking treatment from him earlier, the practitioner is shown scant consideration, due to the in-built prejudices in the Government doctor's mind and the usual dilatory habits. Why?

7.4 Confrontation, Why?

Where is the point of confrontation among these members of continuing health care team—both claim to help the ailing members of the community, both are paid in their own ways. It is not a mere clash of egos. There is a fault in our planning and training.

If the Government conceives them and treats as such, as the equal members of a continuing health care team, the problems would tend to minimise.

As a patient is referred or brought by a practising doctor to a hospital colleague, it is not the duty of the latter to criticize the former—since it would not solve any problem. It is the duty of the hospital doctor to give the advice or treatment for the problem—for which the practising doctor needed help. After doing the needful, the patient must be sent back to the referring doctor. Such a patient is obviously not an encroachment on the hospital—he is even more privileged to seek advice—since it is this patient, who need the hospital attention most, as compares to another, who has come directly, and who may be suffering from a trivial ailment, which may be treated easily elsewhere, say a small dispensary/clinic.

7.5 Patient is a Person

In any case, if a human being falls ill, he does not cease to be a person and hence he has to be treated keeping in view this fact. The hospital doctor or any other staff member cannot arrogate to himself to maltreat anyone of these unfortunate persons who happened to seek help and support from the hospital. Hospital is a public institution, which thrives on public funds and which is designed to serve the public, and the hospital staff is there to be sub-servient to the public.

If the practising doctors undertake to provide all the front line medical and health care and the hospitals are used only for referred cases and the two components of health team work in unison, the coverage of population and the quality of health care will improve.

8. SIXTH SENSE

Examination of a patient involves the employment of the five senses of the doctor. There is a sixth sense to provide information about the patient: the emotional experience evoked (in the doctor) by the attitude and bearing of the patient. This experience is generally excluded while making a diagnosis. It is proper to some extent that this exclusion of feelings should be encouraged. It would be improper for the surgeon to be prevented from performing his technically essential but emotionally brutal function by the intrusion of his feelings during an operation. All doctors spend much of their time in a physical environment of deformity, pus and excreta, and an emotional environment of pain, unhappiness and anxiety. Barriers against the evocation of disgust by the physical environment are, necessary to enable him to tend the patient, but he may also erect other barriers, protect himself from the demands on his Sympathy made by emotion environment. People are made into cases, and feelings we may sway or prejudice judgement are suppressed to obtain objectivity.

When objective findings are equivocal or inconclusive, however, the feelings evoked by the patient in the doctor may be the vital of the doctor's diagnosis and assessment of therapy.

The doctor may experience with his patient, the whole range emotions. He may feel angry, he may feel frustrated, he may feel our important. Similarly, he may feel happy, clever, or important, or he may feel anxious or depressed. Anger is a 'bad' emotion to have towards a patient and is consequently more readily recognized dangerous basis for action. But different patients can evoke the whole range of possible emotions in the doctor and these are regarded as favourable to the patient (for instance admiration) sometimes. It is sometimes easier for the doctor to deal with emotional illness when it presents as a physical complaint because the unravelling of the situation leads directly to its cause. It seems more difficult to deal with, obviously emotional complaint when the patient denies any precipitating cause.

Of all the emotions that can be evoked in the doctor the one likely to be reported to the patient is depression. A depressed does not express himself readily, but easily produces a feeling depression in the people with whom he is in contact. If depression is not talked about, it is because this is integral to the nature of the emotion. A feeling which may be almost as difficult to talk about is sexuality, but this for fear it might not be controlled.

There is an over-riding emotion present in nearly all interviews. This is the doctor's professional anxiety. Patient knows that in the doctor they will have to arouse his professional anxiety. But if the doctor's anxiety is aroused unnecessarily, e.g., unnecessary night can, it makes him angry. What the patient says is often so different from what he feels and wants to convey, the doctor should learn to understand the language of the consultation at the same time as he is learning to the disease. Parallel with the study of Identified Illness, his training, should include a study of the process of interpreting the communication and the underlying cause of the patient attempt to the doctor's professional anxiety.

9. GOOD AND THE BAD DOCTOR

Even the most sympathetic hospital doctors have usually to consider the diagnosis before the person. For the general practitioner the reverse is true. A patient sent to a gynaecologist because of irregular vaginal bleeding will have a dilatation and curettage almost as a routine. It is the practitioner who decides whether or not to send a patient to a gynaecologist, knowing in advance that such an examination will almost inevitably follow. Is the menstrual irregularity of sufficient importance to merit the disruption of family life and difficulties of getting the children care for, or to justify the anxieties which will be created in the patient until the result is known?

A patient sent to an orthapaedic surgeon will rarely receive a decision until X-rays have been taken, but in general practice, however scientifically minded the doctor and however adequate the local facilities, most decisions have to be taken with no more backing than his own clinical acumen. Whereas for the Government consultant such investigations will be routine and taken for granted by the patient. In other words, the Government consultant has to justify his diagnosis by investigation, whilst the private practitioner has to justify his investigation by his diagnosis.

However, some private consultants order a large number of tests, only to earn more money. We may consider the situation when a woman presents complaining of a lump in her breast. The 'bad' doctor will refer her immediately to a surgeon. If the diagnosis is malignant tumour, he must send her to a surgeon. The 'good' doctor will examine her and then have two alternatives. If he diagnoses mastitis he has to consider the alternatives of either sending her to hospital where the consultant will take the responsibility of managing her, or coping with her emotional reaction himself.

10. TRAINING FOR PRACTICE

The practitioner has to take vital decisions before the stage of obtaining laboratory help, it becomes important for him to use all the data that are available for his diagnosis. These include the behaviour and emotional state of the patient and his family, the effects produced on others (including on the doctor himself) and the general environmental situation. Since many of these facts require skill both to elicit them from the patient and to interpret them when obtained, a study of this aspect of patient care must be included in the doctor's training.

Those entering general practice are liable to find many patients suffering from illness they have not been trained to diagnose. On the basis of his teaching, the new entrant is liable to produce some such classification as 30 per cent neurosis, 50 per cent trivial illness, 10 per cent malingering and only 10 per cent of 'genuine' illness.

Due to uncharitable criticism of the practitioners by the hospital doctors, as well as the aggrieved patients, many practitioners, more and more of what they formerly did or participated, refer to hospital. He is no longer the active person producing the catheter from his top hat to give dramatic relief to a case of retention. A case of abdominal pain is no longer followed through; it now becomes a probable appendix to be sent into hospital, and the 'correctness of the diagnosis may only be established by a telephone call next day or the receipt of a hospital discharge a few weeks later.

The technical competencies which doctors bring from hospital training remain unused and unsatisfied, and like the underfed baby whose unsatisfaction with his milk supply turns to dissatisfaction with his mother, many doctors become dissatisfied with practice. The advance of specialist technique has taken from the general practitioner much of the work formerly within his province, and has compelled him to entrust his patient much more often to the care of others.

11. SYMPATHY

The feelings and expression of sympathy is an integral part of the approach to a patient. But sympathy has its pitfalls. The mere expression of sympathy, howsoever genuine and heartfelt, is far front being therapeutic. Sympathy is an emotional response to be used under conscious intellectual control. It may act as a barrier to effective communication between doctor and patient, and secondly, it may be used by the patient for his own ends; the doctor may be manoeuvred into actions which may serve only to foster the patient's neurosis and be the reverse of therapeutic.

Tears are a time honoured weapon in the armoury of a patient, especially female, sometimes used in doctor's chambers to enlist sympathy. Most commonly this is done to avoid discussing unpleasant issues. In these circumstances, they can be a very convenient refuge but they are then a barrier to further communication, diagnosis and effective treatment. The doctor's response may be: 'If you are crying I know you are miserable. If you can talk I will then know why. When we know why we may be able to find out some way of relieving it.'

Excessive sympathy, when evoked, may be used for purposes which would be contrary to the doctor's judgement. Any doctor called in to arbitrate in marital disputes soon learns not to place absolute credence on the story of either partner, at least until he has heard what the other has to say. Indeed, when both husband and wife are in agreement that all the blame should fall on one of them, the doctor must be even more on his guard before accepting this situation at its face value. But most typically the sympathy is used in order to manipulate the doctor like a puppet into serving the patient's ends.

Experiences with such patients lead to doctors withdrawing their sympathy from professional relationships. It is essential that a doctor uses his discretion and thought in such cages. There are no harmful side effects to the administration of sympathy, if it is directed to the correct area of disturbance and if its continued administration is reconsidered each time, the situation alters. Undue and unnecessary sympathy can lead to clouding of clinical judgement and misuse of doctor's precious time.

12. COMMUNICATION

Ideal relation involves a state of communication, in which the doctor and the patient can converse with mutual confidence. It demands doctor's interest, consideration, empathy, friendly objectivity, understanding and the patient's full faith and co-operation. If a doctor clumsily alarms his patient while explaining the treatment or the patient gets frightened, it is a failure in communication. Of the two participants fail to understand each other, either due to language difficulty, lack of vocabulary, wrong use of technical terms, etc. The doctor may fail to understand the idiom, dialect, phraseology or use of words. The patient will either take such a doctor as stupid, in-attentive or uninterested or a snob. Often the patient does not understand what the doctor wants to know and in turn the doctor gets impatient and starts shouting in a loud voice. The problem arises specially when the patient uses medical terms of jargon which he fully believes to be correct. But a doctor who shouts, ridicules or shows indifference would forfeit patient's respect. The doctor has to keep him cool and has to extract the information as to what the patient really means.

13. THE MEDICAL SOCIAL WORKER

The role of social and personal factors in the causation of disease has been well recognised. With changing social and family patterns and the increasing role of underlying stress as a cause of different symptoms, the importance of a person, other than a busy physician, who can serve as a homely worker, is being felt all over—especially to facilitate medical care delivery in the big hospitals. Similarly, the requirement of such a worker is no less in private clinic, where he can supplement the work of the physician and help in the development of community medicine relationships.

In our hospitals and private clinics there has been no provision of a skilled medical social worker. The concept of having such a worker, though not new, has not become a reality in India, either due to lacuna In planning or due to resource constraints. The principal of omniscence and omnipresence is being perpetuated with impunity, with regard to physician, thus burdening him with such non-clinical jobs, which could be easily looked after by others, e.g., ward boys, attendants, nurses and workers.

In our hospitals, a typical social worker, wherever available, is a fashionable middle aged lady (usually the wife of a bureaucrat, keen to enhance her status and trying to look younger than her own daughter), who visits the hospitals at her convenience, when the husband is to office or on tour. Her main function is to make her presence before the hospital—people who matter and interfere with the wherever possible. At random, she may help one or more poor getting medicine, etc. from local red cross, in a ostentious manner exhibit her benevolence, rather than to be really concerned after long-term welfare of that patient. She is not a part of the team of hospital workers, nor is she a link between the hospital and Co. She has no knowledge or interest in the mutual support hospitals and private practitioners to promote the cause of members of the community. In nutshell, she is more often a nuisance, rather than being of any help to the patient, staff, the private practitioners.

When we refer to a medical social worker, we do not worker of the type mentioned above—we mean a skilled worker versed and well-involved in facilitating the health care deliclinics, hospitals and the community (we are not confusing community health worker, as envisaged by Government of India in the year 1977-78). This is neither for fun nor for charity. He is a staff, who has responsibility and accountability.

13.1 The Role

A medical social worker is a friend of the patients, attendants, other visitors and a ready help to the physician, in solving the problems of patients and the community. He relieves the phys of the burden of non-clinical work, as also such clinical work, which can be easily done by other members of the team.

He helps the patient with his personal difficulties and make adjust towards the environmental difficulties which predisposes towards or interfere with obtaining maximum benefits for medical care. A patient in a hospital seeks satisfaction for his very special and emotional needs. Patients are rarely interested in the confusing medical statistical aggregates of a hospital performance. He is only satisfied when he realizes that he has secured maximum benefits and the possible results from his hospital experience, because medical social work furthers this end, it also strengthens the public relations of a hospital (Anand, *et at.*, 1983).

The role of such a worker in discharge planning and continuing care has already been mentioned in the chapter on Hospitals and Private Practitioners—Mutual Support.

13.2 Social Medical Service

This is to provide personalised service, as if in a commercial organisation, so that the patient's medical situation can be inter-related with his personal needs and problems. Interviews with the patient and members of his family and conferences on his behalf with professional persons are the principle methods used. The range of services may vary from concrete suggestions to tide over simple problems to helping in distress situations like fears of permanent disability, disfiguring, handicaps, anxieties and uncertain future. The resources of the patient and his immediate environment are primarily used sometimes, supplemented by hospital or community facilities.

The other factor is referring the patient to the proper department/ doctor/proper clinic. The treating doctor has to recognise the social and personal problems that may affect the natural history of disease and take assistance of the medical social worker to settle them. Health agencies, courts, schools may ask the help of medical social worker for individual help. He has also to supervise record-keeping which is indispensable for follow up. A running account of the patient's social data is available for future references. Records are also used for supervision and for performance measurements. The confidential nature of the record should always be guarded. The valuable information collected can help the hospital administrators, the medical staff, development of services, procedures and in community health education.

13.3 The Recommendations

Anand, *et al.* (1983), grouped activities of medical social workers, as given below:

- (i) Eliciting medico-social data along with their clinical assessment.
- (ii) Organise financial assistance for poor and needy patients.
- (iii) Organise distribution of clothes, blankets, shoes, empty bottles through philanthrophic organisations.
- (iv) Counselling unmarried mothers, and women with family problems broken homes.
- (v) Arrange foster homes for babies.

13.3.1 At Inpatient Level

- (i) Arrange distribution of donation/sample medicines, clothes, shoes, milk, good supplements to needy patients.
- (ii) Arrange financial assistance to needy patients.
- (iii) Elicit case date for the clinicians.
- (iv) Arrange for rehabilitation of patients, in their homes, rehabilitation centres of other hospitals.
- (v) Tend to the emotional and psythological needs of patients;
- (vi) Arrange for patients to leave the hospital when no further active treatment is required thereby facilitating a bed for the next needy patient.
- (vii) Arrange for library and recreational facilities for patients.
- (viii) Sending letters to the relatives of the patients.
- (ix) Arrange for rehabilitation of patients.

13.4 Role in Private Practice

This has been described in the chapter on Hospitals and Private Practitioners—Mutual support. Such a worker can be an important link in the liaison between hospitals and private clinics in the interest of continuing care. However, the role of the medical social worker can be expanded, depending upon the needs and situations in the hospitals/ private clinics. If this service can be well-developed and utilized, it can go a long way to achieve the goal of health for all by the year 2000 A.D.

Hospital care often lags behind in the body of knowledge, advising sensitivity to the emotional needs of the hospitalized persons, as also the attendants looking after him, his relations, children and courtesy callers. Whereas one set of visitors comes and goes after leaving behind their 'get well soon' wishes, the other set has to keep hanging around the hospitals, to look for the patient.

The contact of the visitors and hospital-staff is at several points and starts right from the moment it is decided to seek hospital advice or admission. Generally, the first contact is with the enquiry/reception. This, if well-managed can help a lot to mitigate the subsequent sufferings of attendants and patients and can facilitate a great deal, the dispensing of medical care and the associated services, e.g., registration, OPD service, fee deposit, laboratory services and admission if required. Generally, the failures of hospital administration and its staff start from here and get accentuated as the patient proceeds further in various queues. More often the attitude of the reception staff is impersonal, indifferent, inadequate, curt to impolite. The visitor to this counter is more often dealt away by putting off, rather than by offering him any tangible help. The same culture is perpetuated further, as he moves to get his card made, approaches the lift or awaits in the OPD at the mercy of the peon or a self-styled social worker.

In the OPD where he is waiting anxiously to get attention of one of the doctors or doctor of his choice, he is pushed around, as if in a herd of cattle. His turn to see the doctor becomes a 'mirage', with politicians, VIPs bureaucrats, hospital staff and others who matter not showing only respect for the queue, or the human beings in distress, huddled there.

The waiting in the congested and polluted environment, involving standing for hours, uncertainty of the 'turn' for the patient, with hospital noises, cries, smells and infections all round, prove to be a real test of nerves and physique, for the attendants.

Getting a hospital bed/room is the real measure of one's tactfulness, resourcefulness and manipulation. After passing through the rigmarole of formalities, the serious patient with his worried attendant arrive in the ward, where the hurried nurses receive him with a shower of "get out attendants, do not crowd here, allow us to work for God's sake"—without enquiring as to why the hopeful people are roaming about. Nobody cares to provide them a sitting place or even a glass of water.

When confronted with the job of getting some laboratory investigations done, the patient's relatives face another volley of hostilities.

The sweepers and ward attendants are nowhere to be found and their work is allotted to the attendants of the patient, out of expediency, encapsulated in 'patient's interest'. After depositing the requisite fee for the tests, the relatives wander in search of the laboratories and its ingenious workers. When they turn up in the evening to discuss the report, the replies usually are 'the blood was clotted-send it again', 'culture sterile' or 'shows growth of no significance', 'NAD'. If any figures are reported, they look to be imaginary and often do not seem to have any semblance to the reality of the situation. Repeat samples are sent every day, fees are deposited daily, but nobody bothers about the reports—if they have come and what they are like! Is it due to the overwork alone ? Overwork has something to do—but not all.

The other area of contact between the patient's attendant and the staff, especially the nursing staff and junior doctors is over the implementation of 'drug administration schedule'. While the medicine is entrusted to be given to the attendants, the problem arises over the administration of different types of injections or drip of blood, glucose, saline, etc. While the relative is supposed to keep a close supervision over the execution of 'drug administration' if he points out any failing, he is accused of over-stepping his jurisdiction and told not to step in the shoes of a doctor.

The callers to the hospital, either in their anxiety to enquire after the welfare of the patient or just to mark their attendance as a gesture of goodwill, come under heavy fire. While it is a fact that too many visitors are a menace to the hospital cleanliness, environment or even administration of services to the patient, it is a necessary evil. Wherever a human being is confined to bed, those known to him would come. If their visit could be cut short, but made more comfortable, it would be a better management. Merely shouting at them will not solve the problems.

Let them meet him, explain to them briefly and then they can be asked to bow out. Their visit may satisfy the emotional needs of the patients and hence may help in the treatment.

14.1 Children Visitors

The practice is to strictly curtail visits by young children to a hospitalized parent. But infants and children may visit a hospitalized parent as an integral part of the treatment plan (Levai, 1968).

Two factors cited to support exclusion of child visitors have been demonstrated to be mythic in nature and unsubstantiated by data: (a) the potential for increased infection; and (b) disruption of hurried staff routines and procedures. The literature on an issue which impacts both on patient well-being and hospital administration is scant. Gremillion and others (1980) cite a number of studies which clearly place the risk for infection factor at a minimum. Moreover, simply screening and precautions can assure safety even for the immuno-compromised patient. Second, anticipation of noise and disruption of routines are also not substantiated.

Nonetheless, the argument persists to support exclusion of a child's contact with a hospitalized parent.

The organisation of a play room in hospitals for visiting children has been described as a recent innovation (St. Vincent, 1978). Such facilities are convenient and a step forward. In point of fact, some hospitals have relaxed restrictive visiting rules for children for a number of years with no ill-effects, and obvious benefits. Notable are improved morale of the hospitalized parent as separation from and anxiety about absence from normal parental role functions are diminished. Moreover, the presence of a child actively counters the potentially morbid tone of a hospital environment for other patients infusing the millieu with vitality and a future orientation.

The exclusion of children intensely magnifies the stress of a brief separation imposed by hospitalization for surgery.

The patients confrontation with his health crisis is greatly aggravated by a confrontation with traditional administrative bureaucracy, when the request that the child be allowed to visit her room is refused. A compromise "visit" in a noisy, drafty hospital lobby can leave the vulnerable patient and the overwhelmed baby son frustrated and totally unable to connect emotionally amidst wheel chairs, an attending private nurse, the mother and housekeeper and an intrusive stream of other visitors and staff. A medical social worker's advocacy can help to settle the matters.

We would urge hospital administrators to creatively re-examine policies about children's rights to visit—now rooted more in tradition and myth than any experience. Social work staff sensitized by training to the impact of illness and hospitalization on the patient/family unit can perform a pivotal function in advocating for a revaluation of this issue and creative programme planning.

14.2 Information Exchanges

One unfortunate aspect of contact between the hospital staff and the patient is the barrier in information exchange. While the attending physician and others often shirk to listen to the visitors' narration about the patient's condition or his progress (which are often repetitive and generally not so relevant), they do not like to divulge anything about the patient's condition; diagnosis, prognosis or the plan of treatment. That stone silence (sometime definite arrogance) in response to the visitor's questions give rise to misgivings about the outcome of patient's hospitalization. It would be proper to listen to some of the visitors and give them brief resume of the patient's condition. Though, such an exercise is time-consuming yet not time-wasting. If the relevant facts of the patient's progress or otherwise are given out briefly, it would exhibit staff's involvement in patient's care and allay the anxiety of the relatives, etc. The patient would get a feeling of reasonable attendance and the chances of law suit against the hospital for alleged negligence, would minimize.

While the courtesy-callers and well-wishers, need only regulated flow in and out of the hospital, coupled with some words of wisdom from the 'medical social workers' to quench their thirst for welfare-information about the patient, the attendant involved in patient's care, require organised management for their stay to facilitate their work. After all they are a resource in the patient's treatment plan. If this aspect is ignored they would tend to crowd around the bed of the patient, or the corridors, spread the eatables as well as their body excretions on the floor, look unkempt and fatigued, hence more irritable to the staff—thus polluting the environment and hindering the administration of various services.

Attached to each ward, there should be a visitor's room, where they can sit-when not on duty with the patient, use the toilet facility and give respite to their legs.

Then for the stay of attendants of such patients, who require round the clock care, a room must be made available in the hospital serai. Such rooms should be generously/abundantly available on the medical social worker's or nurse's recommendation. The physician may not be bothered with this aspect. To look after the needs of such attendants, provision of a canteen and recreation room on the pattern of a hostel is essential. They should be given the impression of being a wanted lot and involved in patient's care, rather than being pushed round or shunted out. If they are well looked after, their level of Involvement in the patient's treatment plan would be high.

Politician confronts the hospital administration at every-stage and in a big way, i.e., the conception of the hospital, its setting up, management and the day-to-day functioning. During day-to-day functioning he may appear to be interfering and taxing. But he can be a resource to the hospital development and expansion, if approached rightly. In any case his interference, though sometimes unwarranted, has to be borne with a smile. Showing any neglect or indifference to him, may lead to stress on the hospital administration, including paucity of funds.

Those in power, be it a politician or a bureaucrat, tend to seek it special attention of the hospital services. This may mean seeking advice (either for himself or others recommended by him) for a minor ailment; which could be easily attended outside (by a dispensary doctor or private general clinic) or jumping the queue in the matter of availing various services, e.g., a private room, laboratory tests, consultation discussion with the consultant physician (which is often unnecessary), etc. Some physicians might interpret it as a nuisance and burden and might treat it as a problem to be dealt with. In fact, the politician cannot be shunned away, from its negative or positive role, either in the management of the hospital or its planning and development. It is the measure of the ability of the hospital administrator, how well he accommodates him, without sacrificing the dignity and discipline (of the hospital and it's staff) and in the process how much positive role he could assign to him in the matter of planning and development (without allowing his undue interference in the functioning) of the hospital. In a democracy you cannot put barriers for any section of society, let alone the politicians, who wield power and influence in the Government as well as society.

However, hanging around the residences or offices of the politician/ bureaucrats to unduly please them in a bid to get personal gains at the cost of hospital efficiency and dignity of the staff, can be ruinous for the functioning of the hospital and prove counter-productive for the hospital administration.

The role of medical social worker cannot be over-emphasised, to deal with the politician-bureaucrat combine, so that their nuisance can be reduced and they can be made a resource for the hospital.

Professional, patients are a great menace and an avoidable burden, on the hospital services. Such patients tend to seek repeated and perpetual hospital attention, either in OPD or wards, or wards, out of their anxiety and neurotic traits, addiction, malingering, poverty, insecurity, VIP connection or fun-shake. They make mound from the mole—hole of their illness, which may be incurable, chronic, psychosomatic, trivial, non-disease or non-existent.

They devise ways and means and adopt new strategies by virtue of their knowledge and experience of hospital systems and connections with the staff. Then they manipulate their stay to be longer and longer. Thus, they deprive others who are in dire need, from the services and attention of the physician and others. Medical social worker and nurse should try to analyse and understand the underlying cause of request for hospitalization of such patients and try to help him out of the hospital by neutralizing his resistance tactfully, that will be in the interest of hospital and the community. Whereas, certain factors prompting him to seek hospitalization, e.g., anxiety or psychosomatic factors should be dealt with sympathy, others should be resisted with firmness, politely. Tact and politeness will always be necessary, since such patients can be a source of adverse publicity, public agitation or even legal suits.

A FRAMEWORK FOR PATIENT-PROVIDER COLLABORATION

Supporting patient-provider collaboration with technology requires an underlying framework to facilitate participation. Goldberg *et al.* suggest a framework for patient empowerment and the technical realization of that framework. Such a framework is a requirement for properly designed collaborative healthware applications. This framework consists of core elements essential to facilitating patients' active access to personally relevant credible information, ongoing and facilitated communication, clinical data capture, a reporting and feedback mechanism, and community support. In addition to this framework, other issues must be considered prior to the design, implementation, and evaluation of collaborative healthware.

Such consideration should include:

- What do patients need?
- What do providers want?

- How can the patients' "view" be designed into the system?
- How can prescribed, profile-driven knowledge be delivered?
- What are the best methods of information delivery?
- How can credible data be collected from patients?
- How can the system be integrated into the current work flow?

With widespread adoption of collaborative healthware applications, all patients and their families will come to expect improved access to services, greater convenience, and alternative methods of communicating with their health care providers. Since the emphasis is on the partnership between patient and provider, collaborative healthware will be used to promote informed decision-making, improve patient outcomes, increase patient satisfaction, enhance patient education, lower health care costs, and improve the coordination of care. While collaborative healthware applications have intuitive appeal to diverse groups of health care stakeholders, adoption of such systems will likely depend on their ability to demonstrate positive impact on outcomes.[9]

(I) Confidentiality

The doctor must keep all the information shared by the patient with him as confidential. Patient is afraid of family and society if some adverse information about the patient is leaked. This becomes very important for a psychiatric patient as the stigma is attached with the disease in the society. There are members in society who can take advantage of his secret problems. The doctor must not tell to anybody until and unless it is desirable.

Consumers expect change, and they want to be able to interact with their health care provider and their health care system as they do with their stockbroker or their favorite merchants on the Web. Privacy, the credibility of medical information, and the ability to correctly use that information for decision-making will be essential features of the medical Internet. We must create the environment for consumers to feel at least as secure as they do when transacting business or viewing information from stockbrokers, mortgage lenders, and educational institutions. The Medical consumer is a vital part of the supply-and-demand system that drives the world economy today and into the future. We cannot afford to fail to meet the medical consumers' needs and to empower them to assume a greater role in their care. We need to carefully identify the best approach to these challenges and act on them professionally and responsibly. The Internet will have an impact on how health is maintained and how care is delivered. The authors of the chapters in this section suggests that we are at a crossroads in health care, and we must be careful to effectively and responsibly use the tools that are available to improve consumer access, understanding, and quality of life.[10]

(2) Effective Communication

Communication is the touching of mind by mind, of person with person. It can include conversation, interview, dialogue, visual technique carefully used.

Communication is an integral part of every function of health administration "and that is why it is said to be the bloodstream of an organization." It is a two-way process between people. In communication a message is transmitted and received.

Transmission	→	Reception
Message transmitted is the communication	←	Message received and understood first half of is the second half of the communication

Communication can be transmitted through audio, visual and audio-visual means. Communication plays the same role as the nervous system in a body. Norbert Wiener has rightly observed that "communication is the cement that makes an organization." Communication is central to the exercise of authority in an organization. In the words of Ordway Tead, "Communication is the touching of mind by mind, of person with person, whether it be one man, or a thousand.... it can include conversation, interview, dialogue, visual technique carefully used."[11]

According to Terry, eight factors are essential in making communication effective:

(a) Inform yourself fully;
(b) Establish a mutual trust in others;
(c) Find a common ground of experience;
(d) Use mutually known words;
(e) Have regard for context;
(f) Secure and hold the receiver's attention;
(g) Employ examples and visual aids; and
(h) Practice delaying relations.

Online health consumers are increasingly prevalent and are therefore important to health care providers. Organizations must fulfil their needs for communication, information, convenience, and access to their health records. Patient Site is an excellent way to meet these needs. Both patients and providers have vigorously adopted it, yet the demand on physician time is modest. The system has introduced controversial and interesting issues that we continue to work through. Patient Site is also a useful platform for future projects, such as patient-computer interviewing, disease management, health care quality, and patient safety.[12]

(3) Developing Rapport and Relationships

Building rapport with the client is the first important step as he feels to divulge all his problems frankly and freely. This is also called principle of acceptance.

Sanjay Bhattacharya rightly suggests that the principles of acceptance implies that social workers must perceive, acknowledge, receive and establish a relationship with the individual client as he actually is, not as we wish the individual to be or think he should be. It means that no matter how much our perception of it may differ from his, we must acknowledge and accept him as if we are to help him. In health education one begins from where the client is.

Purpose—to respect, to help, to add, to comfort, therapeutic understanding, acknowledge, receiving, etc. Quality of acceptance-warmth, courtesy, listening, respect, concern, interest, consistent, maturity, fairness, willingness to enter and share life experience, etc. Object—his integrity as a fellow human being, the individual as he is with all his limitation, his real potentiality, etc.

Obstacles to Acceptance

- Insufficient knowledge of human behaviour.
- Non-acceptance of something in self (lack of self-awareness).
- Biases and prejudices.
- Imparting to the client one's own feelings.
- Unwanted assurance.
- Confusion between acceptance and approval.
- Loss of respect for the client.
- Over identification.[13]

Imagine an entire population with access at home to a network that enables people to access information, communicate with providers and other interested parties, and receive some diagnostic and therapeutic services. The home, as a site of health care delivery, is of increasing interest to health care planners and providers. For those individuals whose access to traditional health care delivery is limited by circumstances such as distance and mobility, home-delivered services would be particularly attractive and potentially beneficial. In recent years, major advances in computing and telecommunications technologies, particularly the exponential growth of the Internet, have suggested possible approaches to improving health through the direct provision of services to patients.[14]

(4) Motivating the Patients

Doctors should not discourage the patient about disease. He should rather motivate the patient and create will power, which is basic for any treatment.

They should be motivated to do this job as a part of their medical duties. S.S. Sooch in his Article, "Revamping Health Care," in the *Daily Tribune*, (26th January 2000) rightly remarks that there is a general feeling that most of the health care providers in the government run hospitals are indifferent, apathetic and insensitive and a few even outrightly arrogant in their behaviour. A sense of compassion and human touch is simply missing. A series of crash courses should be arranged to expose the entire staff to the art of public relations.

Health Education is vital to provide health to all in 21st century. This is the cheapest and most effective tool of health care. The success of Health Care in 21st century depends upon the identification of community needs through community needs assessment surveys and later on providing health education to the community so that they can solve their problems themselves.[15]

(5) Doctors must Devote Time and Energy to Solve Patients' Problems in Collaboration of Paramedical Personnel

(a) that the patients are treated as close to their homes as possible in the smallest, cheapest and simply equipped unit such as a sub-centre which is capable of looking after them adequately;
(b) that the medical services should be organized and administered in such a way that the quality of medical care improves gradually;
(c) the medical care services should be organized from the bottom-up and not from the top-down;
(d) that the services planned should meet the needs of the people;
(e) that all members of the health and medical personnel function as a well-knit team; and
(f) that new categories of health personnel such as multi-purpose health workers and community health workers should be given suitable training to provide simple medical care and preventive services to large sections of the community.

In the case of virtual epidemic of behavioural disorders, modern health care must place a new emphasis on solving the human side of medicine. As stated by Maureen A. Backy, "The crucial link between the person providing health care and the persons receiving it, is often very weak indeed. Modern medicine tends to emphasize technical solution and to overlook the value of close personal contact and relationship."[16]

(6) Health Education

The most important aim of Health Education is to alter behaviour, which may have directly or indirectly influenced occurrence of spread of diseases in a given cultural setting. A culturally relevant health education programme can be planned only after understanding the behaviour in all its manifestations. One of the best definitions of Health Education was offered by Wood in 1926; "Health Education is the sum of experiences which favourably influences habits, attitudes and knowledge relating to individual, community, and racial health."[17]

Different authorities have differently viewed the aims of health education. According to one source:[18]

"The aim of health education is to help people achieve health by their own actions and efforts. Health education begins therefore with the interest of people in improving their condition of living, and aims at developing a sense of responsibility for their own health betterment as individuals and as members of families,communities or government."[19]

Another source[20] highlights that, "Health education aims at promoting the greater possible fulfilment of inherited powers of the body and the mind and the happy adjustment of individual to society. It is the educational approach to health problem and as such is concerned with practical measures for the promotion of health and the control and treatment of diseases.

Studies made in different countries of the world have shown that fluctuations in the toll of disease and death depend even more on the level of education than on the social and economic conditions in which people live. Ignorance can be just as much a killer as poverty, and these two often go hand in hand[21].

An excellent examples of the success of health education can be cited from Egypt. Esmut Mansour in his Article, "Egypt Tackles Polio," rightly suggests the role of health education in polio eradication. To quote:

In fact, women in Egypt represent a considerable proportion of all private and public physicians and health service administrators. As in many other countries, the nursing staff are predominantly women and are therefore engaged in the front-line battle to eradicate polio. The nurse's role here is much boarder than the one she plays during clinic hours, and her value to her community and its welfare should not be underestimated.

Not only does she routinely give the polio vaccine, but she is the primary mechanism for dispensing health care information to each child's careers, thus increasing their awareness about the dangers of disease, the importance of vaccination, and any possible side-effects of the vaccine. Therefore, she acts as the first defence line against the disease, and her understanding of the early effects of polio and her ability to recognize the disease is essential.

Egyptian society is particularly blessed by a culture and history that produces strong family ties. So untimely the success of our programme to eradicate polio must also credit the mothers who have listened to the information provided at the official level of health care and who have been convinced that the health of their children is worth all the expense and effort they make.

Egypt's Expanded Programme on Immunization is one of the most effective in the world. Reaching our goal of eradicating polio will be a worthy tribute to the hard work contributed by all of us—women and men together—to protect out children.[22]

Health education does not mean merely removal of ignorance. On the contrary, it involves three important things:

(i) It provides a person with appropriate knowledge to enjoy decent health and also the knowledge about the occurrence and spread of disease thus enabling him to adopt relevant preventive measures;

(ii) It creates in him an interest for the health of other members of his family as well as of those living in his surrounding; and

(iii) It creates in him a desire to support health education programmes in this area.[23]

Health education is an essential component of any programme to improve the health of a community, and it has a major role in promoting:

(a) good health practices—for example, sanitation, clean drinking water, good hygiene, breast feeding, infant weaning, and oral rehydration;

(b) the use of preventive services—for example, immunization, screening, antenatal and child health clinics;

(c) the correct use of medications and the pursuit of rehabilitation regimens—for example, in tuberculosis and leprosy respectively;

(d) the reorganization of early symptoms of disease and promoting early referral; and

(e) community support for primary health care and government control measures.

Despite the potential benefits of health education, existing schemes are often inadequate and ineffective. The key decisions that form the basis for any planning are decisions over what the desired change should be, where the health education should take place, who should carry it out, and how it should be done[24].

We mention here the following points to prove the important role of health education in health delivery system:

(1) Health Education develops a permanent base to support the delivery of health services.

(2) Health Education kindles interest among people about their health.

(3) Health Education, being preventive in nature is cost effective.

(4) Health Education promotes Community Participation in the health programmes of the Community.

(5) Health Education can reduce dependence on health system, as 75% diseases are preventive.

(6) Health Education creates a chain effect as it passes on from individual to family to society.

(7) Health Education removes many mis-conceptions entangled into the minds of people.

(8) Health Education can promote partnership among health professionals and health receives.

(9) Health Education can promote individuals to take timely action to avoid complexities.
(10) Health Education can check the rush for secondary and tertiary health care system.
(11) Health Education being a two-way process can help in providing knowledge to health professionals.
(12) Health Education can help professionals in creating right attitudes among people about their health.

(7) Patient is a Person and not a Statistic: Need of Dedication and not an Earning Machine on the Part of Doctor

To the mechanization of medicine is added the sin of commercialization. This is an age of consumerism where the lure of money—which brings with it power, luxury, comfort and enjoyment of life in all its varied physical forms is paramount. Dreadful as it may sound, medicine is fast becoming a business rather than a profession, and that too,, not uncommonly, a nefarious, corrupt business. What could be more nefarious than charging exorbitant fees from those who cannot afford them? What could be more corrupt than the practice of doctors who on purpose refer unsuspecting vulnerable patients from one specialist to another for no reason other than profit? What could be more corrupt than the unethical practice of commissions demanded by general practitioners from a specialist to whom a patient is referred?

Another major drawback of contemporary medicine is the crippling expense an ill patient often incurs—an expense that is often ruinous to the family. This is partly due to the fact that the physician of today has forgotten the art of medicine and remains solely pre-occupied with its science. His rapport is with machines and not with patients; it is technology that dictates his course of action and not his clinical judgment. History taking is a neglected art; he forgets to use his senses—his eyes, ears and hands, but remembers numbers, equations and formulae. Expensive investigations and expensive modes of treatment result, when simple tests and simpler measures would have sufficed.

Institutionalized medicine has also led to malpractice. Expensive glittering machines and foyers resembling five star hotels are the landmarks of modern institutions. To meet the cost, and, hopefully, make profit, machines have to be fed, and patients become the fodder for these machines. If an audit were to be carried out on the cost-effectiveness of modern day investigations, the result would indeed be shocking.[25]

Commercialization of Medical Education

During recent years we have seen mushrooming of private medical colleges in many states. The trend is towards increasing commercialization. The health industry would like to get quick return for their huge investments at the cost of patients who are required to undergo unnecessary investigations and expensive treatment.

Even though charging capitation fees is punishable under the law the practice continue to go unabated with tacit understanding between different agencies. Through the private medical colleges we are creating a large number of affluent medical professionals from the privileged sections of the society. Having spent a fortune to get medical education how do we expect them to serve the rural population? Many of us feel that the medical degree would be awarded only after two years of service in rural areas irrespective of where the candidate comes from—Government or Private Medical colleges.[26]

(8) Faith in Values of Medical Problems: (Doctors no longer Believes in Values)

Why has there been such a decline in the ethics of contemporary medicine? It is almost certainly related to the decline in the sense of values in our present-day world. This decline is observed in all professions and in the whole of society, perhaps even to a greater extent than that observed in medicine. A burning desire for material gain and wealth dominates life today. It is indeed difficult for a profession to remain an island of virtue when surrounded by a sea of filth and corruption. The island is first eroded and then gradually swamped. But please remember that we have an ancient heritage to cherish and maintain. We must therefore combine and rise to root out the canker eating into the heart of medicine.[27]

(9) Look to the longer Welfare of Patient

The first is clinical iatrogenesis-diseases produced by physicians, either by treatment or investigations, or by the hospital in which patients are treated. But then iatrogenic disease is as old as medicine; it is an inseparable companion of medicine since antiquity. Contemporary medicine is aware of the epidemic of iatrogenesis resulting from the frequent use of potent drugs, sophisticated gadgetry and invasive procedures used in the diagnosis of management of patients. Far too often, the treatment meted out to patients today may be worse than the disease.

The second form of iatrogenesis is social iatrogenesis by which is meant the creation of an environment, which no longer has the ability to allow people in society to look after themselves. People are hopelessly dependent on the medical system and the medical system operates to ensure that this remains so. Medical help is sought for trivial and unnecessary reasons, to the benefit of the medical profession and to the detriment of people in society.

The third form of iatrogenesis, accordingly to Illich, is cultural iatrogenesis whereby institutionalized medicine has sapped the ability of the people to face the reality of the sufferings in life and the inevitability of death. This may be true in the West but is not so in India and many Eastern countries. A patient's, and for that matter a doctor's, attitude to suffering, pain and death is conditioned by socio-cultural and religious factors. Most people in the East accept that life cannot be divorced from suffering and pain, and that each one is apportioned his or her share of pain and suffering in life. It is being increasingly recognized today that modern medicine with its science and technology should relieve suffering but should refrain from prolonging the act of dying. Above all, it should prevent death from being lonely, gruesome, obscene, de-humanized and ruinous to the patient and his family.[28]

(10) Sympathy

'It is necessary to recapture the spirit of humanism and reestablish the special sympathy in doctor patient relationship. To restore the image we need to distance from lure of money, raise the ethical standards and place the welfare and care of patients above all.' It is felt there is decline in values in medical profession. The frustration of patients and relatives is often translated into litigation demanding compensation; to protect himself the doctor falls back on defensive medicine. He over investigates not to miss even a rare disorder. There is need for healthy interaction between medicine and society, which is a two-way reciprocal affair. In India doctor is often brought before a consumer court for any alleged incompetence or offence, The Judiciary in India considers practice of medicine as "Consumer Industry" and services rendered to a patient like "consumer product." It is unfortunate that the doctor with years of study, knowledge, expertise and experience and above all in spite of the care provided to the patient his services are to be equated as consumer product. In most countries the disputes between doctors and patients are decided by duly constituted professional bodies; Lack of Internal audit and control within the profession is responsible for this sad state of affairs. The medical professionals must develop effective public relations and media management skill. These will help in true projection of our achievements, avoid or dispel rumors, respond to criticism, diffuse controversies and project a positive image.[29]

(11) Trustworthiness

Medical professors are the architects and builders of students' behavior using a standard program. They are also the curricular developers and thus have pivotal role in shaping the future medicos. Charka Samhita lays down that the teacher should be one "whose doubts have been all cleared in respect of medical scriptures—possessed of experience—clever in the practice in his profession. Conversant with nature—his knowledge of medical science supplemented with a knowledge of other branches of study—without malice—of a peaceful disposition—capable of bearing privation and pain—well affected towards disciples and prone to teach them—capable of communicating his ideas, etc. (Chaudhary, 1994). The professional temperament of the doctor with capability for clinical training/ educational tutelage is as follows:

Every doctor who is appointed afford clinical or educational supervision for a doctor in training, or who undertakes to provide clinical training and supervision for medical students, should demonstrate resolution to our professional guidance in Good Medical Practice. This will encompass:

- Presuming a high standard of professional and personal values in relation to patients and their care.
- Being available and accessible to patients.
- Maintaining a high standard of clinical competence.
- An ability to communicate effectively.
- An assurance to personal, and professional, development as a doctor.
- An assurance to professional audit and peer review.
- An assurance to team working in a multi-professional environment.
- An understanding of the multi-cultural society in which medicine is practiced.
- An enthusiasm for his/her specialty.
- A personal assurance to teaching and learning.
- Impressionability and responsiveness to the educational needs of students and junior doctors.
- The capacity to promote development of the required professional attitudes and values.
- An understanding of the principles of education as applied to medicine.
- An understanding of research method.
- Poetical teaching skills.
- A willingness to develop both as a doctor and as a teacher.
- A commitment to audit and peer review of his/her teaching.
- The ability to use formative assessment for the benefit of the student/trainee.
- The ability to carry out formal appraisal of medical student progress/the performance of the trainee as a practicing doctor.[30]

(12) See the Patient as Integrated Whole

Improvements in the health status of a population cannot be achieved simply by expanding and developing the health services. The prevention and control of disease and the promotion of health require a concerted effort for the improvement of human well-being as a whole. In this task, what has been defined as "health care" has to be supported by improvements in the social and economic infrastructure, and contributions from various sectors other than health.

Certainly there has been a broad understanding of the linkages between health development and development in other sectors. The health experience of the industrialized countries has contributed significantly to this understanding. We know that the major causes of sickness and death arising out of a large cluster of diseases associated with poor sanitation, illiteracy and low levels of income were effectively controlled in these countries well before the discovery of antibiotics and other spectacular curative "break-throughs." The control of diarrhoeal diseases, tuberculosis and a wide range of communicable diseases was primarily achieved through far-reaching improvements in the urban infrastructure, housing and environmental sanitation, through the changes in health behaviour which accompanied higher levels of education and literacy, and through the improvement in nutritional status as incomes and living standards steadily rose. The positive outcome in health was therefore the result of an intersectoral effort.

The more recent experiences of a few developing countries illustrate even more dramatically the way in which health forms part of an integrated process of development. These countries have been able to achieve high level of life expectancy and have shown remarkable progress in reducing infant and maternal mortality at comparatively low levels of income. The state of Kerala, with per capita incomes well below the average for India as a whole, enjoys a health status—as measured by life expectancy, infant mortality and other health indicators—which is well above the rest of India.[31]

(13) Not Exploitative

Doctor must treat the patients with economy and efficiency. It has been seen that Doctor prescribes large number of tests relating to laboratory investigations and Radiology, which are costly and dangerous. These are prescribed only to get 50-60 per cent commission. Doctor is not interested in treating the patient but exploiting this for material benefits. In this way mind of the doctor gets perverted and he looses self-respect in his own mind. This trend is on the increase. Which should be curbed by Government through some legislation. If the tests prescribed by the doctor are not needed legal action must be taken against the doctor.

(14) Doctor must Treat the Patient on the Basis of Equity

It is well known that Doctor is highly qualified in medicine but this is not sufficient until and unless the doctor treats the patients on the basis of equality and in a dignified way. His diagnosis and treatment would depend upon the information he is able to get from the patient. If the doctor keeps himself on high pedestrian which prevents the disclosure of information and prevents the good rapport between patient and the doctor. Doctor must make the patient feel as equal partner of treatment.

Involving patients in the provision of their own care offers enormous benefits to both the patients and their providers. Physicians recognize that the patient is their primary source of information regarding symptoms and perceived reactions to treatment. They would further assert that the critical factor in the effectiveness of treatments is the patient's compliance with prescribed protocols. So patients already are involved in their own care. "Empowering" patients simply acknowledges their shared responsibility and builds upon the trust that has historically served as the foundation of the provider-patient relationship. The empowerment comes from giving patients greater access to information and from facilitated patient-provider communications. Empowered patients are better equipped to manage their own health, to educate themselves regarding their health condition, and to play an active part in their treatment.[32]

(15) Doctor must be Prompt, thorough and Patient's Friendly

In a poor country like India, there is great rush of patients. How to deal with them? Doctor must be prompt, i.e. not waste time talking to friends, colleagues, etc. He must understand the concept of Time Management, i.e. Time is Money. He must concentrate on patients treatment with dedication and sincerity. In this way he can deal efficiently both quantitatively and qualitatively. He must also deal with the patients sympathetically. Even a single good word to the patient can help the patients in fast recovery.

(16) Medicines must be Prescribed of Generic Nature which are Cheap and Patients can Afford

People in India are poor and they cannot spend much on health care. It has become a fashion to prescribe costly medicines, which make the patients sicker as he has not the means to purchase them. Doctors prescribe them under the pressure of pharmaceutical companies to get some money from them. Medicine is a noble profession; therefore, doctor must attend to the patients as per his need and affordability.

(17) Doctor should Ensure the Satisfaction of the Patient

Doctor must understand the problems of the patients first. After understanding, he must tell him his diagnosis and satisfying the patient with all the questions in his mind. Many questions in the mind of the patient are unfounded but still the doctor must remove the doubts of the patient. When the patient is satisfied, he develops trust in the doctor and at this stage doctor can suggest him both preventive and curative measures.

(18) Doctor must Understand the Art and Science of Counselling Patients

Doctor has to change the attitude and behaviour of patients towards positive health. It is highly difficult as it is easier to destroy the mountains than to change the minds of the people. Counselling requires patient listening and better understanding of patients. Doctors should not use harsh language. He must convey in polite and simple language. It has been seen that some doctors start quarreling with the patients when they do not agree with his viewpoint, which is wrong in principle and practice. He must learn that there is and science of counselling, which can create positive, change in his mind.

Counselling is one of the effective methods used in health education and social work to help individuals and families to require their health problems solved.

A recent English definition may also be quoted for further clarification: "Case work is professional service offered to those who desire help with their personal and family problems. Its aim is to relieve stress and to help the client to achieve a better personal and social adjustment. It proceeds by the study of the individual in his social milieu, by the establishment of a co-operative relationship with him, and by the mobilizing of both his own resources and those of the community to work towards these goals."[33]

Analysis of case studies suggest the following for effective counselling:

(1) A harmonious rapport between the individual and Doctor is the first most important requirement to make counselling effective.
(2) Doctor must be knowledgeable and competitive so that he can take a firm decision.
(3) Individuals must develop trust and faith in the Doctor.
(4) Doctor must keep the individual's problems confidentially.
(5) Counsellor must learn the art and science of communication to be effective.[34]

We must all learn together to see how we are going to communicate in the future. We are at the advent of a new era in health care and medicine in which users; health care providers and practitioners, directors, and managers work together to make efficient use of new information and communication technologies.[35]

Doctors must also attend these patients who do not shown any sign of physical ailments—Patients generally complain of many problems but physically they are fit and fine: How to deal with them? There is a need of advice to the patient to change lifestyle, etc. Doctors must try other methods to improve him rather than sending the patient to a psychiatric department till he shows severe signs of stress and strain.

(19) Ethical Values

Doctors must follow Ethical Values. It has been reported that few doctors misbehave with the patients and even outrage the modesty of women patients. It is highly deplorable act. That is why primary health centers have been provided a post of woman doctor.

Such acts by few individuals create a poor image of medical profession. It is suggested that strict action must be taken against doctors indulging in such heinous crimes.

We have discussed the duties and responsibilities of Doctors to the patients. Let us discuss the duties of patients toward doctor, which would ensure complete integration between the doctor and the patient. Patient should be as good as he wants doctor to be good. Let us discuss some of important qualities inpatient, which can make the doctor a co-partner in the process of treatment and health care.

1. Patient's faith in the Doctor

Patients must have respect for the doctor as well as have full faith in the capability and capacity of the doctor. It has been rightly said that faith begets faith. It is the duty of the patient to have complete faith in doctor otherwise doubt would emerge in the patient which would make his disease more serious. If he has no faith for reasons known to the patient, then he can approach other doctor of his choice and have faith in him. Faith is the first ingredient for the patient in the Doctor for treatment.

2. Patient's Need to Disclose all Problems

Past, Present, i.e. case history—The patient must disclose all the information asked by the doctor correctly without fear as his diagnosis is going to based upon that. There is a tendency among patients not to tell correctly all the information for fear of shame or being let down by the doctor. Even if the doctor does not ask any information; the patient must tell every thing, which is perturbing the mind of the patient. He can get the treatment for all the problems otherwise the treatment can not be effective.

3. Good Behaviour of the Patient

We already discussed that the doctor must have good behaviour with the patient, the same way patients must have good behaviour towards doctor. Patients must understand the limitations of doctors, i.e. number of patients are so large that doctor cannot provide time immediately. Patient must wait for his turn. Good behaviour of patient can make the doctor more careful and attentive to the patient. He should show respect to all medical fraternity who are engaged in a noble profession.

4. Patients need to follow Doctor's Prescription in Letter and Spirit

Disease prevention is possible only if the patient acts on the prescription. Even time schedule of taking medicines, etc. must be followed scrupulously. Some patient for one reason or the other do not follow the prescription and start taking something else, they cannot be treated. So follow the prescription of one doctor only religiously.

5. Diet must be taken as Prescribed

Patients must take diet as prescribed. Indoor patients are given only the diet suitable for them. Outpatients are however advised to take particular diet at home. Diet and disease are related. Patients must take the prescribed diet.

6. Regular Follow-up

The patients must follow-up his treatment as advised by the doctor otherwise the disease can re-appear with more serious threat. Therefore, till the doctor wants follow up, the patients must go and see the doctor.

7. *Be Patient for his turn at every Place*

Whether it is examination by the doctor or laboratory tests.

8. *Respect to Lady Doctor*

There have been some cases where patients have misbehaved with the lady doctors and even sometimes harassed them. Exemplary punishment must be given to patients or their relatives who indulge in anti-social activities. The administration must also be strict to take care of lady doctors so that no patient can dare to misbehave with the lady doctors.

9. *Patients must Bear in Mind about*

The shortage of staff/non-availability of medicine, etc. Most of the hospitals in our country are starved of funds resulting into shortages of men, money and material. The patients must cope up with such situations rather than creating unnecessary trouble. Patients may contact the Government/Health department which is responsible for all these problems. The problems in AIIMS recently were not due to doctors but because of interference of the ministry of Health and Family Welfare.

A basic doctor, to be effective to deliver health care to the country must be an astute clinician, a good communicator, and a sound administrator, so as to effectively lead an ever-expanding health team for a positive health action. Work and action domain of the doctor has crossed the boundaries to drugs and dispensaries and presently extends to a large extent to the families and to the communities—hence the need for the basic doctor to be a community physician. Thus has emerged the need for developing a well-designed and structured programme of education for basic doctors with general applicability, departing from the present MBBS curriculum, and with emphasis on the primary health needs of the country. In addition, human values and medical ethics need to be incorporated as a part of the curriculum. In essence, the National Education Policy in Health Sciences aims at, and strives towards, the production of basic doctors equipped with adequate knowledge, requisite skills and appropriate behavioral attributes to meet the health needs of the country.[36]

CONCLUSION

The success of the medical profession depends to a great extent upon the harmonious relationship between the medical team and the patients. Medical team should not function as machinery but in a human and purposeful way. The medical team should have a sense of dedication, responsibility and be responsive and alert to the aspirations and problems of the patients. Patients on the other hand should also provide meaningful co-operation to medical team. Under such an atmosphere, it would be very easy to implement the patient care activities smoothly.

While endorsement of inefficiency or sheer neglect on the part of a hospital or its staff is uncalled for, it would be prudent to understand the constraints under which the hospitals and the medical personnel have to serve the ever increasing number of critical patients, some of which may not respond to a well proven treatment or the nature of affiction may be incurable or the delays in administration of treatment may occur despite the best efforts of the doctors on duty—due to multifarious pressures and bottlenecks, while judging their performance it is imperative to examine, whether the person was adequately skilled to handle the situation, whether there was intention to help to the best of his capability, whether an all out effort was made to render the service promptly and properly. If the answer to the above questions is 'Yes' no charge of negligence can be made out. It goes without saying that the staff has been accessible, humane, commitment...sympathetic in the hand of stern and grief, which patients and their attendants face in the hospital situation.

A spirit of service and dedication must pervade among the providers of the health care as they are considered second God on earth by the receivers of health care. In the new millennium, we must empower the patients by looking after them carefully and making them feel important.

The progress and achievements of the past 50 years are solid foundations for a healthier and better world. It is already time to build on them. Life in the 21st Century could and should be better for all. We can pass no greater gift to the next generation than a healthier future. That is our vision. Together, the people of the world can make it a reality.[37]

Dr. H. Mahler is very critical about the inability of health workers in contemporary society to influence those social and environmental factors, which truly determine public health. He states:

> "There persist widespread negative attitudes among health professionals towards the health care of the poorest strata in the rural and urban population in the developing countries. Most of these attitudes imply-with a repetitiveness of an old gramophones records caught in a narrow, arrogant, condescending and indifferent groove-that these poor people are too apathetic, too superstitious, too illiterate to benefit from the health care potentially availability to them. Health professionals and those who train them should be much more radicals in accepting a social responsibility for the health needs of the people in these poor rural urban communities so that they can act as agents for change."[38]

Thus, we can say that there is a need to train health administrators and workers in the new art of Public Health Administration so that they can take the benefits of the modern science to the common man and maintain the spirit of Geneva Declaration[39]."

Now being admitted to the profession of Medicine, I solemnly pledge to concentrate my life to the service of humanity. I will give respect and gratitude to my deserving teacher. I will practice medicine with conscience and dignity. The health and life of my patients will be my first consideration. I will hold in confidence all that my patients confide in me. I will maintain the honour and noble traditions of the medical profession. My colleagues will be my brothers. I will not permit considerations of race, religion, nationality, party politics or social standing to intervene between my duty and my patient. I will maintain the utmost respect of human life. Even under threat I will not use my knowledge contrary to the laws of humanity. These promises I make freely and upon my honour."

The same feelings has been expressed in the Tokyo Declaration. To quote the preamble to the Declaration of Tokyo:

> "It is the privilege of the medical doctor to practice medicine in the service of humanity, to preserve and restore bodily and mental health without distinction as to the persons to comforts and to ease the sufferings of his or her patients."[40]

Prof. J.S. Neki has rightly said in this connection that "to help, to heal, to reconstruct, to comfort—and all along the line to act with compassion—all these bear testimony to the moral consciousness of the doctor. Whatever the new strains imposed upon medical ethics, this structure will survive and continue to guide doctors in their professional conduct. Legal and juridical obligations they have, no necessity, to fulfil. But these are not genuine ethics. Genuine ethics has to be ingrained into character and does not have to depend upon external controls.[41]

To err is human, and there is no physician on earth who has not made mistakes. The best-trained faculties may falter in observation, and even in the most experience, errors in judgment must inevitably occur in an art and science which often consists in the balancing of probabilities. Cultivate an honesty of mind which recognizes regrets and proclaims these mistakes. Only then will you learn from them and perhaps not repeat them. Do not hide your mistakes. Only then will you learn from them and perhaps not repeat them. Do not hide your mistakes under a bushel or pretend that they never existed. It you do so, you will tread the unfortunate path of self-deception and delusion and your mistakes will multiply.

Humility is the hall-mark of a true physician. The grace of humility is a precious gift. "Knowledge is proud that he knows so much, Wisdom is humble that he knows no more." Extend your charity, humility and consideration not only to your patients, but also to your colleagues, so that you do unto them as you would have them do unto you.

In my opinion, what distinguishes a great physician from an ordinary one is the power of judgment. Hippocrates said, "Judgment is difficult, and indeed medicine has been defined as the art of coming to a conclusion on insufficient evidence." We can increase our power of observation by constant practice. We can become more knowing and more wise through study and experience, but can we improve on our judgment? To an extent judgment is an inborn faculty; "the result of a union of mind and character, which a man either has or has not, and it is almost as difficult for him to increase it as to add a cubit to his stature."

Perhaps the only way to help improve judgment is to improve our mind, not by scientific training alone, but by an exposure to art, culture, literature, history, philosophy—the other great fields of human endeavour. A broader study of the humanities will enable you to understand Man and his afflictions far better than the detailed study of medicine alone. Dip therefore into the treasures of the world around you. Medicine is the study of Man. Study mankind and you will have enhanced your study of Man.[42]

Notes and References

1. Chandni, Saxena, Role of Ancient Indian Universities in value orientation to the contemporary society in India, in *University News*, 44(05), January 30-February 05, 2005, p. 30.
2. Safran C., The collaborative edge: patient empowerment for vulnerable populations. *Int J Med Informatics* 2002; 1-6.
3. Ferguson T., Consumer health informatics. *Health Care Forum* 1995; 28-23.
4. Brennan, P.F., Ripich S., Use of a home care computer network by persons with AIDS. *Int J Technol Assess Health Care* 1994; 10 (2): 258-272.
5. Brennan, P.F., Health informatics and community health: support for patients as collaborators in care. *Methods Inform Med* 1999; 38 (4-5): 274-278.
6. Tang, P.C., Newcomb, C., Gorden, S., Kreider, N., Meeting the information needs of patients: results from a patient focus group. *Proc AMIA Annual Fall Symposium* 1997; 672-676.
7. Kaplan, B., Brennan, P.F., Consumer informatics: supporting patients as co-producers of quality. *JAMIA* 2001; 8(4):309-316.
8. Tang, P.C., Newcomb, C., Information patients: a guide for providing patient health information, *JAMIA* 1998;5(6):563-570.
9. D. Goldsmith and C. Safran, Consumer Informatics, pp. 9-11 and 17.
10. *Ibid.*, p. 62.
11. Ordway Tead, The Art of Administration, New York, McGraw-Hill, 1951, p. 45.
12. D. Goldsmith and C. Safran, Consumer Informatics, p. 31.
13. Sanjay Bhattacharya, Social Work, Deep and Deep, New Delhi, 2003, pp. 223-24.
14. D. Goldsmith and C. Safran, Consumer Informatics, p. 40.
15. S.L. Goel, Health Care Policies and Programmes, Deep & Deep Publications, New Delhi, Vol. 2, pp. 23-29.
16. WHO, *World Health*, December 1975, p. 6.
17. John J. Hanlon, Principles of Public Health Administration, St. Louis, 1960, p. 402.
18. WHO: Technical Report Series No. 89, p. 4.
19. S.L. Goel, Health Care Policies and Programmes, Deep & Deep Publications, New Delhi, Vol. 2, p. 6.
20. WHO: Technical Report Series No. 156, p. 3.
21. WHO: Etienne Berthet, A new role for teacher, *World Health*, May 1979, p. 23.
22. WHO, Esmat Mansour, "Towards a World without Polio", January-February 1995, p. 27.
23. Dr. S.L. Goel, Health Education: Theory and Practice, "Nature and Scope", p. 93.
24. K. Mahadevan (Ed.), Health Education for quality of life, Delhi, B.R. Publishing Corporation, 2002.

25. Farokh Erach Udwadia, Emeritus Professor of medicine, "Humanity: The Core of Doctor-Patient Relationship", *University News*, 42(34), August 23-29, 2004, pp. 15-16.
26. A. Rajasebram, Radical Changes required in Medical Education, *University News*, 44(23), June 05-11, 2006, p. 15.
27. Farokh Erach Udwadia, Emeritus Professor of medicine, "Humanity: The Core of Doctor-Patient Relationship", *University News*, 42(34), August 23-29, 2004, p. 16.
28. Farokh Erach Udwadia, Emeritus Professor of medicine, "Humanity: The Core of Doctor-Patient Relationship", *University News*, 42(34), August 23-29, 2004, p. 16.
29. A. Rajasebram, Radial Changes required in Medical Education, *University News*, 44(23), June 05-11, 2006, p. 17
30. Vijay Pithadia and Vandana Parmar, Appraisal of Medical Education in India, *University News*, 44(44), October 30-November 05, 2006, pp. 11-12.
31. Aleya Ei Bindari Hammad, Intersectoral Cooperation in Primary Health Care, *World Health*, March 1986, p. 3.
32. D.B. Baker and D. Masys, "Research and Development," Consumer Informatics, p. 67.
33. S.L. Goel, "Health Education with Individuals (Counselling)", p. 299.
34. *Ibid.*, p. 315.
35. R.D. Appel and C. Boyer, "Steps Toward Reliable Online Consumer Health Information, Consumer Informatics, p. 89.
36. Public Health in India's Five Decades, 50th Anniversary of India's Independence, Vol. I, p. 7.
37. S.L. Goel, Health Education, Theory and Practice, pp. 82-83.
38. Text of Address by Dr. H. Mahler, to the Thirteenth Session of Regional Committee of South East Asia.
39. Geneva Declaration.
40. I swear by Apollo by Christian Viedma, *World Health*, July 1979, p. 28.
41. J.S. Neki, Medical Ethics, *World Health*, July 1979.
42. Farokh Erach Udwadia, Emeritus Professor of Medicine, *University News*, 42(34), August 23-23, 2004, p. 14.

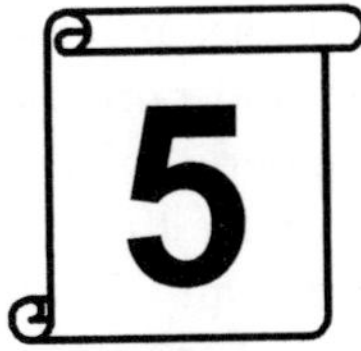

Manpower Planning

A hospital is a complex organization. No where else the need for trained manpower and their degree of training and skill is greater than a well managed hospital. The diversity of duties and expectation of a near perfect outcome from the humans in pain or disability demands that each job is assigned to a person who is well trained in his job-requirement and is also willing to suffer loss of comfort and convenience for the sake of a patient or his relations. A hospital has all those requirements that are needed by any good hotel/hospitality/industry. In addition it has to possess manpower with medical/surgical/nursing and humanitarian skills to take care of the ailing person. It goes without saying that the needs, expectations, sensitivities and reactions of a sick person are for more and far varied than another guest. The need of a new born child patient his mother in labour or post-labor are totally different as compared to an old person suffering from chronic heart failure or cancer. To meet the diverse and varied needs, there is a paramount requirement of manpower planning. This also entails their training and skills top in hospital set-up.

GENESIS AND NEEDS

A developing economy needs high level technical manpower as urgently as it needs capital. A crucial factor in improving the coverage and quality of services is the availability of adequate number of personnel with task-oriented training. Among the three components required for developmental tasks—men, money and material (M^3), it is more the men (or the human element) duly qualified than any other factor which determines the quality and quantity of the performance and output. After all, even the contribution of money and material to performance depends substantially upon their manipulation by the men in an organisation. Human resources are critical for the success of any social activity.

Dr. C.D. Deshmukh in his Article, "Management and Administration—New Trends" published by Department of Personnel in Training Abstracts 17, as rightly said that, "Good management provides the surpluses which on investment nourish the processes of industrialisation and modernisation of society. Good administration furnishes the infrastructure of services which secure the order, stability and social development. Carefully recruited and periodically trained or re-trained top-personnel is needed for both spheres of operation. How to regulate the affairs of the nation so as to maximise the efficiency of both is the supreme challenge to political leadership. Only by meeting it successfully can a democratic polity survive in the not-too-long-run."

"Adding employees haphazardly can create more problems than it solves. It pays to take the time to consider how new employees will fit into the existing organisation and whether they will be contributing to its success" (Industrial Engineering, October 1985/p. 14).

Development is not a mechanical process. It is a human enterprise and its success will depend ultimately on the skill, the quality and motivation of the persons associated with it. Human rather than capital is the key to development. According to Prof. Merle Fainsod 'Improvements in the effectiveness of development administration depends on the quality and training of public servants who man it and on a social and political environment which liberates their energies. Structural adjustments can work no developmental miracles where administrative manpower is inadequate or the will to develop is lacking. The secret of development is not concealed in the interstices of governmental or administrative structure. Development takes place where skill is supported by commitment and the human material resources exist to translate dreams into actualities."[1]

Mr. Stahl in his Article "Managerial Effectiveness in Developing Countries" in *International Review of Administrative Sciences* (Vol. XLV-1979/No. 1/pp. 1-5) has rightly mentioned that "Contrary to many initial assumptions, poverty and low productivity in some societies are attributable not so much to over population or inadequate natural resources . . . The most important resource in any society—rich or poor, advanced or backward—is the mind of man. It is this resource above all, that cannot be protected, developed and fully utilised. Husbanding this precious asset is the most vital single ingredient of any plan for improvement of public administration." Professor Lewis has rightly said that "growth is the result of human efforts."[2] The most valuable investment is that which is invested for improving the abilities and capacities of the people so that they can become competent to bring about socio-economic development. An improvement in the quality of the human factor is as essential as investment in physical capital. If there is under-investment in human capital, the rate at which additional physical capital will be profitably utilised will be comparatively low and as a consequence the process of economic development will be slowed down.

According to Prof. Myint,

> "It is now increasingly realised that many under-developed countries may be held back, not so much by a shortage of savings as by a shortage of skills and knowledge resulting in a limited capacity of their organisational framework to absorb capital in productive investment."[3]

In the developing countries, there is a shortage of skilled manpower which is responsible for poor progress in these countries. Prof. Meir observes in this connection that,

> "While investment in human beings has been a major source of growth in advanced countries, the negligible amount of human investment in underdeveloped countries has done little to extend the capacity of the people to meet the challenge of accelerated development."[4]

It has been rightly said: "that due to the labour-intensive nature of hospital services, it is essential to keep the working environment and employee attitudes in tune with the interests of maximum productivity."

Personnel management in the beginning of this century was based on simple—"carrot or stick" approach. During the last quarter century, organizations have become complex requiring special skills and techniques to produce maximum output. One such technique is that of manpower planning, i.e., ensuring that the requisite staff of desired quality is available at the right time.

Manpower planning is a technique of correcting imbalances between the manpower demand and manpower supply in the economy. Such imbalances can create either the problem of unemployment or shortages. Both situations are dangerous and suicidal for the socio-economic development of a country. Thus, it is necessary to plan the long-term growth and development of highly skilled manpower to avoid the evil consequences. Manpower planning is not only concerned with the balancing of demand and supply of different categories of manpower, but also with overall development and utilisation of manpower resources in a country. Prof. Harbison has rightly remarked in this connection that:

> "in the broadest terms, manpower policy should be concerned with development, maintenance and utilisation of actual or potential members of the labour force including those who are fully and productively employed as well as those who experience difficulty in getting work. The development of manpower is the process of man's acquiring the skills, knowledge and capacities for work—the maintenance of manpower is the process of preservation and maintenance renewal of man's capacities for work. The utilisation of

manpower is the process of matching men and work in accordance with their level of development."[5]

Manpower planning has not received due attention in the public sector inspite of its expansion and diversification. The development of human resources has an importance that can only be overlooked at the cost of survival. An important pre-requisite for improving such situation in any country is undoubtedly the availability of different categories of manpower suitably trained to fulfil the needs of the people and respond to the established and emerging needs of the people. Effective manpower planning is a vital national responsibility because on it largely depends the success of all other activities. Let us now define manpower planning:

> "Manpower Planning is concerned with organising, in systematic fashion, the goals, objectives, priorities and activities of manpower development in order to ensure that the right number of staff with appropriate skills are provided at the right time to meet the requirement of the work to be done."[6]

There should be only one yardstick to judge the effectiveness of Manpower Planning, namely, continuous improvement of the status and the quality of life of the population with the least friction to those who supply the services and the most satisfying to those who receive it. We have to achieve all this with the minimum cost and maximum efficiency.

Thus, Manpower Planning, is the key-stone in the arch of personnel management. Manpower planning, looked at from the statistical point of view, is a process of information collection, analysis and projection to determine the likely effect of existing or proposed manpower policies on the manpower system under study and to present, and advise upon possible course of action to over-come present or future problems. This process is designed to help management to match manpower supply to requirements in accordance with the policies of the country. Manpower planning can help the organization in the development of uniformity and consistency; designing tools of personnel appraisal and developing the standards to avoid the impact of pressures. This would led to effective and sound decision-making relating to personnel in an organisation.

In a broader sense, it can be defined as the process by which an organisation ensures that it has the right number of people and the right kind of people, at the right places, at the right time, doing things for which they are economically most useful. Manpower planning is concerned with organising in systematic fashion, the goals, objectives, priorities, of manpower development in order to ensure that the requisite number of staff with the appropriate skills are provided at the right time to meet the requirements of the work to be done.

While planning for manpower, we may keep the quality also in view. Vernon. E. Mcbryde, in his Article, "In today's market, quality is best focal point for upper management" in *Industrial Engineering* (July 1986) has rightly said that not only must more brainpower be brought into the action, but a synergiotic use of human resources must also be developed . . . The key to unlocking this vast potential is the development of a state of quality awareness on the part of the entire Organisation such that no activity will take place without intense effort to ensure that its consequences promote rather than detract from the firm's cause. Top management pressing need is to determine a strategy for doing this."

Let us now discuss the essential ingredients of manpower planning.

INGREDIENTS OF MANPOWER PLANNING

Manpower planning of technical personnel must take into consideration all the factors which are taken into consideration by Manpower Planning Units in other sectors of development. Besides technical manpower planning units have to take into consideration many other factors which are peculiar to this sector alone. In the present situation, most of the factors are ignored resulting into defective personnel policies and decisions. Let us now discuss all the factors which must be taken into consideration by the personnel responsible for Technical Manpower Planning.

(1) 'Long Lead Time' between the Need and Supply of the Manpower

Manpower consists not only of people but also of knowledge, skills and attitudes acquired through education and formal training. The difficulty arises from the long 'lead time' required to bring about such education and training, e.g., it takes about 7 years after the college education to prepare an under-graduate physician in India. It has been rightly said that: "For a profession such as medicine, even a ten-year planning period is insufficient. Decision made in year one can begin to affect supply only by year eight or nine."[7] Same is true of other categories of technical personnel.

(2) High Cost of Training Personnel

The largest element in the budget of services is cost of training and retention of staff. Data from various sources indicate that the expenditure on the establishments of technical personnel in many countries ranges between 60-70 per cent of the costs of delivering services. The cost of educating a physician ranges between US $ 5,000 and US $ 80,000 depending upon the socio-economic conditions in the country and the level of specialisation of the physician.[8] In India, it is estimated that the cost of training an under-graduate Doctor is Rs. 80,000.

(3) Comparative Cost of Training and Retaining Workers

How to decide about the possible mixes of different sorts of technical workers? We may decide on that mix which can train and retain the manpower to cover the whole of the country and be within the financial limits of the country.

Major economies can be achieved as functions are transferred from high salary to low salary workers, because the main costs in the technical field are for services rather than goods. For example, we must decide about the proper mix of doctors, nurses, paramedical staff while doing manpower planning to provide decent health care to all.

Tamas Fulop has rightly stated in his article, "Who will Care for Health" (published in *World Health*, April 1977):

> "These changes should result in a sound health manpower system which will plan, develop and manage/utilize efficiently the right 'mix' of health personnel within well-conceived health and other services, which will continuously monitor whether they all are functioning properly and which will adjust the planning and 'production' system on the basis of such monitoring, so as to achieve a full health coverage for the entire population in the coming decades."

(4) Migration of Technical Personnel

A large number of technical personnel migrate to developed countries. For example, it was estimated that about the year 1991, there were at least 140,000 physicians and 135,000 nurses working outside their country of birth, citizenship or training. The most affected countries in this regard are India and the Philippines, each with over 10,000 physicians abroad. Other countries suffering heavy losses are Ireland, Iran, Pakistan, Bangladesh and the Republic of Korea, all with over 3,000 physicians abroad. Brain drain from one country to another results in other country's brain gain. What is the impact of this migration on the manpower planning machinery in a developing country? It affects gravely the development in these countries. Therefore, the manpower planning units should discourage the migration through:

(a) Fostering of national loyalties and ideals of service.
(b) Opening of new avenues to retain qualified and competent personnel.
(c) Strict legislation to stop migration.
(d) Raising the status of technical personnel.
(e) Strict legislation to serve in the country while granting fellowships to study abroad.

In this way, the developing countries can save a lot of money spent on the education and training of technical personnel serving overseas.

(5) Individual with Differing Skills may not be Easily Substituted

Technical personnel are highly differentiated. It is not possible to substitute a technical expert in any other's place. They are to be substituted only by the personnel of the same specialisation. One cannot substitute the other possessing different speciality. This becomes very serious in the case of teaching-*cum*-research institutions. The Manpower Planning Units must attend to this difficulty and avoid overgrowth or undergrowth in any branch of specialisation.

(6) Need of Team-Work

Most of the technical workers are working in isolation, i.e., their activities are not co-ordinated properly resulting into lower output of services. According to Antonio Ordonez-Plaja:

> "Team-work requires, among other things, that the members have an image of their team-mates which coincides as precisely as possible with reality. In addition, each member must have a self-image which adjusts to reality as much as possible and thus coincides with the image that other members have of him."[9]

The team-work would develop common practices and shared practices. This would also raise the morale of the personnel working at the grass-root level.

Peter F. Drucker, in his classic, "The Practice of Management" (p. 121) stated the conditions that he considers essential to Organisational effectiveness. One of them is team work.

> "Any Enterprise must build a true team and weld individual efforts into a common effort. Each member of the enterprise contributes something different, but they must all contribute toward a common goal. Their efforts must all pull in the same direction, and their contributions must fit together to produce a whole—without gaps, without friction, without unnecessary duplication of efforts."

The top personnel must have working relationships with their colleagues. They should follow the motto mentioned below:

Be my friend
Don't walk ahead of me I may not follow
Don't walk behind me
I may not lead
Just walk beside me and be my friend

(7) Need of Feedback System

Feedback is important to remove the defects of manpower planning. In developing countries, there is no machinery to develop the manpower plans on scientific lines resulting into the mal-utilization of scarce technical resources. Dr. Gunaratne, Regional Director of the South-East Asia Regional

Office of *World Health* has rightly said that:

> "Coupled with ad hoc attempts at manpower production leads to an ironical situation wherein notwithstanding the existence of sufficient capacity for the training of various categories of health personnel, there is a gross under-utilization of the capacity to produce manpower."

This can be avoided if there is a proper feedback machinery to evaluate the manpower planning system.

(8) Need of the New Patterns and Variety of Approaches

The concept of manpower planning is still in its infancy. We Will have to find new structures, new patterns and a variety of approaches to develop manpower planning suiting the requirements of the developing countries. We must encourage applied researches to find solutions to the problems of manpower development.

(9) Need of Designing an Effective Appraisal System

Though the appraisal evaluates past performance, it should be forward-looking in trying to build for successful performance in the future.

Besides, these peculiar features, there are certain other ingredients which may be kept in mind while development plans for manpower development. Most important of them are mentioned below:

(a) Finding and selecting the right calibre and number of people required to perform the operations of the organisation involved.
(b) Adequate briefing of new employees to the organisation and the job.
(c) Fair, sound and effective terms of employment.
(d) Provision of incentives.
(e) Establishment and maintenance of personnel inventories based on periodic appraisals of the productivity, methods, qualifications and potentials of employees.
(f) Well organised and specific training.
(g) Continuing personnel research.
(h) Management and staff relations based on mutual confidence and respect.

According to P. Ghosh, "Personnel policies should respect personnel integrity, ensure fair treatment for all employees, recognise human dignity, treat the employees as individuals, offer reasonable protection to the employees from economic insecurity. The policies should be so designed as to give proper recognition for work and accomplishment, create safe and healthy working conditions, promote common interests, recognise impact of change on people, encourage employee's participation, recognise the role of trade unions and respect their functions and responsibilities."[10]

DEVELOPMENT OF MANPOWER PLANS

Manpower Planning is a co-ordination of three main elements of manpower development process—Planning, Production and Management. This process needs to be linked with socio-economic planning. The Planners must consider the manpower planning process as a part and parcel of the process of socio-economic planning undertaken by a country, otherwise striking results may not be possible in human resource development.

The success of the efforts at Manpower Planning would depend upon the keen interest of the hospital authorities and the staff members. We may quote here the two eminent writers who have suggested the role each side should play.

The organisational structure of a hospital's medical staff is designed to ensure that the inherent responsibilities of an institution's physicians to its patients, administration, and the governing body are met in a satisfactory fashion.

Maintaining a high standard of medical care for the hospital must be the medical staff's primary concern. In order to meet this primary objective, the staff organisational structure must carry out the following six essential duties:

1. Make recommendations to the Administration and to the governing body of the hospital regarding staff appointments and hospital privileges.
2. Conduct continuing analytical review of all clinical work and practices done within the hospital.
3. Actively support individual members of the medical staff and hospital policies.
4. Insure that adequate medical records are kept.
5. Procure autopsies and monitor the minimum standards (20 per cent to 25 per cent of all hospital deaths) for such activities.
6. Conduct consultations.

Some fundamental objectives must be met by each member of the staff. First and foremost, the physician's responsibility is to the patients under his care. Clearly, the doctor must provide the best care that his intellectual capabilities and the physical limitations of the hospital will allow. Also the physician is responsible to the inner organisation of the medical staff, subject to the adopted standards, rules and regulations set-up by the Staff by-laws. While this situation requires a considerable amount of self-monitoring and monitoring the activities of his colleagues, this mechanism can usually be depended upon to maintain minimum standards for hospital medical care. Third, there is the responsibility to assist in attaining and maintaining the goals set forth by the governing body and administration of the hospital.[11]

In order to ensure their co-operation for decent health care, the writers further add that "As hospital care technology continue its phenomenal growth, a concurrent need for expanded staff training for hospital employees and improved public understanding of health self-help development become a dual challenge for a hospital's long-range educational programming. This double-faceted approach is the key to gaining maximum success in any hospital's plans for thorough education.[12]

An important operational objective for the future is, therefore, to improve personnel systems, develop manpower planning and expand the opportunity for education and training of personnel in the hospitals to achieve the goals of hospitals, as it is the human capacities which transform the resources into active agent of production.

Notes and References

1. Merle Fainsod in Irving Swedlow (ed.) Development Administration: Concepts and Problems, Syracuse, 1963, p. 23.
2. W.A. Lewis, *op. cit.*, p. 23
3. H. Myint, *op. cit.*, p. 173.
4. Gerald, M. Meir, *op. cit.*, p. 599.
5. Towards a Manpower Policy (ed.) by R.A. Gordon, New York, 1967, pp. 136-38.
6. WHO: *WHO Chronicle*, 30, 447-454, (1976).
7. T.L. Hall, Health Manpower in Peru: A Case Study in Planning, Baltimore, Johns Hopkinds, 1969, p. 7.
8. Dr. Alfonso Mejia and Helena Pizukri, The Brain Drain in *World Health*, April, 1977, p. 6.
9. Antonio Ordonez Plaza: Team Work at Ministry level, in *Team Work for Health* (ed.) *op. cit.*, p. 170.
10. P. Ghosh: Personnel Administration in India, Sudha Publications (P) Ltd., Delhi, 1975, p. 100.
11. Benjamin, Robert C. and Kemppairen, Hospital Administrator's Desk Book, Prentice Hall, 1983, p. 4.
12. *Ibid.*, p. 222.

APPENDIX I

NATIONAL HEALTH POLICY, 1983

Introductory

1. The Constitution of India envisages the establishment of a new social order based on equality, freedom, justice and the dignity of the individual. It aims at the elimination of poverty, ignorance and ill-health and direct the State to regard the raising of the level of nutrition and the standard of living of its people and the improvement of public health as among its primary duties, securing the health and strength of workers, men and women, specially ensuring that children are given opportunities and facilities to develop in a healthy manner.

1.1. Since the inception of the planning process in the country, the successive Five Year Plans have been providing the framework within which the States may develop their health services infrastructure, facilities for medical education, research, etc. Similar guidance has sought to be provided through the discussions and conclusion arrived at in the Joint Conferences of the Central Councils of Health of Family Welfare and the National Development Council. Besides, central legislation has been enacted to regulate standards of medical education prevention of food adulteration, maintenance of standards in the manufacture and sale of certified drugs, etc.

1.2. While the broad approaches contained in the successive Plan documents and discussions in the forums referred to in para 1 may have generally served the needs of the situation in the past, it is felt that an integrated, comprehensive approach towards the future development of medical education, research and health services requires to be established to serve the actual health needs and priorities of the country. It is, in this context that the need has been felt to evolve a National Health Policy.

Our Heritage

2. India has a rich, centuries-old heritage of medical and health sciences. The philosophy of Ayurveda and the skills enunciated by Charaka and Shushruta bear testimony to our ancient tradition in the scientific health care of our people. The approach of our ancient medical systems was of a holistic nature, which took into account all aspects of human health and disease. Over the centuries, with the intrusion of foreign influences and mingling of cultures, various systems of medicine evolved and have continued to be practised widely. However, the allopathic system of medicine has, in a relatively short period of time, made a major impact on the entire approach to health care and pattern of development of the health services infrastructure in the country.

Progress Achieved

3. During the last three decades and more, since the attainment of

independence, considerable progress has been achieved in the promotion of the health status of our people. Smallpox has been eliminated; plague is no longer a problem; mortality from cholera and related diseases has decreased and malaria brought under control to a considerable extent. The mortality rate per thousand of population has been reduced from 27.4 to 14.8 and the life expectancy at birth has increased from 32.7 to over 25. A fairly extensive network of dispensaries, hospitals and institutions providing specialised curative care has developed and a large stock of medical and health personnel, of various levels, has become available. Significant indigenous capacity has been established for the production of drugs and pharmaceuticals, vaccines, seraai hospital equipment, etc.

The Existing Picture

4. Inspite of such impressive progress, the demographic and health picture of the country still constitutes a cause for serious and urgent concern. The high rate of population growth continues to have an adverse effect on the health of our people and the quality of their lives. The mortality rates for women and children are still distressingly high; almost one-third of the total deaths occur among children below the age of 5 years; infant mortality is around 129 per thousand live births.

Efforts at raising the nutritional levels of our people have still to bear fruit and the extent and severity of malnutrition continues to be exceptionally high. Communicable and non-communicable diseases have still to be brought under effective control and eradicated. Blindness, Leprosy and TB continue to have a high incidence. Only 31 per cent of the rural population has access to potable water supply and 0.5 per cent enjoys basic sanitation.

4.1. High incidence of diarrhoeal diseases and other preventive and infectious diseases, specially amongst infants and children, lack of safe drinking water and poor environmental sanitation, poverty and ignorance are among the major contributory causes of the high incidence of diseases and mortality.

4.2. The existing situation has been largely engendered by the almost wholesale adoption of health manpower development policies and the establishment of curative centres based on the western models, which are inappropriate and irrelevant to real needs of our people and the socio-economic conditions obtaining in the country. The hospital-based disease, and cure-oriented approach towards the establishment of medical services has provided benefits to the upper crusts of society, specially those residing in the urban areas. The proliferation of this approach has been at the cost of providing comprehensive primary health care services to the entire population, whether, residing in the urban or the rural areas. Furthermore, the continued high emphasis on the curative approach has led to the neglect of the preventive, promotive public health and rehabilitative aspects of health care. The existing approach, instead of improving awareness and building up self-reliance, has tended to enhance dependency and weaken the community's capacity to cope with its problems. The prevailing policies in regard to the education and training of medical and health personnel's at various levels, has resulted in the development of a cultural gap between the people and the personnel providing care. The various health programmers have, by and large, failed to involve individuals and families in establishing a self-reliant community. Also, over the years, the planning process has become largely oblivious of the fact that the ultimate goal of achieving a satisfactory health status for all our people cannot be secured without involving the community in the identification of their health needs and priorities as well as in the implementation and management of the various health and related programmes.

Need for Evolving a Health Policy—The Revised 20-Point Programme

5.1. India is committed to attaining the goal of "Health For All by the Year 2000 A.D." through the universal provision of comprehensive primary health care services. The attainment of this goal requires a ·thorough overhaul of the existing approaches to the education and training of medical and health personnel and the reorganisation of the health services infrastructure. Furthermore, considering the large variety of inputs into health, it is necessary to secure the overall national socio-economic development process, specially in the more closely health-related sectors, e.g., drugs and pharmaceuticals, agriculture and food production, rural development, education and social welfare, housing, water supply and sanitation, prevention of food adulteration, maintenance of prescribed standards in the manufacture and sale of drugs and the conservation of the enrolment. In sum, the contours of the National Health Policy have to be evolved within a fully integrated planning framework which seeks to provide universal, comprehensive primary health care services, relevant to the actual needs and priorities of the community at a cost which the people can afford, ensuring that the planning and implementation of the various health programmes is through the organised involvement and participation of the community, adequately utilising the services being rendered by private voluntary organisations active in the health sector.

5.2. It is also necessary to ensure that the pattern of development of the health services infrastructure in the future fully takes into account the revised 20-Point programme. The said Programme attributes very high priority to the promotion of family planning as a people's programme, on a voluntary basis; substantial augmentation and provision of primary health care facilities on a universal basis; control of Leprosy, TB and Blindness; acceleration of welfare programmes for women and children; nutrition programmes for pregnant women, nursing mothers and children, especially in the tribal, hilly and backward areas. The Programme also places high emphasis on the supply of drinking water to all problem villages, improvements in the housing and environment of the weaker sections of society; increased production of essential food items; integrated rural development; spread of universal elementary education; expansion of the public distribution system, etc.

Population Stabilisation

6. Irrespective of the changes, no matter how fundamental that may be, brought about in the overall approach to health care and the restructuring of the health services, not much head way is likely to be achieved in improving the health status of the people unless success is achieved in securing the small family norm, through voluntary efforts, and moving towards the goal of population stabilisation. In view of the vital importance of securing the balanced growth of the population, it is necessary to enunciate, separately, a National Population Policy.

Medical and Health Education

7. It is also necessary to appreciate that the effective delivery of health care services would depend very largely on the nature of education, training and appropriate orientation towards community health of all categories of medical and health personnel and their capacity fo function as an integrated team, each of its members performing given tasks within a co-ordinated action programme. It is, therefore, of crucial importance that the entire basis and approach towards medical and health education, at all levels, is reviewed in terms of national needs and priorities and the curricular programmes restructured to produce personnel of various grades of skill and competence, who are professionally equipped and socially motivated to effectively deal with day-to-day problems, within the existing constraints. Towards this end, it is necessary to formulate, separately, a National Medical and Health Education Policy which:

(i) sets out the changes required to be brought about in the curricular contents and training programme of medical and health personnel, at various levels of functioning;
(ii) takes into account the need for establishing the extremely essential inter-relations between functionaries of various grades;
(iii) provides guidelines for the production of health personnel on the basis of realistically assessed manpower requirements;
(iv) seeks to resolve the existing sharp regional imbalances in their availability; and
(v) ensures that personnel at all levels are socially motivated towards the rendering of community health services.

Need for Providing Primary Health Care with Special Emphasis on the Preventive, Promotive and Rehabilitative Aspects

8. Presently, despite the constraint of resources, there is disproportionate emphasis on the establishment of curative centres—dispensaries, hospitals, institutions for specialist treatment—the large majority of which are located in the urban areas of the country. The vast majority of those seeking medical relief have to travel long distance to the nearest curative centre, seeking relief for ailments which could have been readily and effectively handled community level. Also, for want of a well-

established referral system, those seeking curative care have the tendency to visit various specialist centres, thus, further contributing to congestions, duplication of efforts and consequential waste of resources. To put an end to the existing all-round unsatisfactory situation, it is urgently necessary to restructure the health services within the following broad approach:

1. To provide, within a phased, time-bound programme, a well dispersed network of comprehensive primary health care services, integrally linked within the extension and health education approach which takes into account the fact that a large majority of health functions can be effectively handled and resolved by the people themselves, with the organised support of volunteers, auxiliaries, para medicos and adequately trained multi-purpose workers of various grades of skill and competence, of both sexes. There are a large number of private, voluntary organisations active in the health field, all over the country. Their services and support would require to be utilised and intermixed with the governmental efforts in an integrated manner.
2. To be effective, the establishment of the primary health care approach would involve large scale transfer of knowledge, simple skills and technologies to Health Volunteers, selected by the communalities and enjoying their confidence. The functioning of the front line workers, selected by the community would require to be related to definitive action plans for the translation of medical and health knowledge into practical action, involving the use of simple and inexpensive interventions which can be readily implemented by persons who have undergone short periods of training. The quality of training of these health guides/workers would be of crucial importance to the success of this approach.
3. The success of the decentralised primary health care system would depend vitally on the organised building up of individual self-reliance and effective community participation, on the provision of organised, back-up support of the secondary and tertiary levels of the health care services, providing adequate logistical and technical assistance.
4. The decentralisation of services would require the establishment of a well worked out referral system to provide adequate expertise at the various levels of the organisational set-up nearest to the community, depending upon the actual needs and problems of the area, and thus ensure against the continuation of the existing rush towards the curative centres in the urban areas. The effective establishment of the referral system would also ensure the optimal utilisation of expertise at the higher levels of the hierarchical structure. This approach would not

only lead to the progressive improvement of comprehensive health care services at the primary level but also provide for timely attention being available to those in need of urgent specialist care, whether they live in the rural or the urban areas.

5. To ensure that the approach to health care does not merely constitute a collection of disparate health interventions but consists of an integrated package of services seeking to tackle the entire range of poor health conditions, on a broad front, it is necessary to establish a nation-wide chain of sanitary-*cum*-epidemiological stations. The location and functioning of these stations may be between the primary and secondary levels of the hierarchical structure, depending upon the local situations and other relevant consideration. Each such station would require to have suitably trained staff equipped to identify, plan and provide preventive, promotive and mental health care services. It would be beneficial, depending upon the local situations, to establish such stations at the Primary Health Centres. The district health organisation should have, as an integral part of its set-up, a well organised epidemiological unit to coordinate and superintend the functioning of the field stations. These stations would participate in the integrated action plans to eradicate and control diseases, besides tackling specific local environmental health problems. In the urban agglomerations, the municipal and local authorities should be equipped to perform similar functions, being supported with adequate resources and expertise, to effectively deal with local preventable public health problems. The aforesaid approach should be implemented and extended through community participation and contributions, in whatever form possible, to achieve meaningful results within a time-bound programme.

6. The location of curative centres should be related to the populations they serve, keeping in view the densities of population, distances, topography, transport connections. These centres should function within the recommended referral system, the gamut of general specialities required to deal with the local disease patterns being provided as near to the community as possible, at the secondary level of the hierarchical organisation The concept of domiciliary care and the field-camps approach should be utilised to the fullest extent, to reduce the pressures on these centres, specially in efforts relating to the control and eradication of blindness, tuberculosis, leprosy, etc. To maximise the utilisation of available resources, new and additional curative centres should be established only in exceptional cases, the basic attempt being towards the upgradation of existing facilities, at selected locations, the guiding principle being to provide specialist services as near to

the beneficiaries as may be possible, within a well-planned network. Expenditure should be reduced through the fullest possible use of cheap locally available building materials, resort to appropriate architectural designs and engineering concepts and by economical investment in the purchase of machineries and equipment, ensuring against avoidable duplication of such acquisitions. It is also necessary to devise effective mechanisms for the repair, maintenance and proper upkeep of all bio-medical equipments to secure their maximum utilisation.

7. With a view to reducing governmental expenditure and fully utilising untapped resources, planned programmes may b devised, related to the local requirements and potentials, to encourage the establishment of practice by professional, increased investment by non-governmental agencies in establishing curative centres and by offering organised logistical, financial and technical support to voluntary agencies active in the health field.
8. While the major focus of attention in restructuring the existing governmental health organisations would relate to establishing comprehensive primary health care and public health services, within an integrated referral system, planned attention would also require to be devoted to the establishment of centres equipped to provide speciality and super-speciality services, through a well-dispersed network of centres, to ensure that the present and future requirements of specialist treatment are adequately available within the country. To reduce governmental expenditures involved in the establishment of such centres, planned efforts should be made to encourage private investments in such fields so that the majority of such centres, within the governmental set-up, can provide adequate care and treatment to those entitled to free care, the affluent sectors being looked after by the paying clinics. Care would also require to be taken to ensure the appropriate dispersal of such centres, to remove the existing regional imbalances and to provide services within the reach of all, whether residing in the rural or the urban areas.
9. Special, well-co-ordinated programmes should be launched to provide mental health care as well as medical care and the physical and social rehabilitation of those who are mentally retarded; deaf, dumb, blind, physically disabled, infirm and the aged. Also, suitably organised programme would require to be launched to ensure against the prevention of various disabilities.
10. In the establishment of the re-organised services, the first priority should be accorded to provide services to those residing in the tribal, hilly and backward areas as well as to endemic

disease affected populations and the vulnerable sections of the society.

11. In the re-organised health service scheme, efforts should be made to ensure adequate mobility of personnel, at all levels of functioning.

12. In the various approaches, set out in (1) to (11) above, organised efforts would require to be made to fully utilise and assist in the enlargement of the services being provided by private voluntary organisations active in the health field. In this context, planning encouragement and support would also require to be afforded to fresh voluntary efforts, specially those which seek to serve the needs of the rural areas and the urban slums.

Re-orientation of the Existing Health Personnel

9. A dynamic process of change and innovation is required to be brought about in the entire approach to health manpower development, ensuring the emergence of fully integrated bands of workers functioning within the "Health Team" approach.

Private Practice by Governmental Functionaries

10. It is desirable for the States to take steps to phase out the system of private practice by medical personnel in government service, providing at the same time for payment of appropriate compensatory non-practising allowance. The States would require to carefully review the existing situation, with special reference to the availability and dispersal of private practitioners and take timely decisions in regard to this vital issue.

Practitioners of Indigenous and other Systems of Medicine and their Role in Health Care

11. The country has a large stock of health manpower comprising of private practitioners in various systems, for example, Ayurveda, Unani, Siddha, Homoeopathy, Yoga, Naturopathy, etc. This resource has not so far been adequately utilised. The practitioners of these various systems enjoy high local acceptance and respect and consequently exert considerable influence on health beliefs and practices. It is, therefore, necessary to initiate organised measures to enable each of these various systems of medicine and health care to develop in accordance with its genius. Simultaneously, planned efforts should be made to dovetail the functioning of the practitioners of these various systems and integrate their services at the appropriate levels, within specified areas of responsibility and functioning, in the overall health care delivery system, specially in regard to the preventive, promotive and public health objectives. Well considered steps would also require to be launched to move towards a meaningful phased integration of the indigenous and the modern systems.

Problems Requiring Urgent Attention

12. Besides, the recommended restructuring of the health services infrastructure, re-orientation of the medical and health manpower, community involvement and exploitation of the services of private medical practitioners, specially those of the traditional and other system, involvement and utilization of the services of the voluntary agencies active in the health field, etc., it would be necessary to devote planned, time-bound attention to some of the more important inputs required for improved health care. Of these, priority attention would require to be devoted to:

(i) Nutrition

National and regional strategies should be evolved and implemented on a time-bound basis, to ensure adequate nutrition for all segments of the population through a well-developed distribution system, specially in the rural areas and urban slums. Food of acceptable quality must be available to every person in accordance with his physical needs. Low cost, processed and ready-to-eat foods should be produced and made readily available. The overall strategy would necessarily involve organised efforts at improving the purchasing power of the poorer sections of the society. Schemes like employment guarantee scheme, to which the government is committed could yield optimal results if these are suitably linked to the objective of providing adequate nutrition and health cover to the rural and the urban poor. The achievement of this objective is dependent on integrated socio-economic development leading to the generation of productive employment for all those constituting the labour force. Employment guarantee scheme and similar efforts would required to be specially enforced to provide social security for indentified vulnerable sections of the society. Measures aimed at improving eating habits, inculcation of desirable nutritional practices, improved and scientific utilisation of available food materials and effective popularisation of improved cooking practices would require to be implemented. Besides, a nationwide programme to promote breast-feeding of infants and eradication of various social taboos detrimental to the promotion of health would need to be initiated. Simultaneously, the problems of communities afflicted by chronic nutritional disorders should be tackled through special schemes including the organisation of supplementary feeding programmes directed to the vulnerable section of the population. The force and effect of such programmes should be ensured by delivering them within the setting of fully integrated health care activities, to ensure the inculcation of the educational aspects, in the overall strategy.

(ii) Prevention of Food Adulteration and Maintenance of the Quality of Drugs

Stringent measures are required to be taken to check and prevent the adulteration and contamination of foods at the various stages of their production, processing, storage, transport, distribution, etc. To ensure uniformity of approach, the existing laws would require to be reviewed and effective legislation enacted by the Centre. Similarly, the most urgent measures require to be taken to ensure against the manufacture and sale of spurious and substandard drugs.

(iii) Water Supply and Sanitation

The provision of safe drinking water and the sanitary disposal of waters, human and animal wastes, both in urban and rural areas, must constitute an integrated package. The enormous backlog in the provision of these services to the rural population and in the urban agglomerations must be made up on the most urgent basis. The provision of water supply and basic sanitation facilities would not automatically improve health. The availability of such facilities should be accompanied by intensive health education campaigns for the improvement of personal hygiene, the economical use of water and the sanitary disposal of waste in a manner that will improve individual and community health. All water-supply schemes must be fully integrated with efforts at proper water management, including the drainage and disposal of waste waters. To reduce expenditure and for achieving a quick headway it would be necessary to devise appropriate technologies in the planning and management of the delivery systems. Besides, the involvement of the community in the implementation and management of the systems would be of crucial importance, both for reducing costs as well as to see that the beneficiaries value and protect the services provided to them.

(iv) Environmental Protection

While preventive, promotive, public health services are established and the curative services re-organised to prevent, control and treat diseases, it would be equally necessary to ensure against the haphazard exploitation of resources which cause ecological disturbances leading to fresh health hazards. It is, therefore, necessary that economic development plans, in the various sectors, are devised in adequate consultation with the Central and the State health authorities. It is also vitally essential to ensure that the present and future industrial and urban development plans are centrally reviewed to ensure against congestions, the unchecked release of noxious emissions and the pollution of air and water. In this context, it is vital to ensure that the sitting and location of all manufacturing units is strictly regulated, through legal measures, if necessary. Central and State health authorities must necessarily be consulted in establishing locational development and urbanisation programmes. Environmental appraisal procedures must be developed and strictly applied in according clearance to the various developmental projects.

(v) Immunisation Programme

It is necessary to launch an organised, nation-wide immunisation programme, aimed at cent per cent coverage of targeted population groups with vaccines against preventable and communicable diseases. Such an approach would not only prevent and reduce disease and disability but also bring down the existing high infant and child mortality rate.

(vi) Maternal and Child Health Services

A vicious relationship exists between high birth rates and high infant mortality, contributing to the desire for more children. The highest priority would, therefore, require to be devoted to efforts at launching special programmes for the improvement of maternal and child health, with a special focus on the less-privileged sections of society. Such programmes would require to be decentralised to the maximum possible extent, their delivery being at the primary level, nearest to the doorsteps of the beneficiaries. While efforts should continue at providing refresher training and orientation to the traditional birth attendants, schemes and programmes should be launched to ensure that progressively all deliveries are conducted by competently trained persons so that complicated cases receive timely and expert attention, within a comprehensive programme providing ante-natal intra-natal and post-natal care.

(vii) School Health Programme

Organised school health services, integrally linked with the general, preventive and curative services would require to be established within a time-limited programme.

(viii) Occupational Health Services

There is urgent need for launching well-considered schemes to prevent and treat diseases and injuries arising from occupational hazards, not only in the various industries but also in the comparatively un-organised sectors like agriculture. For this purpose, the coverage of the Employees State Insurance Act, 1948, may be suitably extended ensuring adequate co-ordination of efforts with the general health services. In their respective spheres of responsibility, the Centre and the States must introduce organised occupational health services to reduce morbidity, disabilities and mortality and thus promote better health and increased welfare and productivity on all fronts.

Health Education

13. The recommended efforts, on various fronts, would bear only marginal results unless nation-wide health education programmes, backed by appropriate communication strategies are launched to provide health information in easily understandable form, to motivate the development of an attitude for healthy living. The public health education programmes should be supplemented by health, nutrition and population education programmes in all educational institutions, at various levels. Simultaneously, efforts would require to be made to promote universal education, specially adult and family education, without which the various efforts to organise preventive and promotive health activities, family planning and improved maternal and child health cannot bear fruit.

Management Information System

14. Appropriate decision-making and programme planning in the health and related fields is not possible without establishing an effective health information system. A nation-wide organisational set-up should be established to procure essential health information. Such information is required not only for assisting in planning and decision-making but, also to provide timely warnings about emerging health problems and for reviewing, monitoring and evaluating the various on-going health programmes. The building-up of a well-conceived health information system is also necessary for assessing medical and health manpower requirements and taking timely decision, on a continuing basis regarding the manpower requirements in the future.

Medical Industry

15. The country has built up sound technological and manufacturing capability in the field of drugs, vaccines, bio-medical equipment, etc. The available know-how requires to be adequately exploited to increase the production of essential and life saving drugs and vaccines of proven quality to fully meet the national requirements, specially in regard to the national programmes to combat Malaria, TB, Leprosy, Blindness, Diarrhoeal diseases, etc. The production of the essential, life-saving drugs under their generic names and the adoption of economical packaging practices would considerably reduce the unit cost of medicines bringing them within the poorer sections of society, besides significantly reducing the expenditure being incurred by the governmental organisation on the purchase of drugs. In view of the low cost of indigenous and herbal medicines, organised efforts may be launched to establish herbal gardens, producing drugs of certified quality and making them easily available.

15.1 The practitioners of the modern medical system rely heavily on diagnostic aids involving extensive use of costly, sophisticated bio-medical equipment. Effective mechanisms should be established to identify essential equipment required for extensive use and to promote and enlarge their indigenous manufacture, for such devices being readily available, at reasonable prices, for use at the health care centres.

Health Insurance

16. Besides mobilising the community resources, through its active participation in the implementation and management of national health and related programmes, it would be necessary to devise well-considered health insurance schemes, on a State-wise basis, for mobilising additional resources for health promotion and ensuring that the community shares the cost of the services, in keeping with paying capacity.

Health Legislation

17. It is necessary to urgently review all existing legislation and work towards a unified, comprehensive legislation in the health field, enforceable all over the country.

Medical Research

18. The frontiers of the medical sciences are expanding at a phenomenal pace. To maintain the country's lead in this field as well as to ensure self-sufficiency and generation of the requisite competence in the future, it is necessary to have an organised programme for the building up and extension of fundamental and basic research in the field of bio-medical and allied sciences. Priority attention would require to be devoted to the resolution of problems relating to the containment and eradication of the existing, widely prevalent diseases as well as to deal with emerging health problems. The basic objective of medical research and the ultimate test of its utility would involve the translation of available know-how into simple, low-cost, easily applicable appropriate technologies, devices and interventions suiting local conditions, thus placing the latest technological achievements, within the reach of health personnel, and to the front line health workers, in the remotest corners of the country. Therefore, besides devotion to basic, fundamental research, high priority should be accorded to applied, operational research including action research for continuously improving the cost effective delivery of health services. Priorities would require to be identified and laid down in collaboration with social scientists, planners and decision-makers and the public. Basic research efforts should devote high priority to the discovery and development of more effective treatment and preventive procedures in regard to communicable and tropical diseases—lindness, Leprosy, TB, etc. Very high priority would also have to be devoted to contraception research to urgently improve the effectiveness and acceptability of existing methods as well as to discover more effective and acceptable devices. Equally high attention would require to be devoted to nutrition research, to improve the health status of the community. The overall effort should aim at the balanced development of basic, clinical and problem-oriented operational research

Inter-sectoral Co-operation

19. All health and human development must ultimately constitute an integral component of the overall socio-economic developmental process in the country. It is thus of vital importance to ensure effective co-ordination between the health and its more intimately related sectors. It is, therefore, necessary to set-up standing mechanisms, at the Centre and in the States, for securing inter-sectoral co-ordination of the various efforts in the fields of health and family planning, medical education and research, drugs and pharmaceuticals, agriculture and food, water supply and drainage, housing, education and social welfare and rural development. The co-ordination and review committees, to be set-up, should review progress, resolve bottlenecks and bring about such shifts in the contents and priorities of programmes as may appear necessary, to achieve the overall objectives. At the community level, it would be desirable to devise arrangements for health and all other developmental activities being co-ordinated under an integrated programme of rural development.

Monitoring and Review of Progress

20. It would be of crucial importance to monitor and periodically review the success of the efforts made and the results achieved. For this purpose, it is necessary to urgently identify the base line situation and to evolve a phased programme for the achievement of short and long-term objectives in the various sectors of activity. Towards this end, the current level of achievement as well as the broad indicators for the achievement of certain basic health and family welfare goals are set out in the annexed tabular statement. These goals, as well as other allied objectives, would require to be further worked upon and specific targets for achievement established by the Central and the State Governments in regard to the various areas of functioning.

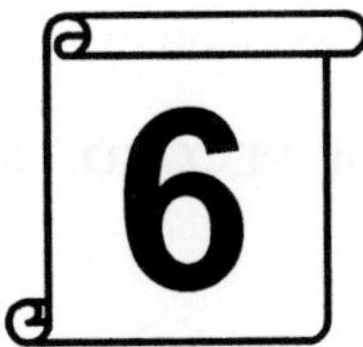

Record Management

RECORDS MANAGEMENT IN A HOSPITAL

Records Management is a programme that involves the functions of creating, administering, retaining, submitting and destroying records. Herbert Hoover has rightly mentioned the advantages of proper records keeping when he says: "A business decision is only as good as the facts on which it is based." Records are the memory of the internal and external transactions of an organisation. By external transaction we mean the correspondence between the organisation and its clients beneficiaries as well as supporters. By internal transaction is meant the dealings on external transactions by persons in the organisations at all levels. Records contain a written evidence of the activities of an organisation in the form of letters, circulars, reports, contracts, invoices, vouchers, minutes of meeting, books of accounts, etc. Thus, the records management is concerned with the retaining, submitting and destroying of records. The proper maintenance of these records in right quantity and quality is the essence of records management. The success of this record keeping would be reflected in the timely availability of all the records. In the context of Medical Records, Dr. McGibony had said, "A chronicle of the pageantry of medical and scientific progress is found in the hospital records. There may be found the running story, disconnected it is true, of the drama, the comedy, the mystery, the miracles of medicines and hospital of the Twentieth Century."

The medical record is a clinical, scientific, administrative and legal document relating to patient care in which is recorded sufficient data, written in sequence of events to justify the diagnosis and warrant the treatment and end results. With the advert of frequent litigations increasing super-specializations, numerous investigations based on technology and patients data swelling by the day, the process of record management is becoming complicated and challenging. A patient history and his data of clinical examination and various tests has to be compiled precisely and stored with care. This has to be available by flick of a finger, within a few hours, to all those who are allowed to access the same.

With the advent of RTI, such a data has to be concise, comprehensive and reproducible. For the data to be clinically useful and legally supportive Management of records assumes a great significance.

ESSENTIALS OF RECORDS MANAGEMENT

I. Comprehensive

The records should be such as can be easily understood when retrieved back for planning, policy-making and decision-making. The language used should be simple and understandable.

2. Properly Planned

The records be screened at regular intervals of time to weed out the information not required for future. In this way, we can reduce the paper work to twenty-five per cent. This would indirectly help us in locating the desired information quickly.

3. Economical

We should manage the records economically so that we may achieve more with minimum efforts.

4. Accurate

The records should be accurate otherwise its utility would be doubtful.

5. Timely

The time taken in reprieving the information should be as short as possible. Reducing retrieval time is essential for effective materials management.

6. Classification

Records must be classified to be of practical use. The classification be done either on the basis of subjects or chronology.

According to Dr. K. Pennathur, Records should:

- Serve specific needs.
- Have specific objectives and purposes.
- Be kept to a minimum with respects to number, scope and content.
- Be designed for least expensive handling.
- Be up-to-date.
- Be worth their cost.
- Be related directly to tabulations and reports that will stem from them.

- Be available when needed.
- Be considered valuable by supervisors and lines management.

CONTENTS OF MEDICAL RECORDS

The medical record is a clear, concise and accurate history of the patients' life and illness, written from the health and medical point of view. The story of the patients illness narrated by the patient, observations made by nurses and the comments and treatment given by the doctors are recorded in the medical record. Thus, the medical record comprises three general sections:

(i) a general section covering administrative and personal data. The socio-economic record of the patient includes. The Name of the Patient, Father's or Husband's Name, Age, Sex, Religion, Income, Patient's Address and the Address of nearest relative. Other administrative information's which are included are—The data of admission, The inpatient number, The name of the nursing unit and bed number. This sheet is prepared in the Central Admitting Office;

(ii) a nurses section wherein are noted the observations of the trained nurses and the detail of treatment administered. This part of the medical record consists of graphic charts relating to Temperature, Pulse, Respiration, Blood Pressure and any other observations maintained, intake output chart and medicine administered; and

(iii) a medical section containing statements on the studies, observations, conclusions and activities of the attending doctors or of the intern or the resident working under him. The medical section of the record consists of the entire medical history of the patient. It contains:

History sheet
Physical examination sheet, Provisional diagnosis
All the investigation reports
Physicians orders sheet
Treatment, medical or surgical
Anaesthesia record
Operation record
Obstetric record
Consultancy report
Progress report
Final diagnosis
Discharge summary
If death—Cause of death, Autopsy report.

CLASSIFICATION

The classification of records would depend upon the nature of organisation. However, it would be useful to classify records into the following four-fold classifications:

(a) Vital Records	Protected and preserved for a long time.
(b) Important Records	Not currently in use but are of high value of retain.
(c) Useful Records	Currently used correspondence.
(d) Transit Record	Useful for only a short period till the subject is alive or active

MECHANISM OF RECORDS MANAGEMENT

There are two basic instruments through which we create and maintain records, i.e., form and files. Let us discuss in brief about these two mechanisms.

Filing

Filing is the process of classifying, arranging and storing records systematically so that these can be easily retrieved. Neuner and Haynes defined filling as 'the systematic arrangement for keeping of business correspondence and records so that these may be found and delivered quickly when needed for reference in future.' George R. Terry defines, "Filing is the placing of documents and papers in acceptable containers according to some pre-determined arrangement so that any of these when required, may be located quickly and conveniently."

Filing Arrangements

- Alphabetical order
- Numerical order
- Geographic order
- Chronological order
- Subject-wise

Many variations and innovations in these five general systems of filing have been developed, e.g., the use of colours, sound and special visual devices.

In the offices of the Government of India and State Governments, filing system is based on subject system. This system has many defects—lack of uniformity, lack of clear-cut demarcation and time-consuming tracing process.

The question of filing system was examined by the Administrative Reforms Commission and they recommended the functional filing system. The proposed system can be elaborated as follows:

(a) The main subjects under the functions, say establishment, common office services, budget, are first listed under functional group headings which are respectively identified by capital letters, 'A', 'B', etc.
(b) Each main subject or main head under each functional group is assigned consecutive Arabic numerals beginning with 'I' which may go upto '99'.
(c) Similarly, the sub-subjects or sub-heads under each main head are assigned consecutive, Arabic numerals beginning with 'II' which also could go upto '99'.
(d) The identifying subject numerals and sub-subject numerals are separated by '0' the group of numerals to the left of '0' refer the main head while that to the right to its sub-head, topic or aspect.
(e) Files opened under the same subject, etc. are given serial numbers 1, 2 and 3 and so on and separated from the groups of numerals by an oblique.
(f) The year in which the file is opened is shown separately from the file number by an oblique.
(g) At the end of each file code number is to be indicated with the abbreviated form of a section or a unit.

File Indexing

File Indexing is a key to locate the files. Index is a reference list used for locating a particular document in the filing equipment. The following types of indexing may be used for locating:

Vertical card indexing
Visible card indexing
Visible book indexing
Loose leaf book indexing

Centralized and Decentralized Filing System

Centralized filing system is one, where all the filing equipments and personnel are located in a single area of the office, accessible to all departments by messengers, controlled by a centralized plan or index of the filing. Decentralized filing system also called departmentalised filing system is one, where each organization makes its own arrangement for filing.

Advantages

Advantages of centralized filing are:

1. It ensures uniformity and standardisation of the filing equipment and procedure which can help in easy and quick location of records.

2. It eliminates the need of duplication and distribution to all concerned sections. It encourages completeness of related documents.
3. It enhances economy of time for both file users and file personnel because there is only one place to send material to be filed, and one place to find it.
4. Control is exercised more effectively since one person or group alone is responsible, which minimises oversights and loss of valuable records.
5. It promotes economy of filing equipment and floor space.

To be most effective a compromise has to be struck between centralized and decentralized filing systems. Decentralized filing should be kept to a minimum.

ADVANTAGES OF RECORDS KEEPING

The records help the management in the following ways:

1. Help in Sound Decision-making

Effective decision-making depends to a great extent upon the adequate information provided by the records and availability of these records in time.

2. Effective Channel of Internal Control

Records are very important to ensure internal control. Records can help in minimising chance of error and prevent occurrence of fraud and corruption.

3. Facilitate Evaluation of Corporate Performance

The records can help in evaluating the performance of an organisation during definite intervals of time and different periods. Besides, records can help in comparing the performance of organisation in the same line.

4. Promotes Efficiency of Operations

The effective operations of an organisation depend to a great extent upon the speed and accuracy of the records. Records keep the wheels of the organisation moving fast.

5. Fulfils Statutory Requirement

Records are also kept in compliance with the provisions of different statutes, e.g., maintenance of statutory books under Indian Companies Act, 1956. Besides, records are needed in the event of litigations, disputes or claims.

6. Futuristic Approach

Analysis of records help in ascertaining future trends which can help in better policy-making and planning.

The fundamental reason for promoting maintenance of an adequate medical record is its utility to good patient care, to the doctor, to the hospital and towards medical education and research. Besides, the legal requirements of the hospital, medical records are also to be completed.

USE OF HOSPITAL STATISTICS FOR MANAGEMENT

The Medical Records Department in a hospital is mainly responsible for the collection as well as analysis of the date to ensure utilisation of the hospital for patient care. Such date has immense value for the day-to-day management of the hospitals as well as future planning of the hospital services. Let us some mention of the important information which is used by the hospital management to enhance the hospital functioning.

I. Death Rates

Hospital deaths include deaths of patients admitted to the hospital Deaths are generally classified into two categories, i.e., the Gross Deaths and the Net Deaths. Gross Deaths include all the deaths of admitted patients while Net Deaths exclude the patients dying within 48 hours of admission. Net Deaths in a hospital is a reflection of the working of the hospital. Net deaths rate is calculated as follows:

$$\frac{\text{Number of net deaths during a period of time}}{\text{Number of total discharges during that period of time}} \times 100$$

In an average net death rates range between 4 to 6 per cent. Any gross variations from the normally expected net death rate indicates an abnormal phenomenon which should be analysed by the hospital management. Such deviation can either be due to natural causes or due to failure on the part of one of the service areas of the hospital. In the case of later event correctives need be applied and death rate brought back to the normal expected range.

The use of net death rates for enhancing the efficiency of the hospital services is not only limited to the overall net death rate of the hospital but also can be splitted up into death rates of various departments and units of the hospital. As such, the hospital management can keep a track of the performance of each and every unit/department of the hospital by keeping a track of their net-death rates. This is being practised in most of the teaching hospitals but not in district hospitals.

2. Average Length of Stay

The length of stay of patients is another important hospital indices. For purposes of calculations, the day of admission of the patient is always taken into consideration and the date/day of discharge is always ignored irrespective of the time of admission or the time of discharge. Through the process of discharge analysis, the average length of stay of patients discharged during a particular period of time is worked out not only for the whole hospital but also department-wise/unit-wise. The aim of this information is to locate the unnecessary length of stay and to discourage it. By reducing the unnecessary length of stay more patients can be admitted to the hospital and provided services. This information, therefore, is not only important from the economic point of view but is also important from the community services point of view, average length of stay is calculated as follows:

Total length of stay of discharged patients during a period of time x 100 Total discharges during that period of time.

3. Bed Turnover Rate

Bed Turnover Rate indicates the number of patients who have been

$$\frac{\text{Total number of discharges during a year}}{\text{Total number of authorised beds}} \times 100$$

given services per bed per year. It is calculated as follows:

Bed Turnover Rate is determined by the Average Length of Stay as well as the time interval between one discharge and successive admissions. This time interval is known as T-interval. Also, Bed Turnover Rate as well as T-interval are important indicators of the planning utilisation of hospital resources.

4. Bed Occupancy Rate

Bed Occupancy Rate gives the relationship between the availability of facilities and their utilisation. Optimum bed occupancy is treated to be between 85-90 per cent. An occupancy of over 90 per cent means stress is on one or another area of the hospital. When the bed occupancy rate is 100 or more than 100 per cent, it is a case of dilution of hospital facilities and lowering of efficiency. Bed Occupancy Rate can be worked out for the whole hospital as well as for each discipline/unit of the hospital, as under:

$$\frac{\text{Average daily census during a period of time}}{\text{Number of authorized beds}} \times 100 \text{ Bed Occupancy Rate}$$

ISSUES AND PROBLEMS OF RECORDS MANAGEMENT IN HOSPITAL

Based upon observation, discussion and analysis we give here the main problems faced by hospitaı authorities in Records Management and suggest probable solution:

(a) Use of Out-dated Forms

Need of Constant Revision: At present, forms being used in most of the hospitals are not in tune with the improvements in new technology and scientific developments. Some of the columns in the forms are obsolete while many important columns are not available. It is thus essential that forms must be revised constantly to keep them up-to-date. The ultimate purpose of tabulating the date from forms becomes insignificant as the forms do not convey the desired information. It must be statutory for every organisation to get their forms reviewed after every three years either by the internal O & M cells or central O & M organisation.

(b) Shortage of Experienced Personnel

Need of Trained Personnel: The hospital authorities do not attach as much weightage to records management as is done to other sources. This gives less emphasis in terms of resources to this activity. There is generally shortage of trained personnel to handle records. It is suggested that adequate experienced personnel may be appointed to take care of records management.

(c) Lack of Planning of Storage of Inactive Records

Need of Effective Storage and Control of Inactive Records: Storage should be done at a proper place where proper conditions of temperature, circulation of air and humidity are provided. Mostly, we find dirt and dust in this area. After storing the records, indexing is necessary to locate the record for retrieval.

We can reduce congestion and cost through the control of inactive records. This would indirectly help us in finding the relevant record immediately. The Secretariat Training School in its report on Work Study (III) suggested the following improvements to make effective control of the inactive records:

(a) Keep a table of the important contents of a file on the cover or a slip. This will facilitate location of contents which the title of the file or its number may not help to locate speedily.

(b) Keep documents like records, separately from the files. This will reduce the bulk of the files and assist speedier location and use of documents not related to correspondence and notes.

(c) Papers containing information may be carried in a third folder separately from notes and correspondence.

(d) Persons dealing with 'information' should compile the vital elements of information and keep it at hand in cabinets for ready reference. Simple 'Home made' devices can be invented to carry such information and reduce dependence on records.

(e) Keep a small alphabetical register of important files, cases, reports and other documents in your personal custody for more purposeful follow up, records location and speedier disposal.

(d) Need of Effective Handling and Processing of Records

Handling and processing of records should be simple and should not consume much time and personnel resources. The expert handling and processing of records would depend upon the design of registry and its place in the office layout, rational and well laid out procedures and the training of the personnel responsible for job.

Evaluation of Records Handling

There is a need to check the records frequently. A random checking can be done with the help of the following two ratios:

$$1.\ \text{Accuracy Ratio} = \frac{\text{Average daily census during a period of time}}{\text{Number of authorized beds}}$$

$$2.\ \text{Accuracy Ratio} = \frac{\text{No. of references not found}}{\text{No. of references found}}$$

If the accuracy ratio is half or one per cent, it is thought to be excellent. If it is three or more per cent, it is in a poor state.

If the activity ratio is below ten per cent, it exhibits that there is too much inactive material. If it is between ten to twenty per cent, it means that there is a need of improvement while it is more than twenty per cent, it shows that the records are in bad shape. Such evaluations can help in improving the records.

(e) Need of Determination of Records Retention Period

There is no hard and fast rule that specific record should be retained for specific period of time. The decision regarding the retention period should be decided by the organisation basing on its needs, requirements and objectives. The records which help in tracing the history of the organisation and help in policy-making should be kept for long. The unwanted records should be destroyed to save time and resources.

Transfer of Records

Transfer of records entail two stages, i.e. (i) Dating of unimportant records for destruction and ultimate disposal, (ii) moving the records from active to inactive files and from there to storage area. In a complex organisation we can make use of micro-films. Micro-films can help in space saving, safe preservation and clean and easy handling. Besides, these reduce the risk of fire hazards and chances of loosing document.

(f) Need of Improving Quality of Medical Records

Quantitatively the system of medical records is fairly satisfactory, but qualitatively the medical records need lot of improvements. It is recommended that more efforts should be made by the hospital management, all clinicians as well as medical records officer towards improving the quality of medical records.

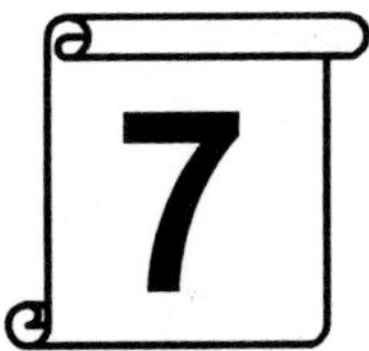

Material Management

With Special Reference to Equipment and Drugs

A. MATERIALS MANAGEMENT

Men, Money and Material are the keys to good management and everywhere, including a hospital development. We generally find that the Chief Executives do not pay the desired attention to the materials management resulting in inefficiency. There are eight primary and seven secondary objectives which can ensure the best performance and use of materials in a hospital. (See Chart 7.1)

Many of these objectives conflict with each other. Balancing of these various conflicting objectives is one of the main tasks before the materials manager. The better this balance is done, the better the efficiency of the materials management.

To quote the Report of the Bureau of Public Enterprises (1984-85), "materials management is one of the key factors for improving performance of any unit. Higher inventories saddle an organisation with avoidable costs besides blocking scarce funds which might be required by the enterprise for its own operations or for some other essential development programmes. Proper Management of materials, therefore, assumes considerable importance in corporate functioning as well as in national economy."

It is not uncommon to find (in a public hospital) that several rooms are full of junk items, equipment or expired/unused drugs. There have been instances when an equipment imported at a cost of crores of rupees is consigned to a junk room for years, either for want of a minor part, screw, trained operator or suitable premises. This may be in the same state for years together and finally becomes useless. Some equipments that are used daily may not be protected from dust, fungus or provided minor repair at the earliest and hence declared out of order. Declaring them out of order

CHART 7.1

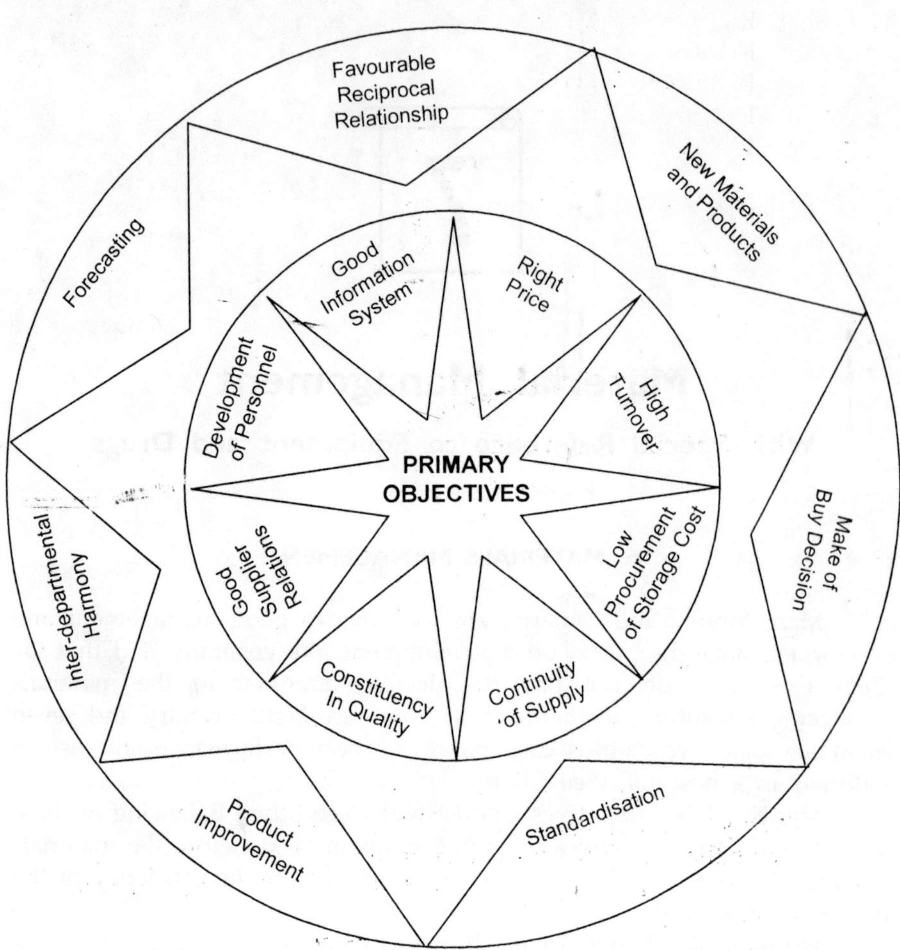

may be deliberate and motivated for extraneous considerations. Similarly, the poor patients may be demised even those medicines, which are available in the stores due to apathy, poor management or selfish designs. It goes without saying that proper management of all the materials viz. liven, instruments, drugs, injectable, sophisticated machines are essential in a hospital for its efficient working.

Essential Principles

Broadly, we can say that there are seven principles of materials management which must be kept in mind to ensure good results. Managers must follow these principles or rights. We can decide about these rights by using the Management Techniques mentioned on next page.

(a) Right item,
(b) Right quantity,
(c) Right price,
(d) Right source,
(e) Right delivery,
(f) Right methods, and
(g) Right people.

Materials can essentially be categorised under three heads, viz., vital essential and desirable. These three categories must determine how much quantity of each item should be in stock for a store-keeper.

Various techniques are available to decide on the right items, quantity, price, source, delivery, methods and people. The techniques are as follows:

	Technique	
(1)	Value Analysis Standardisation Codification	Items
(2)	Purchasing Balancing of Inventories EOQ (How much to buy and when to buy)	(Quantity)
(3)	Cost Price Value Analysis	(Price)
(4)	Market research Purchasing techniques Selection	(Source)
(5)	Procurement technique Follow up PERT/OR	(Delivery)
(6)	Work study System Analysis ABC Analysis Management Information Systems	(Methods)
(7)	Lack of integrity Organizational Analysis Behavioural Sciences	(People)

Essentials

Materials management ensure the fulfilment of the following objectives:

(a) To develop a system of supplies whereby there will be right quantity of stock of Items properly stored, easily retrievable and distributed close to the points of usage, whenever required, at a given time. In case, there is not enough stock, the work in the organisation may have to be stopped and the men and machines will remain idle. On the other hand, if there is overstocking of raw materials, it will unnecessary block capital in inventories.

(b) The reduction in inventory costs-both carrying costs and ordering costs.

(c) To ensure that the resources available are used most effectively and the stores are purchased at the most economical price consistent with the quality.

(d) To bring about co-ordination among the various sections in the organisation, i.e., in a company to bring co-ordination among the financial manager, production manager and marketing manager.

(e) To ensure that the production does not suffer.

(f) To ensure that the sale of finished goods is not effected.

(g) To avoid wide fluctuations in production.

Procedure

To achieve these objectives, the procedures can be enumerated as a cycle, and in sequence of events, as follows:

(a) To determine the categories of stock required in terms of the quantity and quality of each item.

(b) To procure the items necessary from the best, reliable and authentic sources either within or outside the country at most economical prices.

(c) To ensure timely supply from these sources.

(d) To ensure good storage of effective delivery.

(e) To develop an effective control mechanism through good records keeping.

(f) Effective distribution at the points of usage.

(g) To ensure plugging of loopholes of the leakage.

(h) Employment of trained personnel to handle materials management.

(i) Enforcement of performance rather than legal audit.

Principles of Inventory Management

Management has to decide about the following two issues:

(a) Determination of Order Quantity

At the time of placing an order, what quantity should be purchased? That is, what is the most economical quantity to order?

(b) Determination of Re-order Point of Record Level

At what time order should be placed in relation to existing inventory levels?

B. DRUGS MANAGEMENT

Drugs are very important in a hospital and, therefore, these must be used with due care, skill, knowledge and need. The drugs can be dangerous if not administered properly. Wasting of drugs also results in wastage of scarce resources of the hospital. A World Health Publication has rightly summed up the purpose of Drug Management from different angles which are mentioned below.

The purpose of management of drugs is to use drugs wisely and avoid wasting drugs, and therefore to have enough for patient's needs.

Common Causes of Wasting Drugs and Money

- Using too many different drugs on one patient.
- Using expensive, brand-named drugs when cheap or standard drugs are equally effective.
- Using drugs without a proper diagnosis, "just to try it."
- Using a larger dose than necessary.
- Giving drugs to patients who do not believe in them and who throw them away, or who forget to take them.
- Ordering more drugs than are needed, so that some drugs become "expired" on the shelf.
- Not caring for the refrigerator, so that vaccines are no longer effective.
- Exposing drugs to damp, heat or light.
- Giving out (issuing from store) too many drugs at one time so that they are stolen, or used extravagantly.

Educating Staff in the Use of Drugs

Drugs are important, powerful and expensive. For these reasons, all health workers using drugs should be well-informed about them and should develop a mature and responsible attitude towards their use.

A health-worker manager can educate staff about drugs in the following ways:

- Put one or more copies of a simple book on pharmacology in the library.
- Make notes on the common drugs used, explaining their uses and side-effects. Give copies of these notes to all staff.
- Set out the correct doses of common drugs on wall boards.
- Hold staff meetings to discuss causes of drug wastage.
- Inform all staff about the cost of various drugs.
- Make a lecture/discussion programme and discuss one drug each week in the staff meeting.

Educating Patients about Drugs

Very often patients take drugs in a wrong way. They either reduce the dose to make the treatment last longer or increase it hoping for a quicker cure. They use the drugs at wrong times or forget a dose. Patients on long courses of treatment then stop them too soon.

They do his because they do not understand the action of drugs in the body. It is result they are sometimes not cured and the drug is wasted. Health workers should explain very carefully to patients how to take their drugs.

Explaining to Patients the Use of Drugs

They should also explain in a simple way why a drug must be taken in a particular way. Thus, patients could learn that:

- Each drug has a particular action. A drug used for one condition will not help another.
- The size of the dose is very important. If it is too little it acts too weak to cure the condition; if it is too much it may poison the patient. The doses for children are smaller than those for adults.
- Treatment must be regular. This means that the desired level of the drug in the body is maintained.
- The whole course of treatment must be completed. If it is not, the patient may relapse into an even more serious condition than before.
- Drugs must be kept out of reach of small children. They may eat them as sweets and poison themselves.

Special Education

Patients with tuberculosis and leprosy who have to take drugs for many months need a great deal of explanation and encouragement. They must continue to take tablets even when they feel better, in case the disease becomes active again.

Controlling Life-Saving Drugs

Sometimes a patient's condition is so acute, severe or critical that only the immediate use of certain drugs can save his life.

It is of vital importance that such drugs are always in stock. The absence of such drugs is an emergency may result in a patient's death. This is an unnecessary tragedy and a failure of health-service management. Such a tragedy can be avoided by:

- Making a list of vital or life-saving drugs;
- Placing them together on one shelf;
- Checking the shelf frequently or whenever drugs are issued; and
- Ordering a new supply when stocks reach the half-way point (use the A/B or double-shelf system described above).

Pre-packaging Drugs for the Outpatient's Department

This means that a full course of treatment with a certain tablet is put in small envelopes or folded papers, before the clinic or outpatient session. It is ready when the patient needs it. This has a number of advantages:

1. The patient receives the correct and full course of treatment.
2. It saves time and avoids waiting and queuing while tablets are counted.
3. Printed (or duplicated) instructions can be given with the packet or written on the envelope. This tells the patient how and when to take the tablets, and assists his memory. Special signs must be designed for patients who cannot read, e.g., the sun rising on the horizon represents morning.

It is very useful in special clinics where standard treatments are given to every person, e.g., iron and folic acid tablets to pregnant women. It makes it easy to observe and control the issue of drugs.

Besides the Government must streamline the manufacturing of drugs simpler and cheaper through limiting the number of drugs. The World Health Organisation has recommended the manufacture of 295 drugs which can meet the requirements of India while India produces about 60,000 different types of drugs. Mr. S.P. Sharma in his article on Land of Drugs in *The Tribune* dated 24-6-88 has rightly quoted Herbert M. Shelton who says: "It is not illness that is expensive. It is the naive idea that the healing powers of the body require absurd purchasing of "treatment", "reliefs" and other high priced abuses that make suffering a lavish luxury. When man grounds his behaviour in illness on commonsense instead of seeking illusive "cures"—recovery will be far more rapid and without disastrous costs."

C. MANAGING EQUIPMENT

There are five major procedures used in managing equipment, i.e., ordering, storing, issuing and controlling/maintaining and standardisation.

(i) Ordering Equipment

The first important requirement for ordering equipment is to analyse requirements based on past experience and future requirements. This has to be done carefully otherwise this can result into unnecessary purchases and thus leaving less money for important equipment. After this analysis, we may balance the requirements with the resources available so that one can remain within budgetary limits. This process can be facilitated with the help of catalogues which are easily available and this would avoid the chances of forgetting important items. After this, an order or a requisition form is prepared in all details and specifications to avoid later complications.

(ii) Storing Equipment

Equipment must be stored carefully otherwise there is a danger of pilferage or breakage. Equipment can be stored either in a proper store or at the place of use. Inventory of the store must be well maintained and proper accounts must be maintained through stock ledgers. Care must be taken to enter each item in a ledger on a separate page so that the entry for similar new items added or issued can be done on that every page and the stock position can be analysed at a glance.

(iii) Issuing Equipment

Each hospital has many wards, laboratories, etc., where equipment is required. Each ward or unit must be responsible for the equipment issued to them. They should keep liaison with the store to replenish the consumed articles or repairs of some other articles. The person who signs the issue voucher takes responsibility for the care of the apparatus or equipment. Issue vouchers must be filled and a copy kept in the store. It has been mentioned by many stores officers in the hospitals that the various units get the articles issued without requirements and sell these in the markets. There is a need to keep a proper control through surprise checks of the use of these articles.

(iv) Controlling and Maintaining Equipment

This is the most important aspects of equipment management as it has been observed that most of the non-expendable equipment remains out of order for a long time. There have been cases where the machinery remains out of order for years together. Therefore, there is a need to educate the staff in the proper keep-up of the equipment. Besides, there is a need to take immediate action to get the equipment in order if some mechanical defects enter into its working. This is a most serious problem in most of the hospitals. If a list is got prepared of the non-working equipment in health units, it may come to near about 60% which is very serious as it affects the working of these units. It has also been mentioned by some (during Discussion) that the equipment is intentionally made unworkable in connivance with the private practitioners so that the patients can be directed to them for examination.

(v) Codification Nod Standardisation

In any undertaking having a large number of items, codification is essential. It hardly needs any emphasis that codification of items is a pre-requisite for introduction of mechanisation in stock control and purchases and stores accounting. There are two systems which are commonly used for the purpose—Birch System and the Kodak System. The major objectives of the codification are:

1. The classification of items on functional basis to ensure that one item is kept under one code.

2. To bring together the items according to their degree of similarity to reveal excessive variety and the substitutes available.
3. To list item as per National/International standards instead of vendor's numbers wherever possible.
4. To prepare a catalogue indicating the necessary details for procurement action and also which can be used as a reference by the users.

Let us new turn to two important areas of Inventory Management in details, i.e., Economic Order quantity and classification of materials. The dictionary meaning of the word 'inventory' is stock of goods. The classical definition of inventory is that it is an idle resource of any kind having an economic value. It costs money to hold stock. It costs money in terms of storage, space, equipment, personnel, insurance, deterioration, and obsolescence, and above all the cost of capital involved in financing stocks. Inventory management is the procedure and the body of knowledge which can help us in planning to maintain an optimum level of the idle resources. Before this, we may explain briefly some terms which influence Economic Order Quantity.

(1) Ordering Costs (OC)

These are the costs incurred to get the materials into the inventory of an organisation. The costs include the costs on stationery, advertisement, salaries of personnel. If we examine the ordering costs of most of the organisation, we find the major components of ordering cost are salaries. To control the ordering cost, the number of men dealing with purchasing should be kept to the minimum.

(2) Carrying Costs (CO)

All the costs incurred to maintain inventories are termed as Carrying Costs. It is also known as holding costs. The cost is usually expressed as a percentage of the average investment in inventory. The chief components of carrying cost are—cost of capital invested in inventory, cost of storage due to the rents and depreciation changes, salaries to stores personnel, obsolescence, loses due to pilferage and breakages, insurance costs, etc.

(3) Lead Time

It is the period that elapses between placing an order and receiving the same. These can be classified as administrative lead-time, manufacturing lead-time, transporting lead-time and inspection lead time. Any strategy to control lead time must try to control the administrative and inspection lead time. Other, too, can be controlled to a lesser extent.

(4) Buffer Stock

Buffer stock is the quantity of stores set apart as an insurance against the variations in demand and procurement period. This quantity of the item is to be kept as an emergency for unforeseen demands. It is calculated by multiplying the difference between maximum and average consumption rate per day with the lead time for the items.

(5) Reorder Level

This term is used to denote the stock level at which fresh order has to be placed. This is equal to the average consumption per day multiplied by lead time plus buffer stock. By ordering at the time when stock reaches the reorder level we are fairly assured that the chances of 'stock out' are practically nil.

(6) Stock Turnover

Another aspect of inventory control is to see that there is proper turnover of items stocked and to see that the items are used up before the time expiry of the warranty period. Special efforts should be made to issue items on first come first out basis. Expiry date on control sheets to keep a control against keeping out-dated material on the shelf should be maintained. In case, there is no possibility of using the stocks of short life items within the expiry period, efforts should be made to deploy the stock to other institutions so that they could be issued before the expiry time.

Economic Order Equity (E.O.Q.)

The purpose of inventory management is to find the appropriate levels for holding inventories and the ordering sequence and the quantities so that the total cost incurred is minimized. Economic Order Quantity is that quantity at which the cost of ordering the annual requirements of an item and the inventory cost are nearly equal, i.e., when the total of the two costs is lowest. Example: Let us assume that a manufacture will need Rs. 30,000 of a certain raw material in a year. The cost of ordering is Rs. 25 per order and the carrying cost is 20 per cent of the average inventory.

This table clearly indicates that the manufacturer should order 10 times during a year. The ordering quantity is Rs. 3000. Here, carrying cost is Rs. 250 and ordering cost is Rs. 300. The total cost is Rs. 550. We can also determine it mathematically by the formula:

$$Q = \sqrt{2RC_2IUC_1} \text{ or } \sqrt{2RC_2IC_1}$$

(If R and Q are in rupees) where R is annual requirement in units.

C_2 is ordering cost per order.
C_1 is carrying cost in per cent of average inventory.
U is Unit price or Unit cost.
Q is Order Quantity in units.

TABLE 7.1

No. of orders per year	Order size (Rs.)	Average inventory 50 per cent of order quantity	Annual carrying cost	Annual ordering cost at Rs. 25 per order	Total cost
1	30,000	15,000	3,000	25	3,025
3	10,000	5,000	1,000	75	1,075
5	6,000	3,000	600	125	725
10	3,000	1,5000	300	250	550
15	2,000	1,000	200	375	575
20	1,500	750	150	500	650
25	1,200	600	120	625	745
30	1,000	500	100	750	850

Using the data of previous example, we have:

R = Rs. 30,000

C_2 = Rs. 25

C_1 = .2

$$Q = \sqrt{(.2 \times 30000 \times 25) / .2}$$

$$= \sqrt{(.2 \times 30000 \times 25) \times 10}$$

About Rs. 2750 or nearly Rs. 3000.

COST COMPARISON APPROACH

This method has not taken into consideration the discount for bulk purchases. We can use the cost comparison approach. In this method, the total cost of inventory carrying costs and ordering costs using an optimum purchase basis or economic ordering quantity is compared to the total cost of ordering and carrying under conditions which qualify the buyer for the quantity discount.

Re-Ordering System

The main principle of inventory control is that, items for which annual consumption is high, orders are placed frequently so that the inventory level is as low as possible. Items whose annual consumption value is not high, sufficient stocks are maintained and order placed less frequently.

There are two universally organized systems of inventory control. They are:

(a) Cyclic system, and
(b) Bin system.

Let us explain them:

(a) Cyclic System/Fixed Order

This system has a fixed and ordering interval and the size of the order may vary with the fluctuation in demand. Under this system it would be necessary to ensure that the stock could not fall between reviews to a level less than the usage during the lead-time-taking the example just given, less than 20 x 300 = 6000 units. If we assume the stock to be reviewed every 20 days this means it must be above 6000 + 20 x 300 = 12000 units. 50 adding on buffer stock of 700 we have a 12700 ROL.

(b) Bin System/Fixed Order Quantity

In this system, the order quantity is fixed and the frequency of ordering varies and is determined by the fluctuation in demand. Under this system simply multiply lead time by usage per unit of time and add the buffer stock. If, for example, the lead time is 20 days, the daily usage 300 units a day and a 700 units buffer stock is held, then the ROL is = 20 x 300 + 700 = 6700 units

The fixed-order/size system is more suitable for C and low value B items. The Fixed-Order-Interval system with its frequent and careful reviews is suitable for A and high value B items. For a given risk of stock out, the Fixed-Order-Interval system requires more of safety stock as compared with the Fixed-Order-Size system.

METHODS OF CLASSIFICATION

Methods can be chosen from the EXHIBIT depending upon the objective of control, e.g., if we want to control the value or the consumption, we can use the ABC analysis. Besides, we can use some of the methods simultaneously to fulfil the different objectives of inventory control. In this chapter, we shall concentrate on ABC analysis. This approach is simple and helps in selective control. The principle of selective inventory management recognizes that it is impossible to manage and control every item in inventory holding in the same way and still meet the two broad objectives referred to earlier.

Take care of the forest, the tree will take care of itself should be the motto of an inventory controller. Classification of inventory can help in effective control, i.e., concentrating on items which are most important as itself difficult to give equal attention to all the items in the inventory. This is also known as "Management By Exception" which is a system of

TABLE 7.2

Selective Inventory Control Exhibit

Sl. No.	Title	Basic	Main Uses
1.	ABC (Always better control)	Value of Consumption	To control raw material components and works-in-progress inventorial in the noram course of business
2.	HML (High, Medium, Low)	Unit price of the material	Mainly to control purchases
3.	XYZ	Value of items in storage	To review the inventories and their uses of scheduled intervals.
4.	VED (Vital, Essential, Desirable)	Critically of the component)	To determine the stocking levels of spare parts.
5.	FSN (Fast moving, slow moving, non-moving	Consumption pattern of the components	To control obsolescence
6.	SDE (Scarce, Difficult, Easy to Obtain)	Problems faced in procurement	Lead-time analysis and purchasing strategies
7.	GOLF (Government, Ordinary, Local, Foreign)	Source of material	Procurement strategies
8.	SOS (Seasonal, Off-seasonal)	Nature of supplies	Procurement/holding strategies for seasonal items like agricultural products

identification and communication that signals a manager when and where his attention is primarily needed. The primary objective of such a system is to simplify the management process itself, i.e., to enable a manager to identify and isolate problems that call for decisions and action on his part and avoid dealing with less critical problems which can better be handled by those at a lower level in the organisation hierarchy.

ABC ANALYSIS

It is found that in most inventories some items have a much higher annual usage value than others. ABC analysis separates inventories into A, B and C items. In order to make such an ABC analysis, the list of all the stored items and their annual consumption in value is tabulated on the basis of the latest available records. Each individual item and its annual consumption value is listed separately and then this list rearranged in a descending order beginning with the item of highest value and ending with the item of lowest value. When such an analysis is made it is usually seen that the 1st 10 per cent of the items: (a) approximately account for 70-80 per cent of the value. Next 20 per cent of items, (b) 20-25 per cent and the last 70 per cent of items, and (c) only 5-10 per cent of the value.

The analysis can be used as a guide for economizing purchases and controlling stores by having concentrated attention on the inventory control of A and B items. The ABC concept tries to isolate the vital few, 80 that the bulk of resources be devoted to control this.

Procedure

The steps computing A-B-C analysis are:

(a) First we are trying to prepare a list of items and calculate their annual usage in rupees. This can be obtained by multiplying the quantity (number of units) of the item consumed in one year by its unit price.

(b) Arranging all these items in the descending order of their individual usage in rupees. That means the first item in the list will now show the maximum annual usage in rupees, the second item the second maximum, the third item the third maximum and so on. After having done this the total of annual usage in rupees is put at the bottom of the list.

(c) Those items which together form about 70 per cent of the total annual usage may be categorised as A items. Similarly, items which contribute the next 20 to 25 per cent of the aggregate are listed as B items. The rest which contributes 5 to 10 per cent of the total percentage of annual usage are called C items.

(d) Placing of the orders on the basis of this classification.

Example: Let us explain with the help of an example from a public enterprise 'X'. The company has 10 items mentioned in the Table 7.3.

TABLE 7.3

A-B-C Analysis Usage in Rupees

Items	*Annual usage units*	*Unit cost in Rupees*	*Annual usages (Rs.)*	*Ranking*
101	20,000	0.25	5,000	4
102	30,000	0.20	6,000	3
103	10,000	0.10	1000	6
104	500	0.30	150	9
105	50,000	0.20	10,000	2
106	8,000	0.05	500	8
107	60,000	0.40	24,000	1
108	700	1.00	7,000	7
109	9,000	0.50	45,00	5
110	50	2.00	100	10

Table 7.3 shows a representative ABC analysis where 10 items have been studied and annual usage extended by unit cost to get annual usage in rupees. Table 7.4 shows the ranking and assignment of A, B and C categories for items.

TABLE 7.4

(A-B-C Ranking)

Ranking	*Item*	*Annual Usage (Rs.)*	*Cumulative Annual Usage (Rs.)*	*Cumulative Percentage*	*Category*
1	107	24,000	24,000	46.28	A
2	105	10,000	34,000	65.57	A
3	102	6,000	40,000	77.14	B
4	101	5,000	45,000	86.74	B
5	109	4,500	49,500	95.47	C
6	103	1,000	50,500	97.14	C
7	108	700	51,200	98.14	C
8	106	400	51,600	99.51	C
9	104	150	51,750	99.81	C
10	110	100	51,850	100.00	C

Table 7.5 is a summary of ABC analysis showing that 20 percent of the items represent 65.57 percent of annual usage 20 percent of the item represent 21.21 percent of the annual usage, and 60 percent of the items represents only 13.22 per cent of the annual usage.

TABLE 7.5

Summary of A-B-C Analysis

Class	*Item*	*% of items*	*Rs. (per group)*	*Cumulative percentage (Rs.)*
A	107,105	2-0	34,000	65.57
B	102,101	20	11,000	21.21
C	109,103,104 106,108,110	60	6,850	13.22

A items are ordered more frequently and in small quantities (i.e., few weeks requirements) while C items are ordered just once or twice a year to obtain the entire year's requirements. Without A-B-C analysis, the ordering policy of an undertaking may be to order all items once a quarter and position would be somewhat as represented by Table 7.6.

The average total inventory in the above case is 5550 and adding 20 percent carrying cost of the total inventory cost works out to be 5550 plus 1110=Rs. 6660. Now, if A-B-C analysis is applied the ordering policy would

TABLE 7.6

Category	No. of per years orders	Annual Requirements (Rs.)	Quantity ordered each time (Rs.)	Average Inventory (Rs.)
A	4	40,000	10,000	5,000
B	4	4,000	1,000	500
C	4	400	100	50
Total	—	—	—	5,550

be different as shown in Table 7.7 though the total number of orders placed during the year is the same as before.

TABLE 7.7

Category	No. of per years orders	Annual Requirements (Rs.)	Quantity ordered each time (Rs.)	Average Inventory (Rs.)
A	10	40,000	4,000	2,000
B	5	4,000	800	400
C	1	400	400	200
Total	—	—	—	2,600

Average total inventory is now Rs. 2600 and adding 20 per cent inventory carrying cost the total inventory cost works out to be 2600 plus 520 = 3120, which is 3540 lower than the corresponding cost in the first instance.

VED ANALYSIS

VED Analysis is used for spare parts inventory, medical stores, etc. Those items, the absence of which even for very short duration will stop production/work are known as vital products, e.g., life saving drugs. Essential items are those, the absence of which cannot be tolerated for more than a day or so. The desirable items are those which are definitely needed, but with their absence, the work can continue. This type of analysis helps in deciding on the confidence level.

CONCLUSION

A thorough understanding and use of the techniques of materials management would help in ordering supplies when needed, controlling their use, keeping them safely and in working order, and also motivating the personnel in the best use of equipment and drugs. This also prevents the chances of non-availability of equipment and drugs as being out of stock of these reduces the usefulness of the hospital system.

Quality Control of Health Care in a Hospital

MEANING

Quality is of great significance to both the providers of health care and the receivers of health care and in the process builds a solid foundation of health care institutions. Press Reports, personal discussions and observation reveal the poor functioning of health services as there is no emphasis on quality health care. Such situations create unnecessary sufferings to people and even become cause of death in many cases. This situation can be improved by injecting quality in health care system rigorously and meticulously. Talveen Singh in an Article, "What is wrong with Indian Hospitals" in the *Daily Tribune,* May 6, 2000, rightly observes, in India I notice that we are very far from world standards even when it comes to basic things like cleanliness. My room is cleanish but there are visible layers of dust encrusted on the venetian blind and the window panes and the bathroom is less clean than those you find these days. A friend's mother had been taken to the intensive care unit of a smaller Mumbai hospital and I had gone to see her only to find myself in a place of dark, dirty corridors and wards that looked more like prison cells than places of healing. Garbage lay uncollected amid piles of old furniture in forgotten comers. It is also true that you put your life at risk when you go into an Indian hospital for treatment. In Delhi I know personally at least two women who went into hospital for minor gynaecological problems and came out with hepatitis C. I know of a young boy who went into hospital with a broken arm and ended up nearly dying of septeicemia. I know of heart patients at the best hospitals in India who worry not about whether the surgeon will be able to perform their bypass properly but about whether they will survive the aftercare. ORA, AI-Assaf, WHO consultant, defines the concept of quality health care as:[1]

Quality is doing the right thing right the first time and doing it better the next, and that quality is simply the process of incremental improvements. Quality in health care should also be client focused and should emphasize meeting the clients' needs and expectations in the most effective and efficient manner. Quality, however, does not have to be luxurious or expensive. It should also be the responsibility of everyone involved and should be based on a learning environment rather than a disciplinary environment. Quality is simply a process of continuous improvement of the *status quo.*

Quality is described as having eight dimensions: effectiveness, efficiency, interpersonal relationships, safety, technical competency, access, continuity, and amenities. Each of these dimensions should be met at least minimally to meet the definition of quality.

The concept of quality has been defined as "The totality of features and characteristics of a product or service that bear on the ability to satisfy stated or implied needs." The features or characteristics may be: (1) Meeting well defined purposes; (2) Satisfying patients and job satisfaction to health personnel; (3) Complying with applicable standards; (4) Reliability of products/services; (5) Excellence; (6) Complying with safety requirements; (7) Complying with Environment requirements, and (8) Improving health status.

Quality is not obtained by chance. Efforts must be made by everybody at every level and at various phases of health care delivery system. In this context, the concept of total quality management (TQM) which is being adopted by almost all excellent institutions throughout the world appears to be the only hope for establishing quality standards.

TQM may be thought of as a way of organising and involving the whole health institution—every department, every activity and every single person at every level towards achieving excellence, high quality health care and research, growth of institution, patient satisfaction, and finally, moulding doctors of highest calibre. TQM can work well where culture and environment in the institution reflects academic quality as a way of life for all its employees.

Sri R. Venkatraman, former President of India, delivered the Convocation Address at the sixteenth convocation of Gandhigram Rural Institute, Gandhigram. He said,[2] "A quality conscious system has been described as one which produces people who have the attributes of mental agility, efficacy and reliability and, above all, the capability to take initiative and innovative measures to meet situations."

Dill (1992) grouped Deming's fourteen points management into six basic themes in providing a framework for academIc quality management (Williams, 1993):[3]

- The imperative of continuous quality improvement if an enterprise is to hold or enhance its place in the market,
- The emphasis on obtaining consistent quality in incoming resources through careful management of suppliers,

- The active participation of all members of an organisation's productive work force in the improvement of quality,
- The importance of meeting customer needs as the fundamental basis for the improvement of goods and services,
- The need for co-operation and coordination as the basic way in which an enterprise can improve its quality, and
- Quality improvement comes not from inspection but design, that is the establishment of procedures which make it impossible for bad quality to be inducted and encourage the primary aim of continuous improvement.

Murgatroyd and Morgan (1993) defined three quality-related terms:

Quality Assurance

The determination of standards, appropriate methods and quality requirement by an expert body.

Contract Conformance Quality

Some quality standard has been specified during the negotiation of forming a contract.

Customer Driven Quality

Those who are to receive a product or service make explicit their expectations. Quality assurance means delivery of efficient and effective medical care in accordance with the professional standards. The health system need to develop standards of quality in a comprehensive and scientific manner. They should not refer only to the technical aspects. Of effectiveness but to other aspects as well, like compatibility of service and work environment, communication with patients and their relations, and promotion of collective responsibility for medicare and health of the community.

In the context of hospital systems quality assurance has to be understood in terms of entire hospital care system. The concept of quality assurance should not be fragmented for the different aspects of medicare system in a hospital rather the totality of the medical and health care provided to the patients in a hospital should be kept in view.

In Public Administration quality control is also equated with Good Governance. Quality of health services can be achieved only by efficient administration of health services that is by optimising the use of health resources.

NEED

Quality control is essential to make the efficiency of health institutions possible through:[4]

(a) Improvement of existing obsolete processes and procedures.
(b) Improved layout of office and working environment.
(c) Economy in human effort.
(d) Suggesting the best use of money and material.
(e) Improved design of the goods or services provided by the organization.
(f) Improved performance.
(g) Job satisfaction.
(h) Improved flow of work.
(i) Standardisation of processes and products.
Manpower: Brain, skill, morale and effort.
Materials: Inventory, quality, standards.
Equipment: Design and operation.
Services: Communication and information systems.
Space and Building: Availability, design, utilisation.

Environment of Quality Control

Quality control cannot be initiated in isolation. It depends upon a number of factors both internal as well as external to the health system. Let us analyse some of them.

1. An Urge and Desire on the Part of the Personnel in the Health Organisation to Find Better Methods of Quality Health Care through Analysis of Existing Practices

Dr. M.K. Mani, Chief Nephrologist, Apollo Hospitals, Chennai, delivered the convocation address at the third annual convocation of NTR University of Health Sciences, Vijaywada on Thursday the 4th Feb., 1999. He said,[5] "What we get by reading is the distilled wisdom of others. It is necessary, and we must do it, but there is something more important, and that is to learn from our own experience. Reason, Observation and Experience are the Holy Trinity of Science. Why do we not trust ourselves? An important reason is that we do not really know what we are doing. The patients we remember are the spectacular successes or the dismal failures, but they are always the exceptions, and do not represent the true behaviour of the disease. We cannot draw on our experience if we do not record it. Documentation is our Achilles' heel. We must make sure that all our experience is recorded. That is half the task. The other half is to review the records from time to time. This has two advantages. If we make an honest appraisal, we will find deficiencies in our own performance, and can improve on it. The second is that we may make genuine contributions to the world's body of knowledge. The doctors must always examine critically the work they are performing so that they can think better ideas to promote better health care.

2. Need of Requisite Skill, Attitudes, and Ability in the Persons Engaged in Quality Control

Dr. K. Kasturirangan, Chairman, Space Commission and Secretary to the Government of India, Department of Space said that:[6]

> "Medical profession is one of the noblest professions that serve the humanity. It has a rich legacy of countless men and women who, through their selfless dedication and devotion, added new chapters to the long history of medicine."

The future environment is going to be dynamic and you have plenty of scope and challenge to play your part. Our society critically depends upon your contributions—which can make its members healthier, stronger and more prosperous.

Prof. J.S. Bajaj, Member, Planning Commission, Government of India, delivered the Convocation Address at the Second Convocation of the Nizam's Institute of Medical Sciences, Hyderabad. He said:[7]

> "Medicine is now undergoing a paradigm shift from organ physiology and cell pathology to molecular biology and reverse genetics. The recipients of post-graduate and post-doctoral degrees today are indeed fortunate that they would be practicing medicine in the twenty-first century when contemporary fundamental research and resultant basic discoveries shall be transcribed into diagnostic tools and therapeutic modalities of everyday use."

The dawn of the age of aquariums for bio-sciences seems to be tantalizingly close. However, the concern and compassion of a physician, and his inherent capacity to develop an inner vision and in-depth perception, shall always go beyond the hitherto known frontiers of bio-sciences. Indeed, this is where the sublime art of medicine surpasses the narrow confines of the advancing horizons of the science of medicine. This is when a physician attains the divine gift of healing. Yet, how many strive for both? And how few achieve either?

To quote Dr. M.K. Mani again: The medical profession has become rapacious, viewing every sick man as a gold mine.

"Hail to thee, oh physician, brother of Yamaraja, Elder brother, for Yama takes life, but you take life and money too." We need to earn money to live, and to support our families, but we should remember that the source of our money is a human being, and one who is in distress and suffering.

You are fortunate in that your profession enables you to do good to others in the normal course of your work. You need not go out of your way to make opportunities for social service. If there is nothing that pleases you, then make yourself useful. That action is best, which procures the greatest happiness for someone in distress. By giving happiness we will receive it multiplied many-fold.

3. *Need of vision among Medical Professionals to Inject Quality*

Medical profession through Indian Council of Medical Research,

Medical Council of India and other organisations should define the role of the medical profession in the new millennium in the context of social development and improvement of the quality of life of the people.

A nation without a 'Vision' perishes. It is the vision that drives the progress of the nation. More than 500 experts drawn from various fields have prepared the "Technology Vision 2020" document for the country, which was released by the Prime Minister in August 1996. This vision document consists of 17 major technology packages. It deals with agricultural infrastructure and production, food-processing, health care, electric power, water-ways, life sciences and bio-technology, inland transportation, civil aviation, engineering industries, electronics, information and communication technology, material technologies and strategic industries, etc.

The Technology Vision Report aims to develop variety of indigenous technologies to transform India into a developed nation by the year 2020. With effective use of indigenously developed technologies in the next quarter century some of the visible results by the year 2020 will be, enhanced wealth of the nation, abundant production in various areas, well-being of the people and national security.[8]

ICMR should prepare a document for the new millennium to ensure quality health care which should not be second to developed countries so that our people do not rush to the health institutions of advanced countries and waste financial resources and bring discredit to the country. We should develop our own health system which should possess all quality standards.

4. *Need of Initiative and Creativity among Medical Fraternity Gained through Critical Examination*

The critical examination is the crux of the quality control as it helps us to arrive at the true basis underlying each event and to draw up a systematic list of all possible improvements for designing of the most efficient, economic and practical way in which the job could be done. As stated in the report of the Secretariat Training School, Ministry of Home Affairs, Government of India (p. 91):

"Critical Examination is a disciplined questioning technique. The questioning technique attacks the governing considerations of a specified activity under study in a systematic, logical and objective manner." The questioning technique is the means by which the critical examination is conducted, each activity being subjected in turn to a systematic and progressive series of questions.

In short, we can say that critical examination challenges the existing purpose, the resources used, the processes employed, environmental considerations of health organizations, etc. to improve quality health care.

The critical examination is an intellectual exercise and must be used cautiously. It is perhaps worth-mentioning a few points which should be borne in mind:

(a) Facts must be examined as they are, not as they appear to be, or should be, or said to be.

(b) Preconceived ideas, which often colour the interpretation of facts, must be allowed no play.

(c) All aspects of the problem must be approached with a challenging and sceptical attitude. Every detail must be examined logically and no answer accepted until it has been proved correct.

(d) Hasty judgements must be avoided.

(e) Experiment resulting from 'hunches', which should have been immediately committed to paper as they occurred, should be reserved to the appropriate place in the investigation.

(f) New methods should not even be considered until all the undesirable features of the existing method have been exposed by systematic examination.[9]

(g) Details must have persistent and close attention.

We can thus say that the critical examination for its success presupposes the existence of the following ingredients—an analytical mind, freedom from prejudice, absence of pre-conceived notions, willingness to learn, strength of mind to avoid going off a tangent in pursuit of bright ideas, and concrete evidence.

Let us cultivate the valuable resources of creativity to creatively respond to the changing situations and become the 'Masters of Change' in every field.

C = Customer satisfaction leading to customer delights,
H = Honour and dignity to all the people,
A = Accountability from every area of service,
N = New ideas and commitment to innovation,
G = Growth as a continuous discipline, and
E = Excellence expressed as yardstick for performance and evaluation.[10]

The health institutions that will survive and thrive in the future, are those that foster creativity today among their health professionals. Without creativity, health professionals would become junk after a decade or so and would be a liability for the health system and even on themselves. Creativity only can keep health professionals alive in the true sense.

5. Need of High Quality Research Both in the Area of Medical Science and Human Behaviours towards their Health

According to P.V. Young, "Social Research may be defined as a scientific undertaking which by means of logical and systematised techniques aims to:

(1) discover new facts or verify and test old facts;
(2) analyse their sequence, inter-relationships and casual explanations which were derived within an appropriate theoretical frame of reference; and
(3) develop new scientific tools, concepts and theories which would facilitate reliable and valid study of human behaviour.

As stated in the Encyclopaedia of the Social Science, Social Research is systematic method of exploring, analysing and conceptualising social life in order to "extend correct or verify knowledge, aids in construction of a theory or in the practice of an art."

The purpose of research is to discover answers to questions through the application of scientific procedures, i.e. Research Methods. There is no guarantee that any given research undertaking actually will produce reliable, relevant and unbiased results. But scientific research procedures are more likely to do so than any other method known to man. According to Young, "A researcher's primary goal, distant or immediate—is to explore and gain an understanding of human behaviour and social life."

Quality is more important than quantity in research. What is required is an increased quantity of quality research. The institutions must realise that high quality of work is a permanent asset which builds the foundations of science. A healthy climate is necessary for quality research. Openness, enthusiasm, trust, independence and team spirit is essential for the development of a scientific culture.

Prof. J.S. Bajaj, Member, Planning Commission, Government of India, delivered the convocation address at the first annual Convocation of the University of Health Sciences, Vijaywada. He said, "The major goal of the new policy would be to usher in our fellow citizens a positive change in their health status where health benefits are maximised and health hazards minimised, if not altogether eliminated. The new health policy must provide a reliable and relevant framework for not only effecting but also measuring and monitoring the health policy direction during the first quarter of the next century."[11]

Dr. A.P.J. Abdul Kalam, Scientific Advisor to Raksha Mantri and Secretary, Deptt. of Defence R & D, Ministry of Defence, New Delhi, delivered the convocation address at the Second Convocation of the National Institute of Mental Health and Neuro Sciences (Deemed University), Bangalore, he said, "There is an urgent need of unified approach to the planning of health care delivery in our country. Besides traditional medical education and research programmes, the emphasis must be made on poly-clinic level training programmes in clinical technologies. Indigenisation of costly diagnostic and curative equipment to make them cost-effective and establishment of a nationwide maintenance mechanism of medical equipment using indigenous skills and spares is also equally important."[12]

Dr. Myint Htwe and Dr. Stephan P. Jost, in their article, "promoting the Application of Research Findings in Health Development" rightly concludes.[13]

Public Health programmes can be conceptualised as a pyramid. Research knowledge forms the base of the pyramid. Standards, norms, methods or procedures are developed on this basis. The public health information and documentation systems serve as supporting pillars. The top layers are bound by evaluative research. Therefore, research-based practice, whether derived from fundamental or evaluative findings, is a necessity. This is especially true in today's health care climate where increasing demands for high quality and cost-effective health care prevail.

Successful application of research therefore depends upon the interest and commitment of both researchers and users. It cannot be achieved by individuals working in isolation (Bircumshaw, 1990). If the ultimate benefits must be understood and implemented by health managers at all levels of the system. This does not happen rapidly. It requires commitment and willingness to learn because this process is cyclical as well as continuous.

Research utilization is an organizational responsibility. It is best accomplished if there is real commitment to apply research findings at the organizational level. Therefore, translating health research into health care practice is neither easy nor quick (Sheehan, 1986). It remains an enormous challenge.

6. Need of Commitment and Empathy

Quality health care needs team work and mutual understanding. Medical personnel must work in a team to achieve quality health care. S.S. Maricodoss mentions two ingredients of team work—commitment and empathy. To quote him:

> "Commitment is a deep and profound value of emotional intelligence. It means aligning oneself with the goals of a group or organisation. It is applying oneself completely for a cause. People possessing this competence readily make sacrifice to meet larger organisational goals. Hence more than the individual interests, the group's mission or interest takes priority. It is very deep to the extent of sacrificing oneself. It also involves taking sides or taking stance. Emotionally balanced and committed people don't yield to any pressure or threat. Instead they courageously proceed whatever may be the consequences.

Emotionally balanced people are generally empathetic and not sympathetic. Sympathy perpetuates oppression and makes people dependent. Sympathy is a form of judgement. We should therefore avoid being sympathetic towards others. Empathy means understanding the issue or concern that lie behind another's feeling. It is an ability to look at things from others' point of view or to read another's emotions or to put oneself into other's shoes and think from their angle. Avoiding pretension, it enables sensing and responding to a person's unspoken concern or feelings. It can be called the foundation skill for all the social competencies. Empathetic listening is a tremendous deposit in the Emotional Bank Account. Empathy includes understanding others, service orientation, developing others, leveraging diversity and political awareness.[14]

7. Outstanding Leadership and Strength of Character

Health services must also develop the normative linkages, i.e., they must develop professional standards which should help them in their performances. Standards are contagious. Standards depend upon the quality of Leadership.

Eminent Industrialist, Mr. Rahul Bajaj, Chairman and Managing Director, Bajaj Auto Limited and President, CII, delivered the Convocation Address at the 49th Annual Convocation of the SNDT Women's University, Mumbai. He said, "To realize our goals and aspirations, we need outstanding leadership in every field and at every level. Leadership means that there is no substitute for excellence, no tolerance of mediocrity and no compromise with integrity. Leadership is not just charisma, not public relations, not showmanship. Leadership is performance, consistent behaviour and trust-worthiness.[15]

Leadership depends upon strength of character

Honourable Mr. Justice A.M. Ahmadi, Chief Justice of India, delivered the Convocation Address at the thirty-ninth convocation and special convocation of Sardar Patel University. He said, "In the final analysis, what really matters is one's character and not the outward signs of achievement. It requires character to face the unending tests that life constantly puts one through; when faced with a crisis, it is only a person possessed of true character who is able to keep his head steady whilst others around are losing theirs."[16]

Samuel Smiles says in Self Help

Character is the noblest possession of an individual. It exercises a greater power than wealth and secure all the honour without the jealousies of fame . . . Men of character are not only the conscience of society but in every well-governed State they are its best motive power. The strength, the industry and civilization of nations—All depend upon individual character. Mind without heart, intelligence without conduct, cleverness without goodness, are powers in their way, but they may be powers only for mischief. We may be instructed or amused by them. But it is sometimes as difficult to admire them as it would be to admire the dexterity of a pickpocket or the horsemanship of a highway man. Even in the noble medical professions doctors are fleecing the customers to make maximum wealth rather than take pride in the profession.

CONTENTS OF QUALITY

Health care quality encompasses many attributes. It is very difficult to enumerate all of them. Let us discuss the important ones.

1. Effectiveness and Efficiency

Effectiveness is an expression of the degree of attainment of the pre-determined objectives and targets of a programme, institutions, or activity seeking to reduce a health problem or improve an unsatisfactory health situation. This factor depends on whether the various activities and measures undertaken work (efficacy) and the degree to which they are accepted by those for whom they are intended.

Efficiency is an expression of the relationship between the results obtained from a health programme or activity and the efforts expended in terms of human, financial, and other resources, health processes, technology, and time. The reason for assessing efficiency is to improve implementation and gain a better idea of the progress made.

Both effectiveness and efficiency came at the top of the list stressing the fact that quality can only be achieved if processes are performed appropriately and in a cost conscious environment. Only appropriate and necessary care should be provided. Waste, duplication and re-work should be eliminated. Only most economical ways and most effective ways to provide care should be stressed. In a system of higher demands for quality care coupled with the reality of limited resources, prudent decisions regarding best possible combinations of effective and efficient care are required and expected.

World Health Report, 1999 rightly states how lessons learned from past successes and failures can guide a more targeted and pragmatic approach to current and emerging health challenges. It warns of the unprecedented challenges. It warns of the unprecedented complexity of these challenges, and offers strategic directions for tackling them in the next decade. Clear conclusions emerge. Despite recent spectacular progress in disease control and extended life expectancy, more than 1 billion people today have not shared in these gains.

Consequently, health systems can no longer afford to allocate resources to interventions of low quality or low efficacy related to cost. Spontaneous, unmanaged growth in any country's health system cannot reliably ensure that the greatest health needs are met. In defining priorities and selecting interventions, decision-makers must focus their efforts on areas where the return in health gains is demonstrably greatest.

2. Equity

Equity considers the coverage of population groups and geographical areas, distribution of resources and facilities, and effectiveness of services in different areas. Equity in the distribution of health care depends on the extents to which different geographical areas and population groups, according to age, sex, or wealth, have access to essential services.

How will history judge the 20th century ? Will it be seen as the era of mankind's greatest advances productivity or as the era when human development faltered and gave rise to a wave of poverty like some epidemic of medieval times ? As the century draws to a close, I fear that it is the latter image which future generations will hold, unless we take decisive action. The tremendous gains made in health development in the past three decades are at risk because the increasing gaps between rich and poor pose an unprecedented challenge to the health and well-being of the people of the world.

Emphasis in development has for too long been on economic advancement alone, based on a simplistic belief that an increase in national income would, of itself, result in social improvements including health. In effect the world has reverted to a latter-day trickle down theory of development, an approach that was already discredited 30 years ago. Furthermore, the promise of more money for social development, following the end of the Cold War, has not materialized.

Improving the health of nations is therefore dependent on reducing inequities both between countries and between the rich and poor within a country.

The basic elements of our strategy for action need be:

- Ensuring that the poorest and most vulnerable groups of the population have access to primary health care. This means redirecting often scarce money as well as personnel to the front line of the health care system at community and district levels. It also means increasing their access to information about health.
- Protecting the poorest from risks to health which are beyond their control; protection from environmental hazards; protection from crime and violence; access to adequate food, shelter, water and sanitation; and, above all, the ability to earn an income. These are the basic minimum needs for health and development.
- Building strong commitment to health among top political leaders in all countries. This includes assuming responsibility, at the highest level, for monitoring the reduction of health inequities.[17]

There is a need to redirect our efforts to ensure social development, equity and justice in 21st century and remove the imbalance accumulated in 20th century otherwise, this would be a danger to peace and prosperity on this globe.

D.R. Gwatkin proposes two initial actions that professionals can take to begin meeting the need:

- The first is that those concerned with health inequalities and the health of the poor should look beyond the issues that divide them and focus on the much more important beliefs which they share.

- The second is that they work towards the redefinition of health goals, now expressed primarily in terms of population averages, so that the goals refer directly to improving the conditions among the poorer groups and to reducing the differences between those groups and others in society.[18]

The goal of sustainable development cannot be achieved in a society if its peoples suffer ill-health. However, healthy people can contribute to the achievement of sustainable development. Therefore, health is a part of the goal of sustainable development and, in turn, helps to achieve that goal. In this sense, especially in a crisis, health is everybody's business.[19]

The principle of equity should be widely understood as the fundamental tenet of justice, to be incorporated into health policies and programmes of every society, with the particular meaning that whereas all have a right to health care, such care should take into account differential needs, so that the care is in accord with the need. Further, extending care beyond the need is the aspirational goal of reducing disparities in health status, with particular concern for the underprivileged and the needy.

A special area of concern is that of gender equality, which calls for policies and actions that will ensure equitable health care for all, including both females and males at all stages of their lives. While much of the concern for gender equality has risen from discriminatory practices directed toward girl children and women, which must be given priority in policy and programmatic actions, it is also important to acknowledge the importance of equitable care of all people at all ages. A gender perspectives is vital to the development and implementation of equitable health policies and strategies. With increase in life expectancy, creating conditions for healthful ageing assumes a sense of urgency.[20]

3. Patients/People's Satisfaction in the Quality of Health Care

Health Administration is named by people and meant for people. People's interest and satisfaction must be ensured through quality health care. R.B. Jain in his article, "Citizen's Charter—An Instrument of Public Accountability" has nicely explained the key elements in setting of citizens' charters. These are:

(i) Standards

Setting, monitoring and publication of explicit standards for the services that individual users can reasonably expect. Publication of actual performance against these standards.

(ii) Information and Openness

Full, accurate information, readily available in plain language, about how well they perform and who is in-charge.

(iii) Choice and Consultation

The public sector should provide choice wherever practicable. There should be regular and systematic consultation with those, who use services. User's views about services and their priorities are to be taken into account for final decisions on standards.

(iv) Courtesy and Helpfulness

Courtesy and helpful service from public servants who will normally wear name budge. Service available equally to all who are entitled to them and run to suit their convenience.

(v) Putting Things Right

If things go wrong, an apology, a full explanation, and a swift and effective remedy to be offered. Well published and easy to use complaint procedures with independent reviews, wherever possible to be introduced and maintained.

(vi) Value for Money

Efficient and economical delivery of public services within the resources, the nation can afford. And, independent validation of performance against standards.[21]

For democracy to be successful at the national level, the grassroots organisations have to be strong. The local authorities have to respond to the felt needs of the people.[22] The citizens have to have faith in the efficacy of the administrative system so that the distance between people and the government is reduced. The administration, for good governance has to be accessible. In developing countries, it is the government, which initiates and implements development programmes. It must gain support of the people in the discharge of these programmes, particularly at the cutting-edge. Such support would strengthen democracy as well as a positive response of the community to development programme which should be the ultimate goal of good governance.

4. Need of Positive Role of Functionaries of Health

Health functionaries have developed negative attitudes which has damaged the reputation and prestige of health system. M.K. Gaur has rightly said: Goodness of governance emerges from positive developmental roles of functionaries, underpinned with a summation of positive values—including morality, ethics, accountability, transparency, etc. in a Weberian model of public administration operating in a democratic context. A true democracy visualises, decentralization and delegation of political power to realise true people's participation, who are the ultimate beneficiaries of all administrative activities relating to law and order, development, social welfare, etc. Assertion of this angle is clearly visible behind the demand for enforcement of people's charter.

Persistence in negative tendencies, in a gradually increasing proportion over the decades, has caused serious and widespread damage not only to the capability of Indian administration to be an effective vehicle of good governance but also its very credibility to discharge even the minimal functions of regulatory nature, let alone the demanding development ones. The situation is desperate and any piecemeal or patch-work approach will not work. Hence recasting Indian administration in a new mould is the crying need of the hour.[23]

Advances in the patterns of health development cannot proceed unless the human resources that lead, plan, staff, monitor and evaluate health-related services and programmes are enlightened and enabled to define and respond to societal needs. Given the evolving understandings of health problems and the changing dynamics of health system development, there must be a close and continuous interaction between educational, research and health system development to ensure relevance of education to need.

The commitment to equity must be imbedded in the educational process. Thus, population-based education and training will include learning the skills for assessing the needs of populations, including differential needs of vulnerable groups, and responding with care in relation to need. The relevant skills include the social sensitivities for interacting with patients and populations, for defining their individual and collective health problems, for determining the appropriate clinical and health-care response, and for leadership of or participation in health teams in providing such response.[24]

5. Need of Change of Attitudes of Health Functionaries

Time has come for a strong message to be conveyed that administration is for the people and not for the public servants themselves. There has to be a change of attitudes, and public servants should realise that efficiency will be measured not in terms of what the services purport to offer, but in terms of public satisfaction. Simultaneously, there has also to be a cleansing of the services and codification of the ethics, value systems and the interface with the politicians.

There is a need for:

1. Making administration accountable and citizen-friendly,.
2. Ensuring transparency and the right to information, and
3. Taking measures to cleanse and motivate Civil Services.[25]

6. Need of Developing Positive Values for Health Functionaries and Ensure their Practice

Employees in public services should avoid wastage and extravagance, ensure effective and efficient use of public money within their control, and endeavour that the benefits of schemes for disadvantage and poor sections of society are not wasted or diverted for the benefit of others. They should avoid ostentation and set examples of austerity for others.

All employees in public services should promote and exhibit public and private conduct in keeping with the appropriate behaviour and standards of excellence and integrity. They should support the juniors in the latter's efforts to resist wrong or illegal directives and in abiding by the Code of Ethics. At the same time, they should reward good work and punish any dereliction of duty or obligations, based on objective and transparent criteria.[26]

7. Setting up of Work Improvement Teams

Another innovative measure designed to achieve higher productivity in public organisations is introduction of Work Improvement Teams (WITs). Adapted from the Japanese experience of Quality Control Circle, the WIT is essentially a small group of employees in the same work area or doing similar type of work who voluntarily meet regularly for about an hour every week to identify, analyse and resolve work-related problems. Through participation of the grass-roots level, the scheme seeks to generate higher employee morale, improved productivity and reduction in cost.[27]

8. Need of Congenial Environment to Provide Decent Health Services

There are a number of factors within the health organisations which must be attended to achieve best health care. To quote WHO report, "Of course in a system that strives for quality other dimension must be fulfiled. Personnel interaction is important in providing quality health care. Health care is provided by highly educated and sophistically skilled individuals but these individuals cannot provide a holistic care to the patient without relying on teamwork. Interpersonal relationships therefore, play a tremendous role in shaping the processes of care and ensuring a positive outcome to the patient. Just think of a scenario where a highly specialized hospital with all the gadgets and whistles of technology and technical competence of its staff but without real care teams. Each provider is working on his own without regards to others in the system. No coordination of activities and no collaboration between providers. Probably a total chaos! How would the care be delivered then? It would almost be impossible to deliver any care let alone quality care. Such an environment is not conducive of quality processes and this hospital is doomed to failure. Effective teamwork is a must for health care quality, health care quality is a process not a programme. A programme has a beginning and an end but a process has no end. It is continuous. Another issue in regard to quality is that care should be provided in a continuum. That is to say, care should be initiated, rendered, evaluated, improved, and continuously monitored even after the patient is cured of his present illness. Care is extended to include well ness, health promotion and disease prevention. Additionally, care that is started by one provider should be continued and followed by the other provider in cases of transfer to ensure continuity of care. Fragmented care and disconnected system is not a quality system and health care quality may never be achieved in such a system.

Finally, it is always more pleasant to have a care provided in an aesthetically acceptable environment. A facility that pays attention to the minute details of its customer's comfort and well-being is certainly a quality facility. Whether it is cleanliness, decor, or service, health care quality can only be enhanced with such a valuable dimension.[28]

Good governance, however, is not a finished product. It is a dynamic concept. It encompasses fast-changing political, social and economic milieu, along with international environment and conditions of operational governance. Hence, the need for periodical rethinking on and even remodelling of the concept and institutions of governance. The search for good governance has to be a continuing exercise.

9. Need of Medical Audit

Medical Audit is defined as the evaluation of medical care in retrospect through analysis of medical records. It is a review of the professional work in the hospital or in other words the quality of medical care; i.e. we try to see how far the clinicians have conformed to the norms and standards of defined medical practice while treating the patients.

According to Sana Zaro some 30 years ago any auditing usually took the form of chart review. This is now regarded as highly inefficient and unproductive use of physicians time, leading mainly to biased judgement. Today perhaps we need constant and recurrent medical audit. Even such review committees like hospital. Tissue review committees' findings and feedback to professionals had lead to dramatic reduction in rate of tonsillectomy as reported. The form of medical audit which have since evolved now uses explicit written criteria for judging whether care provided meets the standards of performance of the staff.

The Medical Audit is now well established as a formal activity in most of the hospitals in west. The assessment of quality 1M care depends upon the quality and reliability of medical records being maintained and the nature of criteria that are being used.

The medical records are of value to patients, the physicians and the hospital and also for teaching and research. The quality of medical records reveals/reflects the quality of patient care and since the main objective is good medical care, it is inevitable that the physicians should assumes the primary responsibility for the quality of the medical records compiled on patients under his care. Therefore, a good medical record section becomes an essential pre-requisite for medical audit. It may be emphasized here that medical audit is not a one time activity. The medical staff of the hospital and administrators realise and appreciate its potential in improving the quality of patient care in hospitals. Besides it is going to be of tremendous professional value to hospital doctors. Keeping all this in mind it is necessary that the medical audit must be carried out as an on-going activity. This could be facilitated by putting the hospital data on computer and having necessary software for medical audit of various diseases.

Pre-requisites of Medical Audit:

(a) To be carried out by fair and impartial clinicians who are thoroughly conversant with the current practice of medicine.
(b) The impetus must come from the medical staff themselves, realising the benefits to the patients and themselves.
(c) A good system of medical record keeping and a trained medical record librarian.
(d) Well defined disease-related criteria.

The purpose of Medical Audit is to evaluate the factors impinging on patient care. All the deaths in a hospital where cause of death are not certain are investigated by the Mortality Review Committee. This improves the knowledge of the medical personnel and enhances their capability of handling such cases in future. The Health Survey and Planning Committee (1959-61) recommended the use of medical audit in all hospitals. The Delhi Hospital Review Committee headed by Dr. K.N. Rao (1968) also recommended the appointment of a Medical Audit Committee in each hospital. Such committee will ensure specific checks on the quality of work performed in the hospitals. We have found the following drawbacks in some of the hospitals where such committees are functioning:

(1) Poor recording of a case history
(2) Sketchy documentation
(3) Operation notes not properly recorded
(4) Lack of inter-departmental coordination
(5) Incomplete case-notes
(6) Not proper follow-up by the senior faculty members.

Either mortality committees have not been set-up in hospitals or function irregularly. The Public Accounts Committee also mentioned that:

> "Although the recommendations of the review committee to carry out hospital mortality review periodically was accepted by the Government in February 1970, it was only after a lapse of six years (May 1976) that the mortality review committee started functioning in Willingdon Hospital (Rammanohar Lohia Hospital).

The conditions are worse in hospitals under the control of State Governments in this regard. Thus, there is a need to set-up such committees to ensure efficient and effective medical audit.

10. Need to have Transparent and Honest Administration to have Good Quality Administration

We mention here some ingredients of quality administration which can help in providing decent health care services:

1. Openness in the sense of having wide contact with men and matters.
2. A sense of justice, fair play, impartiality in dealing with men and matters.
3. Sensitivity and responsiveness to the urges, feelings and aspirations of the common people.
4. Securing the honour and dignity of all human being, however humble he or she might be.
5. Humility and simplicity in the persons manning the government machinery and their easy accessibility.
6. Creating and sustaining an atmosphere conducive to development, growth, and social change and honesty and integrity in thought and action.

PROCESS OF QUALITY CONTROL: SETTING STANDARDS

Standards of quality health care are not fixed as these would vary from organisation to organisation depending upon the quality of inputs. However, efforts should be made to reach standards which are international so that people can get the quality health care in their own country. Government and private resources are wasted in getting health care from advanced countries which can be made available within the countries themselves through the application of quality standards in our health institutions. This is not going to be expensive but only require hard work and dedication on the part of the health experts and sincerity on the part of Governments. Talveen Singh in an Article, "What is lorany with Indian Hospitals" has rightly said (May 6, 2000).

Meanwhile, until our governments are able to provide decent standards of health care to the average Indian we should seriously consider a ban on any politician or bureaucrat being allowed to travel abroad for treatment at taxpayer's expense. When they and their families can no longer be treated free at the best hospitals in the world we can be sure that things will start to improve. We now mention the steps for quality control.

(i) Select/Identifying a Function or System/Activity

It can be a study of OPD, ward, emergency, OT, etc. It is essential to select the activity in the context of economic, technical, human, social and psychological consideration. For example, let us select the problem—How many patients old and new can be seen by an ENT specialist in an OPD with quality in focus. Standard of quality could need be developed separately for each activity like laboratory services, X-ray, Wards, Nursing Services, etc. These would depend on many factors and hence would be flexible. Therefore, Standards should be set keeping in view the profile of the organisation.

After the selection of the problem, it is necessary to get a formal approval of the sponsoring organization. This formal approval or terms of reference should define clearly the purpose of the assignment, time dimension for completion of the study, cost involved and the inherent technical or organizational limits. This formal approval must be distributed among all the employees of an organization whose quality is being studied so that they can properly appreciate the significance of it. Besides, the organization must ensure cordial atmosphere for the study team to ensure fruitful results. We must always keep in mind that the quality control is not only job of the team but a joint venture where success would largely depend on the support, ethos, attitudes and interest of key personnel of the sponsoring organization.

(ii) Recording of Data

The next and an important step in the quality control is the recording of facts relating to the existing Methods/Procedure/Practice. While collecting data by any method, scientific attitude is very important. To be sure, a scientist avoids personal and vested interests. The success of the quality control greatly depends on the accuracy with which the facts are recorded.

The main aims of recording are:

(a) To obtain adequate and accurate information.
(b) To present the facts in a concise and comprehensible form for analysis.
(c) To submit proposals to management in a way which is easily understood.
(d) To provide, eventually, detailed operating instructions for the use of supervisors and operators.

(iii) Critical Examination

The examination is conducted by means of the sets of detailed questions: the primary questions to indicate the facts and their underlying reasons, and the secondary questions to find the alternatives and the best methods of improvements. The questions pertains to the purpose of the operation, the place where it is carried out and the means by which it is carried out. Both primary and secondary questions are asked for each aspect before passing on the next.

In order to carry out the critical examination in a scientific way, a sheet of standard layout is used. The outline format of this sheet is reproduced on next page.

While examining the factors impinging upon the operational efficiency of purpose, means, sequence, place and person, there is no set sequence to be followed. However, we must initiate with the purpose as other factors would be considered only provided the study of purpose is justified.

The success of the critical examination depends upon the scientific attitude of the investigating team. The aim of all critical examination is the

Facts	*Factual data*		*Creative Thinking*	
	Reasons	*Alternatives*	*Implication*	*Selection for Development*
Purpose What is being achieved?	Why is it achieved?	What else can be achieved?	What are the advantages and disadvantages of each alternatives?	What can be selected for development?
Means How is it achieved?	Why that way?	How else can it be achieved?	What are the advantages and disadvantages of each alternatives?	What can be selected for development?
Place Where is it achieved?	Why there?	Where else can it be achieved?	What are the advantages and disadvantrages of each alternative?	What can be selected for development?
Personal Who achieved it?	Why that person?	Who else can achieve it?	What are the advantages and disadvantages of each alternatives?	What can be selected for development?

furtherance of the quality control philosophy – there is always a better and effective way.

(iv) Develop

The critical examination will suggest a number of alternative solutions to the various aspects of the problems in hand. Besides, the critical examination does not indicate the improvement of the total situation. Therefore, there is a need to devise a composite plan, integrating all the elements, to improve quality. All the elements should be combined through the building of "Family Tree" of all variables. This would provide the integrated plan to produce total quality improvements rather than in a particular area which can create problems and thus produce negative results. Development may be compared to the development of a photograph from an exposed film or negative. The picture needs touching with chemicals to make prints of desired quality.

(v) Define/Set Standards

Apriori, quality cannot be considered as absolute concept but is a multi-dimensional dynamic entity. It is also not a unitary concept but a phenomenon determinable by relating with the excellent or the best in the field. Consequently, for judging quality, a yardstick or standard needs to be established which is otherwise called 'benchmark'.

Through standards, an organization defines what it expects for the inputs, processes, and outcomes of the health services it provides. They are an instrumental part of monitoring the quality of health care and identifying problems and measuring improvements in health care service delivery. Through periodic updating and modifications, they become a part of an organization's cycle of continuous improvement.

(vi) Installing the New Standard

Words written or spoken are of no use unless put to action. The actual implementation is the responsibility of health management. The study team can only play an advisory and supportive role. The implementation can be successful if the top health management has developed faith and interest in the new plan and can motivate the personnel down the line. What has been seen mostly is that such schemes are shelved on one pretext or the other. Installation can be divided into five stages, namely:

(a) Gain acceptance of the change by the supervisors.
(b) Gain approval of the middle management.
(c) Gain acceptance of the change by the employees and their representatives.
(d) Train the employees to operate the new methods.
(e) Maintain close contact with the progress of the work until satisfied that it is being done as intended.

(vii) Maintaining the New Standard

Human behaviour is averse to change. Therefore, Management must see that once a standard has been installed it should be maintained as designed and that the workers should not be allowed consciously or unconsciously to slip back into old methods. As already mentioned, the top management must be innovative to handle any situation which may prevent the working of the new model. The top leaders must learn the art of dealing with interest groups and the pressure groups who may oppose the running of the new methods on flimsy grounds.

(viii) Reviewing the Standard

The main aim of reviewing is to discover whether there are any discrepancies between the authorized quality and current practice at the time of review. Reasons for any variations in the quality must be investigated. Any changes that have occurred for valid reasons should be accepted and the operating instructions amended accordingly. Where the review reveals that there are undesirable variations in the quality, measures should be taken through supervision to ensure that the quality follows the authorized procedure.

The ultimate purpose of standard should be the aim of integrating quality into normal management process so that search for improvement becomes a matter of accepted practice in an organization. We must also ensure that standard of quality is feasible, probable in the overall frame of administration.

CHALLENGES TO SETTING STANDARDS

In spite of a large resource of existing standards to adapt to specific needs and the growing interest in establishing standards by various country health organizations, there still exist certain challenges to this process:

(1) Reliance on Explicit Criteria

Physicians, nurses, and other health care professionals may resist on the basis that standards impinge upon their subjective judgement that they have developed through their practice. Some professionals contend that medicine is partly art, partly science, and that standards may require them to diagnose and treat without allowing them to use their professional judgement. Others may fear that standards will be used in a punitive manner, to identify and punish professionals who don't perform within strictly defined limits. These are legitimate concerns and require the organization to address them in some constructive manner before developing or implementing standards.

(2) Identifying Appropriate Resources, Human, Physical and Financial

Developing or adapting standards takes time and resources. Sometimes the organization must go outside its staff to use experts in the field. Throughout all this the organization will incur certain costs that should be evaluated before hand to determine if the effort is worth the costs.

CONCLUSION

WHO in its Report of WHO Inter-country meeting on quality assurance in health care from 16-20 Dec. 1996 at Indonesia suggested the following for improving quality health care for South-East Asian countries:

(1) Ensure that quality of health care is an integral part of health services delivery at all levels of health care covering public and private sectors;

(2) Organize advocacy/awareness workshops on quality assurance for policy-makers, administrators and the leadership of health care to get their commitment for quality assurance;

(3) Establish a coordinating mechanism for quality assurance activities at national level through the nomination of focal point(s) and constitute a multi-disciplinary task force of national experts to provide advice on technical aspects of quality assurance;

(4) Initiate quality assurance of health care in selected hospitals and in primary health care through the district health system approach, document the experiences and expand gradually to more health care facilities;

(5) Organize national strategic planning workshops with technical assistance from WHO;

(6) Formulate guidelines to set standards and select national key indicators on quality assurance to monitor compliance and measure performance;

(7) Invest on building local capacity in health care quality through the creation of a critical mass of expertise within the country;

(8) Mobilize potential resources from within the country including support from international agencies; and

(9) Ensure that orientation on quality assurance be integrated in both basic and in-service training programmes of all health care professionals.

Implementation of TQM in health institution calls for a total change in culture in terms of customs, practices and improvement by creating increased sense of caring brought about by improved communication, involvement and training. It involves the integration of all functions, processes and personnel within an organization in order to achieve continuous improvement in the quality of health care delivery systems.

By following TQM principles we can bring about harmony and quality working style in all the facets of the health institution and help it gain the top position and maintain it.

Finally, TQM consists in doing for the institution what should be done as a matter of course. The fruits of implementation of TQM may not be available instantly, like magic tree, but it is sure to show improvements in health standards over a period of time.

Notes and References

1. *Daily Tribune,* May 6, 2000.
2. *University News,* March 11, 1996. p. 14.
3. G. William, Total Quality Management in Higher Education, Panacea or Placebo, *Higher Education,* 25, 1993, pp. 229-37.
4. S.L. Goel, Modern Management Technique, Deep & Deep Publications Pvt. Ltd., New Delhi, 1995, pp. 375-76.
5. *University News,* Aug. 2, 1999, p. 18.
6. *University News,* Sept. 6, 1999, pp. 21-23.
7. *University News,* Feb. 23, 1998, pp. 13-16.

8. *University News,* March 2, 1998, p. 12.
9. R.M. Currie, Work Study, 2nd Ed., London, Pitman, 1963, p. 92.
10. S.J. Mariadoss, Creativity-Competitive Resource and Core of Excellence, *University News,* No. 29, 1999, p. 13.
11. *University News,* Feb. 3, 1997, p. 18.
12. *University News,* Dec. 15, 1997, p. 10.
13. Dr. Myint Htwe and Dr. Stephan P. Jost, Research Development.
14. S.L. Maricodoss, Emotional Intelligence: Tool of Credibility, in *University News,* March 20, 2000.
15. *University News,* March 13, 2000, p. 17.
16. *University News,* Feb. 17, 1997, p. 8.
17. Hiroshi Nakajima, "Growing Equity is a Matter of Life and Death", in *World Health,* Nov.-Dec., 1994, p. 3.
18. D.R. Gwatkin, "Health Inequalities and the health of the poor: What do we know? What can be done?" in *Bulletin of the WHO,* Vol. 78, No.1, 2000, p. 15.
19. Robert Kim Farley and Mark Books, "Role of World Health Organisation in the Economic Crises" in *Regional Health Forum,* WHO, SEARO, New Delhi, Vol. 3, No. 1, 1999, p. 1.
20. WHO: SEARO: Declaration on Health Development in the South-East Asia Regions in the 21st Century, New Delhi, 1977, pp. 20-21.
21. Quoted in R.B. Jain, "Citizens Charter—An instruments of Public Accountability" in *IJPA,* July-Sept., 1998, No. 3 (Special Number on "Towards Good Governance", p. 367).
22. A.P. Barnbas, Good Government at Local Level, *IJPA,* July-Sept., 1998, p. 453.
23. M.K. Gaur, Political Stability and Good Governance, in *IJPA,* July-Sept. 1998, pp. 410-411.
24. Declaration on Health Development, *op. cit.,* p. 45.
25. Action Plan for An Effective and Responsive Government, Document 1.
26. *Ibid.,* Appendix IX.
27. *Ibid.,* Document 2.
28. WHO, SEARO, Quality Assurance in Health Care, New Delhi, 1996, p. 20.

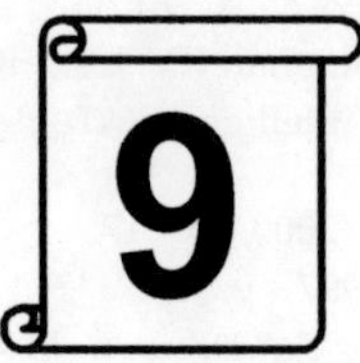

Modernising Health Administration

A. NEED AND NATURE OF MANAGEMENT IMPROVEMENT

People of advanced countries get their health services as much for granted as the essential utility services like water, electricity, public transport, etc. Despite the magic bullets of the modern medicine, the health services in the developing countries are far from satisfactory. The people living in the developing world, and especially 70 per cent of them living in rural areas, have little or no access to modern medical and health care resulting in high rates of morbidity and mortality from diseases which are preventable. If we want to reach the objective of providing decent quality health care to all by the first quarter of 21st century. We will have to introduce innovations in technical and administrative fields. It has been recognized by health experts in all the countries that the difficulties in meeting the health needs of the community are largely dependent upon the capabilities to design and manage the health care delivery system. The management of health care system can help in the greater achievement of goals through the optimum utilization of resources available—men, money and material. Indian rank in Human Development index is 128 as per Human Development Report 2000. To quote Dr. Chi-Yuen Wu of UNDP:

> "To create administrative capabilities, commensurate with requirements, developing countries must be able among other things, to use modern management techniques more, effectively than in the case of the industrially advanced countries."

Joginder Singh in his article, "Reducing Government Flab—Time to drain the swamp" in *The Tribune*, March 16, 2000 rightly observes that it is amazing that the government is always emphasizing on its employees to function with full coordination and assist the citizens with the quickest possible response. Notwithstanding all the instruction/orders of the government, the position on the ground remains anything but people-oriented. The responsive administration to the people who matter is individual-oriented. There is hardly any response where the common good matters, unless powerful interests back it.

The need of the hour for our country, burdened with poverty, illiteracy, backwardness and rampant corruption, is effective and dynamic governance. Good governance and effective management can provide the panacea for all the ills and stumbling blocks in the system. Transformation of the country is possible only when the necessary changes are brought about. We need a revolution of a different kind led by the right-thinking and right-acting leaders, who should not only prepare but also implement a blueprint for future development in a fixed time schedule.

Unfortunately, present management systems are not functioning well as these are managed by untrained personnel. This is the common management challenge faced by those in charge of the health services. To quote a recently published book:[1]

> "In the field of health, we rarely have consciously trained executives . . . We have expected a vast army of professional care givers to fill individual human needs, mainly on a *laissez faire* basis, mostly without planning, without coordination, without providing sufficiently for (those) who either do not look for care, cannot afford it or cannot get to it."
>
> "With little or no formal training, administrators . . . have arisen from our midst willy-nilly, too few through natural ability, too many by virtue of their staying-power on particular job, lack of available competition, or the administrator's uncritical need for power and control . . . "
>
> "In health administration, there are few theoreticians, few training centres, few books, and an almost absolute dearth of strict scientific investigations."

Thus there is a great need to improve the functioning of health care management with the help of modern management techniques. A modern management system is one which is designed to make the existing health care delivery process effective and efficient. Modern management methods and techniques are in reality, only techniques for improving this process by making it more accurate and reliable, by making the process respond faster, or by giving the health-manager the ability and capability to manage better.

Health administration in a country is a part of the total administration and thus influences and is influenced by this general administrative culture. Let us have a look at the general administrative apparatus prevailing in developing countries. In India, for instance, the administrative machinery has not been adequate to handle the tasks of economic and social development. The administrative inadequacies in a national government has a retarding influence on economic and social development. This lack of efficiency in administration equally holds good for the health organizations as well. The widespread feeling of inefficiency of the administrative machinery was rightly sensed and expressed by Mrs. Gandhi in a broadcast to the nation shortly after assuming the high office of the Prime Minister. She said:

> "In economic development as in other fields of national activity, there is a disconcerting gap between intention and action. To bridge this gap, we should boldly adopt whatever far-reaching changes in administration may be found necessary. We must introduce new organizational patterns and modern tools and techniques of management and administration. We shall instill into the government machinery greater efficiency and sense of urgency and make it more responsive to the needs of the people."[2]
>
> In the health sector, it was emphasized that "better management of health services is essential if higher standards of health care are to be achieved . . . that progress . . . today is to a higher extent dependent on education and development of the management, than it is on medical research and increase of material resources."[3]

The development of public administration remains an essential prerequisite for successful economic development of the country. Therefore, far-reaching improvements in public administration are required if the objectives of planned socio-economic development are to be realised. Before we analyse the meaning, nature, scope and application of management techniques for administrative improvements and reforms, let us be clear about the concept of administrative improvement first.

Administrative improvement means the act or the process of improving the administration. As stated in a United Nations Report:

Management improvement comprised the planning, Implementation and evaluation of various measures conducive to the increase of organizational effectiveness and efficiency."[4]

Administrative reform is still widely regarded as a special type of improvement activity, even when it is often closely connected with other activities. The concept of the "administrative reform", as it is applied in practice, also has its weakness. In a report by the Secretariat of the United Nations Programme in Public Administration for the period from 1950 to 1966, it is stated that:

> "Efforts at administrative reform too often stop with the preparation of reports or promulgation of law."[5]

In a number of countries the word 'reform' has also a close relationship to political concepts and attitudes, which makes it less suited for general use than the broader concept of 'improvement' or 'effectiveness'.

The techniques of administration in any country cannot remain static over a period of time. There are always scientific, economic, political, social, cultural and other changes taking place in a country. Health organizations like other organizations, must adjust themselves to these changes in order to be effective and responsive to the needs of the people. Peter Drucker, an expert in the field of management has said: "Social awareness is organizational self-interest. The needs of the society, is left unfilled, turn into social diseases. No institution whether business or hospital or University or Government agency is likely to survive in a deceased society." The need of apply modern management techniques in a hospital set-up is the greatest of all.

The design of an administrative system is a basic aid to the achievement of its primary objectives; if the design is unsound, the achievement of objectives is likely to fall short of expectations. Therefore, there is a great need to improve the structure and functioning of the administrative organizations.

Most of the economic and social progress in the developing countries is halted because, the administrative apparatus in these countries is not upto the mark. Therefore, there is an urgent need of administrative improvement in these countries. H. Paul Appleby has rightly remarked that the full success of the plan, therefore, turns rather exclusively on administrative reform to make the Government as an organism equal to its identified goals.

The administrative capability of a Government and the manner in which the development programmes are likely to be carried out are intimately related. On the other hand, administrative inadequacies in a national Government have a retarding influence on economic and social development. These deficiencies prevent the vast flood of money, talent and material from achieving their objectives. As early as 1950, the Secretary General of the United Nations pointed out that, "Any systematic effort towards economic development must be preceded by or coupled with efforts to make more effective the functioning of Government machinery."[6]

During the last few decades, phenomenal changes are taking place at a fast rate in the field of science and technology as well as administration also, which today, has to shoulder multifarious task designed to fulfil the rising aspirations of the people. In the words of Prof. Waldo, Public Administration is, "a part of the cultural complex, and it not only is acted upon, it acts." It is a great creative force. There is an urgent need to re-orient (improve) the system of public administration to cope with changes in technology and social behaviour and maximise opportunities for raising productivity, and thus the standard of living *of* the people.

According to Sir Isaiah Berlin, "It is certainly a reasonable hypothesis that one of the principal causes of confusion, misery and fear is blind adherence to outworn notions, pathological suspicion of any form of critical examination, frantic efforts to prevent any degree of rational analysis of what we believe, we live by and for."

Thus, public administration including health administration must be recreated, renewed and revitalised to produce the predesigned changes and output in the modernization of societies. This necessitates a different trend and magnitude of administrative culture and capability.

Scope of Management Improvement

If the need for change and effectiveness is to be fulfiled, management improvement must be considered to be an organization wide continuous activity. This important function must embrace the total needs based on the objectives and goals of the public administration and the resources available. The improvement efforts must be regarded as a whole involving a spectrum of different types and levels of activity. There is, in principle, no reason why 'administrative reform' and 'organization and methods' should be set-up as separate and isolated activities and other new activities should rather be merged and coordinated into a total, carefully planned, and organized "management improvement programme" involving the whole organization. The needs require centrally planned improvement programme, and for coordination purposes decentralized programmes in different ministries and institutions. Each agency or institution of importance, should be responsible for its own programme, planned in cooperation with the central authorities.

As the implementation of significant changes in organizational structure and behaviour is complex and time consuming task and is closely related to the long-term development planning of the country, improvement programme must be planned on long-term (from ten to fifteen years), medium-term (from four to five years) and short-term (yearly) basis.

Strategies and Policies in Administrative Improvement

As stated in a UN publication, the following strategies and policies are necessary to bring about administrative improvement:

(a) Improvement work must be a systematically planned organised activity with specific work programmes, a continuous activity, and it should be based on long-term planning and development.
(b) Classification of objectives and goals is necessary to be able to measure or evaluate the effectiveness and manage the improvement work.
(c) Improvement work must be recognised as a responsibility of the management; and in planning and organising improvement projects, participation and involvement of management in the organizations affected by possible changes are of great importance.
(d) Special resources must be allocated to the improvement projects including the support of professional staff of high quality with special qualifications in the management fields.
(e) Improvement work must be based on the concept or the

organization as a socio-technical system where human and social factors are of primary importance.

(f) Training and development of the members of organizations—both management and staff, usually constitute one of the most important parts of improvement work.

(g) Improvement projects should form the beginning be oriented towards implementation and change, step by step, and not only towards writing reports and giving recommendations. Such projects should include specific implementation plans.

(h) As a rule, there is need for both centralised and decentralised (though coordinated) improvement programmes. It is advisable first to build up a strong, central activity.

(i) An improvement work programme should be formalised as an obligation for the public administration institutions and tied with long-term development plans, and budgeting and accounting control procedures.

(j) The improvement project organization should be flexible. A task force, under a responsible project leader and a Steering Committee, is often a usual type of organization.

(k) In larger projects, pilot studies of the implementation of new organizational structures in a limited part of the administration are often necessary and useful to demonstrate effects and results.

(l) Improvement projects must be planned in terms of activities, time and resources. The setting of deadlines or time-limits in the work programmes has frequently proved most helpful in the effort to obtain a high level activity and results.[7]

After explaining the concept of administrative improvements, let us discuss the need, type and utility of management techniques as an instrument of administrative improvements and reforms.

B. NEED FOR MANAGEMENT TECHNIQUES

In a developing country, such as ours, there is a great haste to achieve maximum growth and progress in the shortest time possible. It is felt that the scope of experimentation is a costly and slow process. As such, we need to learn from the experience of others and use their results to help achieve our goals. A word of caution at this point is in order. Nothing succeeds like success. So too is the case of the glamorous instances of technology and management techniques and their tall claims of progress and development. Such a philosophy has done more harm than good. A few years before, modern management techniques were thought to be a panacea for all problems. Some problems did get solved while a host of others took birth as a result; many of the over popular techniques have found their graveyards whilst a lot of organizations which should have gone to the graveyards for not putting into use the 'over popular' techniques, have passed the test of time and resistance. In this context, Ernest Dale and L.C. Michelon observes that:

> "Today's manager lives in a world of rapid change, and yet the rate of change is likely to increase in the years ahead. Unless, he can keep up with this change, he is likely to find himself obsolete—perhaps unpromotable or even unemployable."[8]

Thus, there is a great need to enhance the administrative capability of health administrators so that they can use these techniques profitably. Administrative capability is an important means of converting or processing programme inputs into outputs such as goods and services. It has been mentioned by Gabriel that, "What makes the leadership variable so crucial in implementation process, is its dynamic, not passive quality, i.e., its capability to act and react on these critical inputs. It is this manipulative and transferring quality of leadership that could significantly determine the administrative capability of implementing organisation."[9]

Administrative capability is the capacity to obtain intended results through organizations.[10] Katz says: "Administrative capability for development involves the ability to mobilize, allocate and combine the actions that are technically needed to achieve development objectives."[11]

Organizations are not simply structures but action-oriented system and the success and failure of the organizations are to be measured in terms of this action system. Action system is a structured device in which resources are mobilized and transformed by use of certain skill and technology to produce pre-designed output all taking place by the influence of administrative capability within an environmental context.

Health administrators should facilitate the accomplishment of desired objectives with the least friction and the most satisfaction to those for whom the task is done and those engaged in the enterprise. Thus, there is a need to understand and portray the management techniques in all its various facets.

Management techniques are of added significance for the health sector as this sector deals with preventive, promotive, curative and rehabilitative aspects of health care activities and uses the services of Government, private and voluntary agencies. Most of the practitioners, academicians and political elite are not happy with the performance of this sector as the majority of people in the developing world do not have access even to rudimentary health care. After personal discussions with some of the health experts and other health functionaries, it was revealed that the present administration was in a bad state and needed radical reforms. It was confirmed by personal visits to some of the health institutions and their field establishments, as also by the health and medical personnel at District and Block levels. This is resulting in huge wastage of resources. There have been a large number of administrative problems which account for the unsatisfactory working of the health administration. These problems have already been examined the earlier chapters. Some of the specific problems which need immediate solutions can be mentioned as:

(a) Absence of effective health policy to meet the need of the people.
(b) Absence of coordination between the health and socio-economic sector; between Western and indigenous system of medicine and among Government, Private and Voluntary administration.
(c) Lack of effective planning, monitoring, implementation and evaluation machinery.
(d) Lack of an effective manpower planning resulting in the concentration of health services in the urban sectors.
(e) Absence of people's participation in the health care delivery operations.
(f) Absence of decentralisation resulting in inefficiency of operations.
(g) Disproportionate investments for secondary and tertiary health care.
(h) Top heavy administrative set-up.
(i) Defective organisations and procedure – an obstacle in the way of efficient services.
(j) Lack of interest to improve administrative structure and procedure, i.e., absence of innovative leadership.

In reviewing the management of health services, the delegates who came to attend the 25th Regional Committee meeting of the South-East Asia Region of WHO, noted the following considerations and constraints.[12]

(a) lack of a clear development policy and clear objectives for health services in relation to socio-economic development;
(b) inadequate understanding of health problems and the problem of tackling it from the viewpoint of consumers and provides of health care;
(c) poor utilisation of existing resources and inadequate harnessing of potential resources, human and other for health;
(d) inadequate coordination and integration between different authorities and organizations providing health services in the same geographical areas;
(e) inadequate or no integration of preventive, curative and family planning services;
(f) the increasing cost of health services and their inequitable distribution, with the result that the basic health needs of all the people were not being met;
(g) the participation of communities in the promotion of their own health and in contributing to health services policy-making, financing and decision-making;

(h) the need to find ways of developing new types of health manpower, including local multipurpose health workers, and of employing them on a wider scale;

(i) the need to develop an organization in the countries of the region for improved delivery of health services within the existing constraints—both financial and manpower—for the masses in rural areas, which alone constitutes about 80 per cent of the population; and

(j) meager allocation of fund (3 to 5 per cent) for health in the overall socio-economic development plans in most countries of the Region.

C. NATURE AND CLASSIFICATION OF MANAGEMENT TECHNIQUES

Nature

In order to understand the meaning of 'management techniques' we must be clear about the two concepts, namely, 'management' and 'techniques'. In simple words, management is the handling of tools and techniques to achieve a desired goal. In other words, management infers planning, organising and controlling of human and other resources to achieve specified goals. A technique is a set of procedural steps which may be loosely or rigorously stated, which embody a multiple idea content and which are concerned with doing work to achieve an objective.

In other words, we can say that management technique is a set of procedural steps which may be loosely stated, embodying a multiple-idea content and which are either concerned with decision-making in general or with decision relating to planning, organizing or controlling of human and/or other resources with a view to achieving the specified objectives. Management techniques make positive efforts to analyse the situation in a systematic and scientific manner and provide a rational basis for decisions. Adoption of these techniques would encourage greater professionalism in administrative activities. If a new administrative culture is also developed side by side, it would be possible to make optimum use of available and potential resources. According to one of the ILO publications, management techniques are systematic procedures of investigating, planning, controlling and supervising which can be applied to management problems.[13] Thus, modern management techniques, in actuality, are the techniques for improving the management process by making it more accurate, by making the process respond faster, or by giving the manager greater control. From the above discussion, we can say that management techniques have the following features:

1. They are a set of procedural or formal steps. This is basic for any management technique. Procedural or formal steps lead to 'systematic' approach which has been the highlight of any scientific method, the root of all sound modern management

theory. They take us from the known facts to the unknown parts of the problem.

2. They have a multiple-idea content. They do not have a single idea, but a number of them though related ones.
3. They help in decision-making in general or with decisions relating either to planning, organising or controlling or to any combination of these three processes of planning, organising and controlling of human and/or other resources with a view to achieving certain specified objectives.
4. They give the idea of efficiency which, according to Clay, can further be broken into five components:
   (a) economy of efforts in terms of money and other resources;
   (b) speed;
   (c) quality;
   (d) stability; and
   (e) aesthetic or rhythmical approach.

   They are consistent in their results.
5. Functional Classification of Management Techniques.

Functional Classification of Management Techniques

Management techniques can be classified in different ways. For example, they can be grouped according to the outlet and the department in which they are applied as, for example, preventive techniques, promotive techniques and curative techniques. This does not, however, cover all techniques. For example, where would we place the techniques of brain-storming or critical examination? An alternative can be classification according to parent discipline. But it is more an historical approach than a current use, because many of the techniques are developed in one field but later on used in a number of fields. Clay gives a classification which is based on the objective of the technique, i.e., what does the technique hope to achieve? He mentions the following eight objectives which various management techniques attempt to achieve.[14]

1. Detection (To find out or discover something e.g., what is happening or what is wrong?)

We can include such technique here as input-output Analysis, Attitude Survey, Production Study, Activity Sampling, Critical Examination, Break-even Analysis.

2. Evaluation (To measure or estimate the value of an item)

We can include such techniques here as Job Evaluation, Work Measurement, Work Estimation, Performance Appraisal, Cost-Benefit Analysis.

3. Improvement (To improve performance)

We can include such techniques here as Management by Objectives, Method Study, Value Analysis, etc.

4. Optimization (To optimise performance)

We can include such techniques here as Linear Programming, Ergonomics, Operations Research, etc.

5. Specification (To specify a desired value or situation or action)

Here we can include such technique as Layout Planning for Offices and Plants layout, designing, etc.

6. Control

Here we can include such techniques as Cost Control, Credit Control, Labour Control, Inventory Control, Production Control, Budget Control, etc.

7. Communication (To communicate information)

Here we can include such techniques as Visual Aids, Suggestion Schemes, Report Writing, Communication Theory, Information Theory, Management Information, etc.

8. Demonstration (To demonstrate something)

Here we can include such technique as Programmed Learning, Job Instruction, Management Development and Training, etc.

This achievement criteria tells us that these techniques can help us in discovering or finding something in evaluating the performance, in improving the performance, in optimizing the performance, in specifying a desired value or a situation, in controlling a variable, in communication or in demonstration.

The management techniques can also be classified in terms of various resources employed in an organization, viz., human, material, machinery and equipment, money and time. As such, some of the techniques which can be applied to bring about increased managerial capability, efficiency, effectiveness and productivity can be categorized as under:

Sr. No.	*Source*	*Management Techniques*
1.	Human Resources	Organizational analysis Job Evaluation Training Incentive Schemes Suggestion Schemes Method Study Work Measurement
2.	Material	Inventory Control Value Analysis Material Handling Standardisation ABC/VED

3. Machinery and Equipment	Method Study Value Analysis
4. Space and Building	Labour Planning Method Study
5. Money	Cost Benefit Analysis Budgetary Control Performance Budgeting Management Accounting
6. Time	Method Study Work Measurement Network Analysis (PERT/CPM).

Before we proceed to discuss the systematic applicability of management techniques according to the level of activities of management, let us discuss in brief the meaning and utility of some of the important techniques.

O&M

It is generally used to describe the activities of groups of people in Government or other public bodies or in private institution who asked to advise health administrators or question on the question of Organization and Method so as to increase the efficiency of work for which they are responsible, either by providing a better service, or a cheaper one or both.

PERSONAL ADMINISTRATION

Participative Management and Organizational Development (OD)

The health of an organization is measured in terms of its capability to adjust with internal and external environmental challenges. We find now-a-days that in big health organizations like hospitals, there is a lot of friction amongst the experts and other staff generating an atmosphere of frustration and low morale, resulting in the overall inefficiency. We can introduce the technique of OD in such large hospitals to maintain the healthy atmosphere in health institutions. A comprehensive definition of OD has been given by Backhard. According to him:

> "Organizational Development is an effort: (1) Planned; (2) Organization wide; (3) Managed from the top to; (4) Increase organization effectiveness and health through; and (5) Planned interventions in the organizations; Processing using behavioural science knowledge."[15]

OD depends upon the purely internal initiative of the employees of an organization. The present emphasis in health administration is only on structural changes but structural changes without personnel dedication and capabilities would be of no avail. It is high time that we introduce OD in all our big health institutions to ward off the bureaucratic attitudes which result in low output and stagnation. We have also the other technique to achieve this objective, e.g. Management by Objectives, Participative Management. We must try to integrate all these techniques for optimizing the efficiency of personnel in an organization.

The most important task of Personnel Department must be to give abundant evidence of its belief that personnel in an organization are key to development. This requires proper motivation of the employees. Motivation is of utmost importance as it constitutes the base for the management functions of planning and organising. It has been noticed that the performance of the personnel either as individuals or members of a group is less as compared to their capabilities in terms of skills, abilities, and capacities. Finer, for example, states that demonstrated performance generally never exceeds more than fifty per cent of the individual's ability to perform.[16] Most individuals tend to balance their efforts around an assessment of relative costs (time and energy) and benefits.[17] A climate of creativity must be developed and maintained by management. Maier and Hayes say that the optimal climate for creativity . . . in whatever human conditions is optimal for individual freedom and self-expression in social setting.[18]

It is the duty of the officers of such units to make the employees feel that their work and their association with a given organisation represent a vehicle which will accelerate the achievement of personal goals as well as the achievement of goals of the organisation. This would require the active participation of the employees in the decision-making process of the organisation.

> "Participation is . . . an individual's mental and emotional involvement in a group situation that encourages him to contribute to group goals and to share responsibility for them."[19]

Management Information System

The significance of information for administration can be compared to what Napoleon said about the army: "an army marches on its stomach, any administration marches on information. As the universe is saturated with information, health administration must select pertinent information for their programmes otherwise it is difficult to make any rational policy or decision. This technique is tailored to provide such information to the decision-makers which is most relevant, accurate, complete, concise, timely, economic, reliable and efficient.[20] A good information system provides data for monitoring and evaluating the programmes and gives the requisite feedback to the administrators and planners at all levels.[21]

The development of a suitable technique for a health information system would improve the capacity of health administrators to make appropriate policy-decisions. The information system may not serve the purpose if the health administrators are not committed to use the information constructively. The health administrators should use the available information sensibly and logically rather than construct complex information system which may not be used.

ABC Analysis

It is a technique which would enable a busy executive to chase those activities ardently which would quicken the wheels of administrative machinery. By arranging his work into an order of priorities, he can decide on which items to concentrate first, which others to deal later, and yet which others to delegate to his assistants. When done more systematically and in quantitative terms, this system of building up priorities of work is called the ABC Analysis. ABC Analysis can be of great use in dealing with materials management in hospitals. Forty to sixty per cent of the total expenditure of an organization is generally spent on materials. The other form of ABC Analysis is VED, i.e., arranging the activities in the orders of Vital, Essential and Desirable.

Network Analysis (PERT/CPM)

Both the Critical Path Method (CPM) and Programme Evaluation and Review Technique (PERT) emphasize efficient performance and temporal dimensions of a project. In the simplest form of PERT, a project is viewed as a total system and consists of setting up of schedule of dates for various stages and exercise of management control, mainly, through project status reports, on its progress. The CPM is basically a technique to reduce the time required to implement a project. By breaking the project into activities that must be undertaken for its implementation and by determining their time sequence, it is possible to isolate the most critical activities in the project and to compute the critical path schedule for their implementation. Network planning provides the basis for both CPM and PERT.[22]

Moder and Philips enlist the following key advantages of using PERT:

1. It encourages logical discipline in planning, scheduling and control of projects.
2. It encourages more long-range and detailed project planning.
3. It provides a standard method of documenting and communicating Project Plans, Schedules and Time and Cost Performance.
4. It identifies the most critical elements in the Plan, thus focusing management attention on the 10-20 per cent of the project that is most constraining on the schedule.
5. It illustrates the effects of technical and procedural changes on overall schedules.[23]

The application of PERT/CPM can be profitably utilised in the

Programmes and Projects of Health, e.g., construction of Hospitals, Eradication of Communicable Diseases, Family Planning Programmes, Administration of Environmental Programmes, etc. Care should be taken that the cost of the PERT/CPM should not take away large resources of the Project.

Cost Benefit Analysis

This technique is designed to consider the social costs and benefits attributable to the project. The benefits are expressed in monetary terms to determine whether a given programme is economically sound, and to select the best out of several programmes. Its advantage lies not in making decision-making simpler, but in its possibilities for systematic examination of each part of a problem in hand, for putting diverse decision on a para and following logical sequence.[24]

Cost-Benefit Analysis is an aid to systematic thought and helps the planners to decide as to what should be done—on the relative merits of different programmes. How far, for example, should resources be devoted to health education or maternal and child health services or immunization against particular disease? Any given budget for health may be distributed between programmes by including, first, those with the highest ratio of benefits to cost, then those with the next larger and so on, until the budget is fully allocated. The limitation of this method in the field of health administration is that it is difficult to express the benefits in monetary terms. We must encounter this limitation by making our tools of research methodology perfect.

Cost-Effective Analysis

Cost effectiveness methods are those that search for the least costly way of achieving a defined result. Cost effectiveness analysis are easier to make as the aim is clear. It helps the health administrator in managing his health resources at the local level. The problem is to find the way of achieving the objective at lowest cost, e.g., to find effective ways of treating patients without sending them to hospital. Linear Programming can help in this direction.

Systems Approach

A system is an integrated assembly of interacting elements, designed to carry out cooperatively a pre-determined function. There are five major elements in a system approach—selecting objectives, desiring alternatives, building models, weighing cost against effectiveness and the application of suitable criterion. It can be represented with the help of a diagram.

The application of systems analysis is useful in health management in that it provides for:[25]

1. consideration of all variables, over and above the biological and technical, that affect health intervention programmes;

2. a planning approach that relates input to output;
3. an emphasis on quantification;
4. rigour in analytical methods;
5. orientation towards health problems rather than towards categories of service;
6. communication with key governmental decision-making centres that utilised comparable methods;
7. early attention to planning and priority setting;
8. improved inter-disciplinary collaboration; and
9. the use of wide range of analytical models and methods of considerable power.

Application of Management Techniques for Administrative Improvement and Administrative Reforms

Having discussed the importance and utility of some of the important Management Techniques, we shall explain the application of the management techniques at different levels of management to situations' covering time horizons with the help of a chart.

The chart reveals that one technique or the other is applied in the form or the other at all the three levels of management. Because the lowest level has to perform operational functions, management techniques like: World Study, Network Analysis, Capacity Utilisation Studies are adopted. At the middle level, where the policy is executed, some more important techniques like Manpower Planning, Cost Benefit Analysis, Statistics and Forecasting, etc., are applied to effect improvements. The top managements uses more strategic techniques like Technological Forecasting, Performance Budgeting, Operational Research Studies, etc.

Utility and Limitation

Utility

Let us explain the use of these techniques in improving the health services with some examples:

1. In a case study, a 750-bedded hospital (Medical Institute) was facing acute shortage of nursing personnel. The study of the utilisation of nursing personnel in this hospital revealed that 33 per cent time of the nurses was being spent on non-nursing duties. Besides, there was 25 per cent turnover of the nurses. There was a great delay in appointing the new incumbents. The study suggested that if the nurses are not given non-nursing duties, a saving of rupees three lakhs can take place. This was studied with the help of the techniques of organizational analysis.
2. A study was conducted by the writer of a University Health Centre where there was a problem of pilferage of drugs. The

Chief Medical Officer of the Centre was finding it very difficult to plug this loop-hole as he himself was busy in examining the patients for all the duty time. It was suggested that the whole stock of the medicine may be classified on the basis on the cost with the help of the technique of ABC analysis. It was suggested to the Chief Medical Officer to keep N category of drugs under lock and key to be issued only under his signature. He could check for other drugs once a month concentrating only on A and B categories. This helped the Centre to save about Rs. 25,000 annually.

3. A study was carried out by C.R. Prasad on the 'Application of Quantitative Methods in Hospital Management'. He studied the problems of patients who were wasting a lot of their time to get the prescriptions, (to pay the cash and to receive the medicine). The patients had to stand in line for about 45 minutes. Prasad applied Sampling Techniques and used Simulation Procedures. He was able to suggest a model by which the average time of waiting could be reduced to 16 minutes from 45 minutes.[26]

The examples of the use of other techniques would be taken up in the relevant chapters.

Thus, we find that there is an ever-increasing array of methods and techniques available to assist the management for the acceleration of socio-economic development, with stated policies, objectives and priorities. Further, the impact of interdependence of the management techniques solely depend upon the development of improved management. But it is generally acknowledged that the availability and application of modern management skills do not meet the needs that are felt to exist.

Shortage and difficulties for the grater development and application of management skills are always encountered. Some of them are as under:

1. Shortage of experts in management techniques, and especially of those with knowledge and experience of the special problems of the health sector;
2. Difficulty in recruiting staff to specialise in health management and managerial technologies because of working conditions or lack of career prospects for personnel other than physicians;
3. Shortage of general management capability, together with lack of appreciation of 'systems thinking' and orientation to modern management on the part of doctors and health administrators;
4. Insufficient ability to identify situations in which the available consultants and other sources of expertise could best be used;
5. Lack of a form of organization that can fully utilize the available management skills;
6. Shortage of staff of various kinds (not just those with specific management skills);

7. Shortage of teachers in management for medical schools, etc.; and
8. Insufficient development of management methods for dealing with such difficulties, characteristic of health services as: defining objectives, public participation, coordination, motivation and supervision.

From the above, it is inferred that there is a room for improvement to make simultaneous progress on several fronts by:

(a) spreading the determination to overcome the difficulties mentioned and establishing confidence in using techniques;
(b) general management training and experience for health professionals;
(c) production of management specialists of various kinds, especially those with a broad experience in addition to their specialist skill;
(d) organisational changes necessary to utilize management skills and provide appropriate career and working conditions for their practitioners; and
(e) research and development to adapt management techniques to the health needs.[27]

No doubt, the theory of management techniques in the context of administrative improvement and administrative reforms can be learned in a classroom, from a text-book or through correspondence, but, these cannot replace the practical experience, only through which one acquires the skill of the technique.

CRITICAL APPRAISAL OF MANAGEMENT TECHNIQUES

Although the needs for modern management technology differ from country to country and from situation to situation, it is not to be expected that these differences will always be accurately interpreted, or that the most appropriate techniques will automatically be invoked. In fact, technique like most other things, as susceptible to the influences of fashion. Their value depends on the circumstances in which they are applied. In other words, the use of management techniques, just as the exploitation of any other resources, have to be subject to continuous feedback and review.

There have been many instances when in a hurry to borrow from West, we blindly adopt the management techniques/technology in the 'as-it-is' form without even taking into consideration their limitations. John Argenti in one of his papers observes that "after all, many of the sophisticated techniques have not been employed by a great number of organizations in U.K.—we should not blindly employ the technique. We should be sure of its potentialities and also skilled in its use." This means that suitable technology has to be devised to provide for decent health care to the people much more economically than the affluent and advanced countries. Thus, there is a need to evolve appropriate management techniques and technology to suit our environment.

Modernizing Health Administration requires outstanding leadership. Eminent Industrialist, Mr. Rahul Bajaj, Chairman and Managing Director, Bajaj Auto Limited and President, CII, delivered, the Convocation Address at the 49th, Annual Convocation of the SNDT Women's University, Mumbai. He said, "To realize our goals and aspirations, we need outstanding leadership in every field and at every level. Leadership means that there is no field at every level. Leadership means that there is no substitute for excellence, no tolerance of mediocrity and no compromise with integrity. Leadership is not just charisma, not public relations, not showmanship: Leadership is performance, consistent behaviour and trust-worthiness."

We are in a hurry; we wish to achieve much; we cannot afford the luxury of wasting our resources for experimentation. What is, therefore, needed is a proper identification of opportunities, setting out of priority areas and accordingly, continually devising technology and techniques appropriate to our set-up, our value system and technologies that are compatible. The call is, therefore, to stress on the 'know-why' rather than just on the 'know-how' of techniques and technology. This can materialize only when we bear in mind the following motto:

THE RIGHT TECHNIQUE/TECHNOLOGY
AT THE RIGHT PLACE
AT THE RIGHT TIME
AT THE RIGHT COST
BY THE RIGHT METHODS/MEANS
BY THE RIGHT PERSONNEL

Notes and References

1. Milton Greenabitt, Myron Sharaf R. and Evelyn Stone M, Dynamics of Institutional change, Pittsburgh University Press, Pittsburgh, 1971, pp. 239-40,
2. All India Radio Broadcast, June 26, 1966; Selected Speeches of Mrs Indira Gandhi, January 1966 to Aug. 1969, Publication Division, March, 1971.
3. W.H.O.: Public Health Paper, 55, p. 68.
4. UN: "Inter-regional Seminar on Administration of Management Improvement Services", Vol. I, Copenhagen, Denmark, Oct. 1970, p. 24.
5. UN: United Nations Programmes in Public Administration (E/4296-ST/TAO/M/38), pp. 11-12.
6. UN: Official Record of the Economic and Social Council (E.1708), Agenda Item No. 10, p. 3.
7. UN: Inter-regional Seminar on Administration of Management Improvement Services.
8. Earnest Dale and L.C. Michelon, "Modern Management Techniques", Penguin Books, 1974, p. 9.

9. Legisias V. Gabriel: College of Public Administration, University of Philippines, "Administrative capability as a neglected dimension in the implementation of development programme and projects", Seventy General Assembly and Conference of EROPA on Implementation, the Problem Achieving Results, 24-31 October, 1973, Vol. III, pp. 3-14.
10. Saul M. Katz: A Methodological note on apprising administrative capability for development" (UN Publication, Salr No. E-69 II. 4-2), p. 8.
11. *Ibid.,* pp. 99-100.
12. World Health Organisation, Regional Office of South-East Asia, New Delhi (SEAI RC/26, pp. 31-32).
13. ILO: "Introduction to Work Study, Geneva, 1969, p. 26.
14. M.J. Clay, General Theory of Management Techniques, Part I, in Work Study and Management Services, London.
15. R. Bechhard: Organization Development: Strategies and Models, Addison-Wesley, 1969, p. 9.
16. H. Finer: Theory and Practice of Modern Government, p. 106.
17. Eli Ginzberg: "Perspectives on Work Motivation", *Personnel,* Vol. 31, (No. July), 1959, pp. 48-49.
18. Norman Mairer, R.F. and Hayes John, J., Creative Management (New York: John Wiley and: Sons, Inc. 1962), p. 36.
19. Davis Keith: "The Case for Participative Management"; *Business Horizon,* Vol. 6, No. 3 (1963), p. 141.
20. Walters, Albert F.: "Management and Motivation: Releasing Human Potential", *Personnel,* Vol. 39, No. 2 (March-April, 1962), pp. 8-16 as reprinted in Harold Koontz and Cyrill O'Donnel, Management: A Book of Redings (New York: McGraw-Hill Book Company, 1964), pp. 382-83.
21. For details refers: Information Systems for Modern Management by Murdicks Robert G. and Ross, Joel E., Prentice-Hall of India (P) Ltd., Delhi, 1977.
22. For details see: PERT and CPM—Principles and Applications by Srinath, L.S., Affiliated East-West Press, Delhi, 1975.
23. J. Joseph, Moder and Cecil, Phillips R.: "Project Management with CPM and PERT" (New York: Reinhold, 1(4), pp. 5-6.
24. For details see: Cost-Benefit Analysis in Administration by Trevor Newton, George Allen and Unwin, London, 1972, and Weisbrod, B.A., "Concepts of Costs and Benefits," in Chanse, S., Problems in Public Expenditure Analysis, Washington, D.C., Brookings, 1968, pp. 257-62; and Williams, A., "The Cost-Benefit Approach," *British Medical Bulletin,* 30, 252-56 (1974).
25. WHO Technical Report Series, 596, "Application of System Analysis and Health Management", 1976, pp. 7-8.
26. *World Health,* Paper 55, *op. cit.,* p. 61.
27. William Newman, H. *et. al.,* The Process of Management, (Englewood Cliffs, N.J. Prentice Hall, 1976, pp. 338-45.

10

Organisational Structure and Working of AIIMS: A Case Study

INTRODUCTION

The All India Institute of Medical Sciences (AIIMS) was established by an Act of Parliament in 1956 as an institution of national importance. Its main objectives are to develop patterns of teaching in undergraduate and postgraduate medical education in all its branches, so as to demonstrate a high standard of medical education to all medical colleges and other allied institutions in India; to bring together in one place educational facilities of the highest order for the training of personnel in all important branches of health activity; and to attain self-sufficiency in postgraduate medical education.

For pursuing academic programmes, the AIIMS has been kept outside the purview of the Medical Council of India. The Institute awards its own degrees. The AIIMS continues to be a leader in the field of medical education, research and patient care in keeping with the mandate of the Parliament. The Institute is fully funded by the Government of India. However, for research activities, grants are also received from various sources including national and international agencies. While the major part of the hospital services are highly subsidized for the patients coming to the AIIMS hospital, certain categories of patients are charged for treatment/services rendered to them.

Institute Body

It consists of 20 members with Health Minister as Chairman, Two Members from Lok Sabha, one member from Rajya Sabha, Secretary Health and Family Welfare (Ex-officio), Director-General of Health Service (Ex-Officio), Additional Secretary and Financial Adviser (Ex-officio) Ministry of

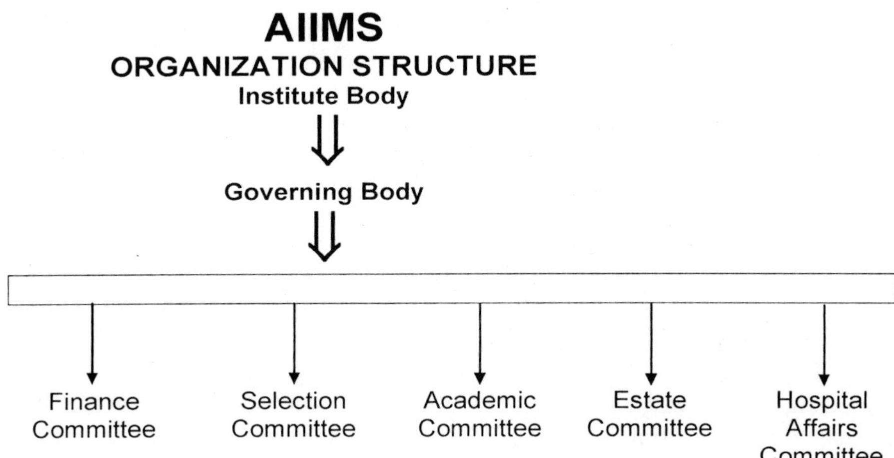

Health and Family, one Joint Secretary, Ministry of Health and Family Welfare, Sectary of Department of Biotechnology, Secretary Secondary and Higher Education and other Experts from AIIMS and other places. From the composition of AIIMS Institute body it appears that the body is dominated by Ministry and other Government functionary. Its composition should reflect top persons of health who can contribute to the development of the Institute. Minster of Health and Family Welfare, GOI, should not be put as Chairman as in his presence, other members' freedom is limited. Since this is top body of the Institute, it should be occupied by eminent persons in different areas of medicine. Same should apply to Governing Body and its Committees.

Governing Body has 10 members with Health Minister as the Chairperson with 9 other members including Director as Member Secretary. All the committees have nine members.

The Organizational structure of AIIMS appears to be under strict control of the Ministry of Health and Family Welfare. The development of such an apex institution of national importance need be granted autonomy otherwise there can very less innovation and creativity without which AIIMS cannot grow to International standard. The Ministry of Health and Family Welfare should exercise policy control and not interference in day-to-day affairs.

FUNCTIONS

1. Undergraduate Education

Academic section handles post-admission formalities for new students, develops and revises curricula, and administers teaching programmes including internal assessment of undergraduate students. The courses include MBBS, B.Sc. (Hons) in paramedical courses such as Medical Technology in Radiography and Ophthalmic Techniques, and B.Sc. Nursing (Post-certificate) and B.Sc (Hons) Nursing courses.

Every year 50 students are admitted to the MBBS course. Out of 50 seats, 5 seats are reserved for foreign nationals and the screening and admission for these 5 seats is done on the recommendation of the Ministry of External Affairs, Government of India. For the remaining 45 seats (7 for Scheduled Caste, 4 for Scheduled Tribe and 34 general category candidates), students are selected on the basis of their performance in an All-India entrance examination. Further, 3% seats are reserved for orthopedic physically handicapped candidates on horizontal basis. During 2006 there were 52,798 applicants and 38,516 candidates appeared in the entrance examination for these 45 seats. The total number of undergraduate students as on 31 March 2005 was 260 including 54 interns.

In addition, 17 Students of B.Sc. Nursing (post-certificate) course including one foreign national, 51 students to B.Sc. (Hons) in Nursing course including four nationals, foreign 12 students to B.Sc. (Hons) in Opthalmic Techniques including one foreign national and 7 Students to B.Sc. (Hons) in Medical technology in Radiography including one foreign national student.

The MBBS course is spread over five-and-a-half (5½) years, dividing the period to one year for pre-clinical, one-and-a-half (1½) year for para-clinical and two years for clinical subjects followed by one-year rotating internship. Para-medical courses like B.Sc. (Hons) in Nursing, Ophthalmic Techniques and Medical Technology in Radiography continued to be popular and attracted students from other countries also. The curricula of these courses are under constant scrutiny by the faculty of the Institute for purposes of improvement.

2. Postgraduate Education

The Academic Section looks after all activities pertaining to admission, selection and training of postgraduate students including junior and senior residents. It also deals with all service matters relating to senior residents. It handles all activities of the Ph.D., DM, M.Ch, MD, MS, MDS, MHA, MSc and MBiotech courses in different disciplines.

The admission to all postgraduate courses is done by an All India entrance examination that is held twice a year. Foreign nationals are also admitted through an entrance examination. Postgraduate students from Nepal are admitted under a bilateral agreement between the Governments of India and Nepal.

During 2006-07 session (i.e. for the courses commencing in January 2006 and July 2006), 333 students were admitted to various postgraduate, post-doctoral and superspeciality courses, i.e. MD, MS, MDS, MDA, Ph.D., M.Ch, DM and M.Sc. in various specialities. 24 candidates belonging to Scheduled Caste, and 9 candidates belonging to the Scheduled Tribes got admission to the postgraduate courses. The Institute provides full time postgraduate and post-doctoral courses in 57 disciplines. In the year 2004, 193 postgraduate students including DM/M.Ch for various degrees in December 2006 and May 2006 and 29 students qualified for Ph.D. degrees from October 2005 to September 30, 2006. The guiding principle in postgraduate training is to train them as teachers, researchers and above all as competent doctors to manage and treat the patients independently. 290 candidates from various organizations and State Government received short-term training at various departments of the Institute during the year.

Following are the important departments of Excellence:

1. Dr. R.P. Centre for Ophthalmic Sciences.
2. Department of Neuro-Radiology
3. Dr. B.R.A. Institute Rotary Cancer Hospital
4. Department of Psychiartry
5. Department of Radio-Diagnosis
6. Department of Forensic Medicine and Toxicology
7. Department of ENT
8. Department of Obstetrics and Gynaecology
9. Department of Urology
10. Department of Pediatric Surgery
11. Department of Pediatrics
12. Department of Orthopaetics.

3. Continuing Medical Education

The Institute organized a number of workshops, symposia, conferences and training programme in collaboration with various national and international agencies during the year. Professionals from various institutions all over the country participated in these seminars and workshops and benefited with updated knowledge. Guest and Public Lectures were organized by visiting experts and faculty of AIIMS.

4. Short and Long-term Training Programmes

The Academic Section handles activities regarding training programmes of short-and long-term duration for both medical and paramedical personnel. During the year, the Institute had 464 short- and 10 long-term trainees. In addition, 14 short-term trainees under the WHO fellowship programme and 18 foreign trainees and 53 (out of 72 candidates) fellows under the WHO In-Country Fellowship (2004-05) were imparted training in various departments. The elective posting of foreign undergraduate medical students is also handled by the section. During the year, 56 foreign undergraduate medical students underwent elective training.

5. Training for Scheduled Castes (SC) and the Scheduled Tribes (ST)

The SC and ST candidates are given due consideration and weightage in accordance with the Government of India guidelines in all selections. During the current year 32 SC/ST candidates were selected for various undergraduate courses, i.e. MBBS, B.Sc. Nursing (Hons), B.Sc. (Hons) Radiography. 33 SC/ST candidates selected for various postgraduate courses, i.e. MD, MS, MHA, M.Sc. (Nursing) and M.Sc. in various other disciplines during the year 2006.

6. Research

The All India Institute of Medical Sciences is a leader in the field of teaching and research which are conducted in 50 disciplines, having more than 1300 research publications by its faculty and researcher in a year 2005-06, besides publishing books. Over 385 research projects are continuing during this period. Research grants totaling to Rs. 8.20 crores (Approx.) has been received from various international and national funding agencies during the year 2006-07 (w.e.f. 01.04.2006 to 30.09.2006).

7. Patient Care Services

AIIMS being a premier tertiary care hospital caters not only to the patients from India but also from neighbouring countries like Nepal, Bangladesh, Sri Lanka, Bhutan and other Asian Countries. At present it has an OPD attendance of over 16,30,479 inpatients admission of over 83,559 and conducts more than 86,081 surgical procedures in a year (2005-06).

8. Budget

During the year 2006-07 the Institute has been provided Rs. 205.86 crores under Plan and Rs. 283.00 crores under Non-Plan. Hospital is administered by Medical Suptd., Professor, Additional Professor and Associate Professor.

The AIIMS has been highly appreciated for contributing to the advancement of medical sciences. Dr. Uton Muchtar Rafei, Former Regional Director for WHO SEARO remarked that WHO in General and the South-East Asia in particular has had a long, productive and cherished relationship of close collaboration with AIIMS. Certainly the fact that we are located in the same great city helps. But the reason of our partnership goes for beyond this. We recognize AIIMS as one of the prestigious and eminent institution on medical education, health care and in health research. Several departments with AIIMS have been designated as WHO collaborative centres where research on "cutting edge" issues is called out in active collaboration with WHO. We are also working on a number of projects in Nutrition. All of these will have significant effect not only for AIIMS and India, but for the entire region and in most instances, for the people of the whole world.

Inspite of some cases of negligence as the operation of a worng eye, leaving a place of cloth in stomach after operation in a woman's stomach, and others, there have been appreciation from all sections of society. Recently the AIIMS was in limelight because of the controversy between the Director and the Minister of Health, Govt. of India. However, AIIMS can still reach the heights of academic excellence and maintain international standards, we suggest the facts and suggestions.

OUTPATIENT DEPARTMENT AND SPECIALTY CLINICS

A total of 16,30,479 patients attended the general outpatient departments and specialty clinics of the main hospital. The details of the outpatient load profile is given in Appendix III.

Inpatient Services

The hospital had maintained its tradition of services and quality of patient care in spite of the ever-increasing number of patients that come to this hospital from all over the country as well as abroad. A total of 83559 patients were admitted during the year in the various clinical units of the hospital. 86,081 surgical operations are performed. Due to non-functioning of computers, some parameters such as unit-wise average length of stay, etc. could not be compiled. The state-wise and department-wise admissions are given in Appendices IV and V. The number of surgical procedures performed during the year in different surgical disciplines is given in Appendix VI.

General Information

Total number of beds	986
General ward beds	861
Private ward beds	125

Hospital Performance Indices

	Current year	*Past year*	*Comments*
Average length of stay (days)	5.2	5.4	Indicates effective utilization of beds.
Average bed occupancy rate (%)	83.2	80.5	Indicates fair occupancy
Net death rate (%)	2.7	2.8	Indicates a low mortality rate despite the fact that a large number of critically ill patients are admitted to the hospital
Combined crude infection rate (%)	8.92	9.5	

Note: Please see Appendices I and II for details.

AIIMS is known all over the world for medical education, research, training, consultancy and tertiary health care. International specialized agencies like World Health Organisation, World Bank and other bilateral agencies have rated AIIMS very high and that is why these agencies have made AIIMS their regional centre in many areas of medical sciences.

A landmark in Delhi, the Institute attracts 9,000 patients a day in OPDs and specialty clinics. It has 50 OPDs and 152 specialty clinics (Monday to Saturday) open 300 days a year. The emergency is open 24 hours round the year and caters, on an average, to 500 to 600 patients a day. A study done by AIIMS in 2003 inferred that 26,500 vehicles are parked in the Institute everyday.

Expansion plans

As part of its redevelopment plan, the administration wants to go in for a multi-storey parking lot. The bed capacity of 2200 will be increased to 4500 when additional specialty centres come up. In the pipeline are centres for geriatric care, renal diseases, liver diseases, genetic and molecular biology, besides a surgical block and the school of public health.

AIIMS also runs a comprehensive rural health project in Ballabgarh to train MBBS students and resident doctors in community health. It also runs the National Drug Dependence Treatment Centre in Ghaziabad.

Rated as the best teaching institute among the medical colleges by two magazine surveys, AIIMS enrolls 50 MBBS students every year from the total of more than 75,000 who appear for the MBBS entrance examination. Of these, five seats are reserved for foreign nationals and 13 are reserved. In the postgraduate entrance examination, about 30,000 doctors appear for 270 seats.

CRITICAL APPRAISAL

I. Eminent Faculty Members feel Frustrated and Disenchanted Leaving the Prestigious Institute: Need of Retention

AIIMS claims to publish 1300 to 1400 papers in national and international journals and 25 to 30 books every year. In its glorious days, till mid-1970s, AIIMS was compared to Mayo and Cleveland Clinic. Professor S.N. Mehta, former Head of the Department of Surgery at AIIMS says, "The Parliament and the government should take some concrete measures to preserve AIIMS. Such institutes are made once in the life of a nation."

A large number of poor and semi-literate patients, in the words of a former faculty member, "are kicked around", though the hospital administration insists that the hospital is pro-poor. They cite *Newsweek's* report of October 2006 describing AIIMS as "an oasis for India's poorest," which says that 3.5 million patients were treated in AIIMS in 2005.

A former faculty member whose association with AIIMS is as old as the institute says, "AIIMS is still the best. There is overcrowding because we are paying the price for our popularity, credibility and professionalism. The image has suffered because of the number of patients. It has reached a saturation point in terms of the number of patients attending the OPD, emergency and the hospital for surgeries."

On the burden on AIIMS, Anoop Saraya, Convener of the AIIMS Front of Social Consciousness, says: "It is up to the government to create proper infrastructure at the periphery so that people don't come to the Institute for minor ailments, otherwise this tertiary care centre will crumble under the workload. Around 8,000 to 10,000 patients come to the Institute every day. At times, I examine 100 patients a day stretching the OPD till 3 pm. So do other doctors."

In the last three years, more than half a dozen senior faculty members have left AIIMS. Last summer, three senior, high-profile doctors associated with AIIMS for nearly three decades, left. They left because they were disillusioned with the system.

Professor V.S. Mehta, Chief of Neurosciences Centre, and Dr. Anoop Misra from the Department of Medicine, bid adieu to the institute in April last year. Four months later, Professor S.N. Mehta, Head of the Department of Surgery and Chief of Kidney transplant services quit and joined Indraprastha Apollo Hospital as a senior consultant. He said, "I had ceased to enjoy my work for almost two years and decided to consider the offers that were coming my way. In my 27 years of association with AIIMS, I had never seen an administration that was so indifferent to the needs of the department and the institute." In May 2005, Dr. Sabyasachi Bal, lung surgeon quit his job as he felt he had not got a fair deal from AIIMS. Professor V.S. Mehta, Director of Neurosciences at Paras Hospital, Guragon left AIIMS on April 1 last year as he was "disgusted with the work environment." Dr. Sandeep Vaishya, Additional Professor, Department of Neurosurgery, left AIIMS in March last year after 14 years of service to join Max Super-Specialty hospital in Saket as Senior Consultant, Neurosurgery and Spine Surgery. "I wanted a fresh challenge. The gradual change in the work environment at AIIMS was disheartening." Dr. Anoop Misra, Director, Diabetes and Metabolic Diseases Department, Fortis Hospital, Saket, quit the Department of Medicine. "When I joined AIIMS as an undergraduate in 1978, it offered a very good learning platform. The students were very bright. The caliber of students is now second rate. The best students are no longer opting for medicine."[1] We suggests here the following:

1. Faculty is the life of the Institute. AIIMS is known by its eminent faculty. The Ministry of Health and Family Welfare should provide incentives to faculty to retain their services.
2. Faculty should engage itself in its work and not engage in politics and try to be favorate to politicians and their relatives.
3. Faculty must attend to their teaching assignment whole heartedly so that excellent doctors can be prepared.
4. Faculty should inculcate ethical values in students as medical profession is coming under great criticism because of its material approach.
5. Faculty should keep themselves upto date and take the patient care seriously.

6. Faculty should not try to be popular with MD, MS students but should make them work serious as they would imbibe the approach taught to them.

2. No Political Interference

The medical experts working in AIIMS do not belong to any party except their discipline and specialisation. The faculty of AIIMS must be allowed to carry out their work without any political interference. Since AIIMS is located in the capital city of Delhi where VVIPS are in large number. There is no harm in giving best treatments to them but they should not ignore the poor patients who have come from long distances with some hope which should be fee filled otherwise AIIMS would become only a tertiary hospital of VVIPS. It is suggested that the personnel working in AIIMS must keep themselves away from politics and concentrate on their specialisation in theory and practice.

Politicians in India interfere in the day-to-day work of such an institution of national importance. Political interference demoralizes the Director and employs and ultimately ruin the institution and act as road blocks in the progress of the institution. During the last two years, AIIMS has been in the news and there has been bad news daily about the institute. Even courts have to interfere to protect the institute from deteriorating. However, political interference went on increasing causing a great damage to this institute.

A Case Study of the Director of AIIMS

For a long time, Health and Family Planning Minister, Government of India was determined to remove Director AIIMS on whimsical grounds. However, he failed to do so because of the intervention of the Court.

The bill was moved following a Delhi High Court ruling of March 29, 2007, which held that the appointment to the director's post was a tenure appointment and could not be curtailed except for justifiable reason and with prior notice to the director.

The court had also directed the centre and the AIIMS's governing body to formulate a policy covering the various facets and conditions of service of its employees, including the director, in accordance with law and to uniformly apply such policy in the future.

The Congress-led UPA government today forced its way and got the AIIMS Bill passed, which indirectly seeks to remove AIIMS director Dr. P. Venugopal, passed in the Rajya Sabha amid pandemonium and strong protest from the opposition.

Rajya Sabha Deputy Chairperson K. Rahman Khan had to adjourn the House twice as vociferous opposition members trooped into the well of the House to prevent the bill from being passed.

The opposition members belonging to the BJP, AIADMK, TDP and the Trinamool Congress shouted that the government was trying to destroy the premier medical institution by pushing through such a bill.

However, when the House reassembled, Khan allowed union health minister Ambumani Ramodass to seek the passage of the bill through voice vote amid pandemonium and slogan shouting by opposition members.

The AIIMS and the Post-Graduate Institute of Medical Education and Research (Amendment) Bill, 2007 has now got the Parliamnet's nod as the Lok Sabha has already passed it.

The bill, seeking to amend the AIIMS Act, 1956 and the Post-Graduate Institute of Medical Education and Research, Chandigarh Act, 1966, was introduced in Parliamnet on August 17.

Justifying the bill, Ramadoss who made his statement amid persistent slogan shouting from the opposition members said the bill would streamline the functioning of AIIMS, New Delhi, and the PGI, Chandigarh.

Earlier as soon as the House reassembled at 3.10 p.m. after two adjournments, opposition members rose on their feet, raising slogans: "Loktantra ki hatya band karo" (stop the killing of democracy), "sansad mein manmani nahi chalegi" (whims and fancies of government will not be allowed in parliament).

Amid din, Samajwadi Party leader Amar Singh, who heads the Parliamentary Standing Committee on Health, regretted that the bill was introduced without consulting the committee.

"I am not opposed to the bill. I am only opposed to the manner, in which the bill has been introduced in the House," he said, and sought the protection of the Chair to ensure that it did not turn into a precedent.

Even as Ramadoss continued his reply on the bill, BJP member from Orissa Rudranarayan Pani moved menacingly towards the health minister, forcing members of treasury benches to stop him. He tore the copy of the bill. Some AIADMK members even tore off the copy of the bill.

The bill seeks to fix the term of the director for five years or till he/ she attains the age of 65, whichever is earlier.

Dr. Venugopal turned 65 in July this year, and with the director and the health minister not having a cordial relationship amongst each other, the bill has become an utmost priority for Ramadoss.

Once this bill becomes law, it will also empower the central government to terminate the services of the director even before his term expires for the sake of public interest[2].

AIIMS docs to resume strike, OPD shout today.

Hindustan Times, Thursday, November 29, 2007, Jaya Shroff, November 28, New Delhi, said in his article:

"If the bill is signed, entire AIIMS will be paralyzed," said Dr. Harsh Kumar, president, RDA. "The situation is worse than Pakistan. There was a lot of resistance in Lok Sabha at the time of passage of the bill. Only selected information was made available to the public. Who says we are a democratic nation?"

Over 10,000 patients may have to return without treatment from the All India Institute of Medical Sciences (AIIMS) on 29th November 2007, as the Out Patient Department (OPD) will be shut.

The emergency ward too will close down when the AIIMS bill, seeking to limit superannuation age of directors of the institute, is passed in the Doctors Association (RDA).

"It is an unfortunate situation as the battle between two individual is going to affect thousands of helpless patients. But strike is absolutely inevitable." Said a senior doctor of the institute.

Hindustan Times Live Chandigarh, November 28, 2007 "AIIMS, PGIMER Bill: Things Calm" at PGI observed:

"Everybody knows that the Bill is extension of an individual's whims and fancies and we extend support to our counter-parts at AIIMS.

On a clause of removal of Directory by the government if he is not acting in public interest, Dr. Banerjee, said this would end autonomy of two premier institutes of the country. "Director would not be able to function properly since he would always feel a sword hanging over his head."

In an Editorial of *The Tribune*: Targeting a doctor.

When ministerial pique becomes a policy.

The ostensible purpose of the All-India Institute of Medical Sciences (AIIMS) and Post-Graduate Institute of Medical Education and Research (PGIMER) Bill, 2007 passed by the Rajya Sabha on Wednesday and the Lok Sabha earlier may be to fix the age and tenure of the directors of these two premier medical institutions situated in Delhi and Chandigarh, respectively. But the real purpose is only to fix the head of AIIMS P. Venugopal by law or otherwise at the instance of the recalcitrant Health Minister A. Ramdoss who has been engaged in a running feud with the eminent surgeon. When nothing else worked, the minister has managed to bring in a Bill which will ensure that the heart surgeon will have to bow out. What is worse is that the minister, who is unable to swallow his pride bordering arrogance, and is hell-bent on throwing out Dr. Venugopal. That should be the first time that a Bill has been brought in to show the door to an eminent doctor who has given new life to thousands of people. That is a dangerous precedent unfit for a democracy. Dr. Venugopal has challenged the decision, saying that it smacked of mala fide and arbitrariness.

Politician's depredations have played havoc with the nation's leading institute. The only way to bring it back on the rails is by giving it autonomy, freeing it from ministerial whims. It should be run by professionals and the government should have nothing to do with its day-to-day affairs.

But the new Bill is a step in exactly the opposite direction. It will push AIIMS even further under the thumb of the minister who is not going to be in the saddle all the time. That is an unacceptable situation, particularly when the minister happens to be as erratic as Dr. Ramadoss. The PMK representative is not likely to understand on his own that AIIMS is not his personal fiefdom. The Prime Minister may have to intervene to ensure that an institute like AIIMS does not suffer. The doctors of the institute are agitated. But they too should not do anything, which inconveniences the public[3].

S.S. Negi, Legal Correspondent, *The Tribune*, Chandigarh on Friday, November 30th, 2007, "Venugopal Moves SC against new law",

NDA boycotts proceedings in RS observed:

The BJP-led opposition NDA today boycotted proceedings in the Rajya Sabha for the entire day in protest against the manner in which the Bill fixing the age of retirement of the director of the All India Institute of Medical Sciences (AIIMS) was introduced and then passed yesterday.

Immediately after the House met for the question hour, deputy leader of the opposition in the Rajya Sabha Sushma Swaraj said her party was boycotting the day's proceedings in the House in protest against the Bill passed yesterday, fixing the age of retirement of AIIMS director at 65.

The NDA decision came despite chairman Hamid Ansari's assurance that the members could raise the matter after the question hour.

The passage of the Bill paved the way for the removal of present AIIMS director P. Venugopal, who has been at loggerheads with health minister Ambumani Ramadoss over various issues.

There seems to be no end to the face off between AIIMS director P. Venugopal and health minister Ambumani Ramadoss as the noted surgeon today in a swift action moved the Supreme Court to challenge the new law curtailing the fixed five-year tenure of the directors of AIIMS and Chandigarh's PGIMER.

The powerful doctors body, Faculty Association of AIIMS, also in a separate petition challenged the AIIMS and PGIMER Amendment Act, 2007 passed by the Rajya Sabha yesterday after the Lok Sabha had passed it last week.

Both the petitions were filed in the Supreme Court Registry amid hectic activities by the lawyers of Venugopal and the faculty association of AIIMS governing body, which virtually went on tracking their move.

In a bid to strengthen his case, the noted doctor cited two rulings of the apex court pertaining to the AIIMS director's tenure in 1992 and 1996 holding it was a fixed tenure of five years.

Similarly, he also cited the two orders of the Delhi High Court of July 7, 2006 and October 18, 2006 while staying Ramadoss-sponsored AIIMS governing body's order sacking him.

Physicians, heal thyselves.

In what appears to be a personal vendetta against All India Institute of Medical Sciences (AIIMS) Director Dr. P. Venugopal, Union Health Miniser Dr. Anbumani Ramadoss has once again thrown the health facility into turmoil. The bone of contention this time is the AIIMS Amendment Bill, 2007, which the minister has pushed through in both Houses of Parliament. The Bill sets the age limit for the director at 65 or limits him to five years in office. When the President clears the Bill, the eminent cardio thoracic surgeon, who will be 66, will lose his post, something the minister has been agitating for. The Bill also provides for the removal of future directors of AIIMS with three months notice. Dr. Venugopal has already moved the Supreme Court challenging the Bill. The result of this standoff would have been the closure of OPD facilities at the institute and enormous hardship to thousands of patients had Dr. Venugopal not appealed to the doctors to refrain from disrupting work.

The Delhi High Court has taken a very serious view of the situation and warned doctors that it will not stand by if patients are harassed. The Health Minister, who should be occupied with far more pressing issues relating to the health system, has been obsessed with wresting control of AIIMS. No one can have a grouse with a government facility dictating the retirement age of its director. But after the unseemly wrangle between the director and minister, it is difficult to believe that the amendment was motivated by professional considerations. The fact that there has been little political opposition to the minister's efforts could lie in the politics behind all this. The minister is the son of S. Ramadoss, the head of the politically powerful Patali Makkal Katchi party in Tamil Nadu, which is wooed by both the major parties in the state, the DMK and the AIADMK. In the era of coalitions, no one, not even at the Centre, can alienate regional satraps like Ramadoss senior.

The minister must realize that after these shenanigans, there will be less incentive for doctors to work in the public health system, even in urban areas. All talk of attracting doctors to work in the rural health system becomes meaningless. We are rightly proud of foreigners flocking to take advantage of Indian health facilities. But when it comes to the health of our own citizens, it would seem that the government's medicine is just not working. A bitter pill that we are forced to swallow.[4]

The Case of Dr. Venugopal

It's nothing but vendetta gone wild.

Ordinarily, poets, writers, doctors and intellectuals should be treated with respect in every democratic country. The sacking of Dr. P. Venugopal from the post of Director of All India Institute of Medical Sciences within minutes of President Pratibha Patil giving her assent to the AIIMS (Amendment) Bill, however, cannot do the nation proud. Union Health Minister Anbumani Ramadoss can have the satisfaction that he could push his Bill through both Houses of Parliament to see the back of Dr. P. Venugopal. In the process, he has caused harm to the medical profession and thrown to the wind all niceties in minister-AIIMS relations. It is, perhaps, the first time that an individual-specific law has been enacted by Parliament. Even if there was a case for fixing the retirement age of the Director, the government could have implemented it with prospective effect and not focused it on Dr. P. Venugopal for satisfying the ministerial arrogance.

The heavens would not have fallen if Dr. P. Venugopal, one of India's topmost cardiac surgeons, was allowed to complete his full term of five years for which he was appointed. But to expect such etiquette from Mr. Ramadoss was not to understand the minister, who has been at the Director's neck for no other reason than that Dr. P. Venugopal did not allow ministerial interventions to scuttle the autonomy enjoyed by the premier medical institute of the country. On the other hand, the minister expected the Director to dance to his whims. The standoff between the two has been adversely affecting the functioning of the AIIMS. Yet, the Prime Minister could not take any step to rein in the minister because of the compulsions of coalition politics, much to the annoyance of the staff, students and patients of the AIIMS.

Had the MPs, who gave their nod for the controversial Bill, cared to find out the minister's motive in introducing it in such a hurry when many other issues concerning the Health Ministry do not engage his attention, they would not have fallen for it. The lack of medicines and staff in government hospitals, the pathetic health delivery system in the countryside and the death of a large number of children even before they complete five years and the prevalence of HIV/AIDS are some of the issues the minister should have ideally been tacking. Alas, he was obsessed with getting rid of Dr. P. Venugopal so that he could sleep well. That the Supreme Court will go into the question is one silver lining in the otherwise sad saga. But Parliament suddenly changing the law might cramp its inclination for justice.[5]

SC sore with Centre over Dr. P. Venugopal's hasty removal.

Describing the removal of AIIMS director Dr. P. Venugopal as "very unfortunate", the Supreme Court on Monday shot searching questions at the Centre, asking what prompted it to rush through the controversial law fixing 65 years as the age of superannuation.

"Why such a reputed person is humiliated in this way", a Bench comprising Justices Tarun Chatterjee and Dalveer Bhandari asked while questioning the motive behind bringing out an amendment to the AIIMS Act when Dr. P. Venugopal's tenure as direct was coming to an end after six months in June next.

The Bench, which was inclined towards the arguments of Dr. P. Venugopal, however, said there was "difficulty" in staying the operation of the law passed by Parliament. "Was there any necessity of bringing the amendment at this stage?" the court asked when the Centre justified its act by saying Dr. P. Venugopal was on contractual appointment and it was addressing the concern of Delhi High Court which wanted that the ambiguity in the appointment be removed by way of regulation or a statute. The Bench's annoyance over the turn of the events was further evident at the fag end of an hour-long hearing when it said, "on the facts of the case we are with Dr. P. Venugopal."

The case came up before the apex court after a bitter turf war between Dr. P. Venugopal and health minister Ambumani Ramadoss over the control of the prestigious institution. The Bench found strength in many of the arguments put forward by senior advocate Fali Nariman and Arun Jaitley, who appeared for Dr. P. Venugopal and Faculty Association of AIIMS. The advocates alleged that the amended law as "hostile" and "discriminatory" against the distinguished cardiologist.[6]

However, subsequently Dr. Venugopal was reinstated and was able to retire on completion of his term, due to judicial intervention.

3. Need of selection of the Director Purely on Merit to Provide the Leadership to the Institute

The Director of Institute should be selected on merit which is in the interest of the institute and no other extraneous considerations. It has been rightly said about the Chief Executive, "Put a good man in a bad set-up, he will make the things go through, Put a bad man in good set-up he will make the mesh of the situation." The Director must be a person who can exhibit quality of leadership to lead the institution to academic excellence.

Swami Chinmayananda feels that it is scarce to find real leaders in today's world. To quote him: But the rare few that develop a universal love and constantly engage themselves in activity under the guidance of their superior intellect, are called "man-men" and they alone can claim the prestige, dignity and glory of man. The core of the human personality is the consciousness, which is the life centre around which all the activities of the body, mind and the intellect revolve. It remains ever changeless and immovable like an axle in the wheel, but causes all changes and movements to occur. When men succeeds in identifying with this changeless, immovable conscious principle within him, he is no longer victimized by the changing phenomena of perceptions, emotions and thoughts, but becomes the Supreme Lord of them all. The intellectual pursuits, emotional attachments and physical cravings of such a man naturally wither and fall away like petals of a flower when the fruit emerges.

According to A.H. Maslow: Self-actualizing people are without one single exception involved in a cause outside their own skin in something outside of themselves. They are devoted working at something, which is very precious to them—some calling it vocation in the old sense, the priestly sense. They are working at something which fate has called them to somehow, which they work at and love, so that the work-joy dichotomy in them disappears.

Swami Chinmayananda says that a life organized for the discovery of the potentialities already exists within ourselves, and the ordering of our behaviour so as to nurture and nourish them, is a life well spent. Herein our success depends upon the amount of transformation we can successfully bring about in our personality and character. The vital question is not how many talents each one of us has, but how much of our existing talents are we capable of exploring, developing and exploiting. An individual may have many talents, and yet, he can be a miserable failure in life. That person is successful who makes a practical use of at least one great talent that he possesses. Our present and future welfare thus mainly depends upon ourselves. Let us never look outside ourselves for help. Let us not fall into the delusion that the influence of others would enable us to do better or accomplish more. All our success entirely depends upon ourselves. Let us realize these fundamentals. We must.

Eminent Industrialist, Mr. Rahul Bajaj, observes, "To realize our goals and aspirations, we need outstanding leadership in every field and at every level. Leadership means that there is no substitute for excellence, no tolerance of mediocrity and no compromise with integrity. Leadership is not just charisma, not public relations, not showmanship. Leadership is performance, consistent behaviour and trust worthiness.[7]

We must remember that it is the top men in each department who set the tone of the administration. It is they who set the example for those under them to emulate. When the acts of those at the top become tainted, when their reputation becomes shady, they will not be able to enforce high standards of integrity in those below them. It is, therefore, imperative that men at the top should exhibit the highest standards of personal integrity, probity and rectitude. As Sir Ivor Jinnings observed, the most elementary qualification demanded of a minister's is honesty and incorruptability. It is, in addition, necessary not only that he should possess this qualification but also that he should appear to possess it.

4. Need of Personnel Motivation

The most important task of an organization must be to give abundant and constant evidence of its belief that personnel in an organization are the key to development. This requires proper motivation of the employees which provides a base for the management functions of planning and organizing. It has been noticed that the performance of the personnel either as individuals or members of a group is less as compared to their capabilities in terms of skills, abilities and capacities. Finer, for example, states that demonstrated performance generally never exceeds more than fifty per cent of the individual's ability to perform. Most individuals tend to balance their efforts around an assessment of relative costs (time and energy) and benefits. A climate of creativity must be developed and maintained by management so that the performance levels know no bounds and growth becomes a way of life.

B. Rattan Reddy opines that there is no doubt that Indian Administration needs a strong core of dynamic values to transform its ethos at all levels. Laws can be enacted and rules framed to this end. Enforcement agencies can prosecute and the system can punish. This will have an impact. Nonetheless, enforcement of morality through law will largely remain an external process that can at best delineate a framework for public behaviour that should not be transgressed. But beyond that, laws or rules have inherent limitations in addressing the question of societal and individual change. As such, lasting public morality and ethics can not be forced from outside. These must take roots and grow within the system itself. People have to understand and accept it so that change becomes organic.

Motivation is a tendency which keeps a person attentively and purposefully engaged to achieve his formulated goals. This, a sense of commitment occurs only when the enterprise becomes a perpetual vehicle for the satisfaction of the dominant needs of the employees, so long as the employees strives fully to achieve the goals of the enterprise. From the above discussion, it is clear that motivation as such cannot be observed, rather it is a concept derived to cover a number of relationships having their immediate point of origin within the organism.

5. Not Effective Administration: Need of Good Governance

Though the progress in harnessing scientific and technological potentiality is good but not sufficient. There is a need of Good Governance to optimize the use of scientific and technological potentialities. Good governance can make India a knowledge super power. A brief description of scientific and technology development reveals that India is rich in her resources but these are not reaching the people and are not making much difference in enriching the life of the poor. Why? India lacks good governance and good government which cause poor delivery. The need is to promote good governance which can improve the growth of scientific and technological progress as well as can accelerate their reach to people to improve their standard of living.

A senior parliamentarian (Prof. Hiren Mukherjee) speaking of politics generally, bemoans. IT will not be far wrong to say, sorrowfully, that there never was a time in living memory when politics and politicians were, almost rightfully, as denigrated, even degraded and sometimes detested, in the eyes of our people as they are at the moment.

The work and conduct of the legislature both at the Union and State level is increasingly becoming a matter of great shame for the legislators as well as the citizens who elected them. It has taken a more serious turn as citizens are viewing their performance on T.V. The legislature passess the law relating to good governance like Right to Information Act, 2005, Consumers Protection Act, 1986 and other Important bills which are supposed to smoothen the life of the people. What can be the impact of the legislature when the members composing it are highly indiscipline, and possess no moral conduct and values? This is not specific to any party and individuals. The same behaviour is observed from the opposition to whatever party it may be.

6. AIIMS was supposed to set the standards of under-graduate and post-graduate medical education but have not been able to achieve the same so far. Need of designing the curriculum as per the need of the country

The objective of a good medical education should be to produce general practitioners, specialists, teachers and research workers. The factors governing this are the curriculum, medium of instruction, duration of course, admission qualifications, the examination system, teachers-students relationship, prospects of teachers and, students, etc. Besides, it may be mentioned that the medical education should fit in with the needs of the country and the conditions prevailing there. For instance 70 per cent of the population of India live in rural areas. The training given to the doctor should enable and motivate him to carry on his work among the vast masses in the villages. We have been designing out undergraduate and postgraduate medical education which can fulfil this basic aim. There has been a big gap between aims and fulfilment. J. Gallagher, Regional Officer for education and training, WHO Regional Office for Europe has expressed concern about inadequate communication between educational systems for health personnel and the health administrations that use the products of these systems. There is very little understanding of how the manpower training and development needs of health administrations can be met in a systematic way."[8]

The Government of India launched the Re-orientation of Medical Education Scheme in 1977 with the objective of involving the various medical colleges in the country in the direct delivery of health care services to the rural and semi-rural population. Under the scheme, each of the 106 medical colleges in the country is to accept in the first instance, the total responsibility for promotive, preventive, curative health services in three Community Development Blocks in the districts in which the institution is situated. 318 mobile clinics at the rate of 3 per college have been provided to the medical colleges to render quality services nearest to the rural population. The objectives of the scheme are:

(i) To expose the Medical faculty, residents in terms and the students to the Rural Community;
(ii) To train the students, interns and Residents in Community Organization and Community Participation; and
(iii) To render comprehensive health care services to the villages in collaboration with the local Primary Health Centres.

It has been expressed in the Fifth Plan document that teaching in medical colleges still requires a radical change for its orientation towards the need for community care. Medical education over the years, has been urban biased. It is hoped that in the Sixth Draft Plan (1978-83), it would be possible "to produce medical graduates who are aware of the health problems of the community, who have a sense of compassion and motivation to serve the public and who have ability to effectively meet the urgent needs of the health care problems of the rural masses and the urban-poor."

According to the Estimates Committee: "The National Policy should indicate in unmistakable terms the goals to be achieved and the method of accomplishment.... Such a policy especially in the context of health being a State subject will help in maintenance of the requisite standards of medical education throughout the country in keeping with the needs of the people."[9]

The Government of India has announced the National Medical Education Policy. There is a need to set-up a Health Care Medical Service Commission responsible for planning of medical manpower, medical education, research, training of all para-medical personnel would be a step in the right direction. This commission when appointed should use Health and Medical Educational Planning as a means of rationalizing the education of health manpower. Besides, the Commission may encourage the health administrations to provide the policy and planning backgrounds required for this purpose.

Medical Education must have Public Health Orientation—The pattern of medical education guided by market economy has concentrated on biological causes of the diseases and curative actions based on hospital care, drugs, surgery, etc. without any recognition of the socio–economic and environmental status of the population. Health problems in a country like ours cannot be solved only through marketing medical therapy and interventions with a curative bias by neglecting the preventive, promotive, environmental health and the community need orientation. The lack of a holistic and community-based approach to disease control over the years has further led to over emphasis on quantity rather than quality of health care resulting in erosion of trust on the quality of health care services provided by the public sector and increasing dependence of the population on the private sector. Thus, during the past five decades, despite the quantitative growth in terms of hospitals, health centres, health manpower, infrastructural support services and number of health and family welfare programmes, the public health situation has remained a cause of great concern as reflected in the mortality, morbidity, health status, urban-rural differentials and health seeking behaviour patterns of the population. This calls for re-orientation and health seeking behaviur patterns of the population. This calls for re-orientation and reorganisation of our medical and health education system with emphasis on holistic and community-based health care as well as effective and efficient administration and management of health care delivery services. Keeping in view the national needs priorities and goods for health for all, it is essential to upgrade the managerial, technological and professional skill of health manpower through appropriate changes in the course curriculums of medical and health education institutions at different levels with greater emphasis on epidemiology, computer and management disciplines.[10]

Even Health Policy 2002 reiterates:

In any developing country with inadequate availability of health services, the requirement of expertise in the areas of 'public health' and 'family medicine' is markedly more than the expertise required for other clinical specialties. In India, the situation is that public health expertise is non-existent in the private health sector, and far short of requirement in the public health sector. Also, the current curriculum in the graduate/post-graduate courses is outdated and unrelated to contemporary community needs. In respect of 'family medicine', it needs to be noted that the more talented medical graduates generally seek specialization in clinical disciplines, while the remaining go into general practice. While the availability of post-graduate educational facilities is 50 percent of the total number of qualifying graduates each year, and can be considered adequate, the distribution of the disciplines in the post-graduate training facilities is overwhelmingly in favour of clinical specializations. NHP-2002 examines the possible means for ensuring adequate availability of personnel with specialization in the 'public health' and 'family medicine' disciplines, to discharge the public health responsibilities in the country.

Health policy 1983 also stressed:

It is also necessary to appreciate that the effective delivery of health care services would depend very largely on the nature of education, training and appropriate orientation towards community health of all categories of medical and health personnel and their capacity to function as an integrated team, each of its members performing given tasks within a coordinated action programme. It is, therefore, of crucial importance that the entire basis and approach towards medical and health education, at all levels, is reviewed in terms of national needs and priorities and the curricular programmes restructured to produce personnel of various grades of skill and competence, who are professionally equipped and socially motivated to effectively deal with day-to-day problems, within the existing constraints. Towards this end, it is necessary to formulate, separately, a National Medical and Health Education Policy which (i) sets out the changes required to be brought about in the curricular contents and training programme of medical and health personnel, at various levels of functioning; (ii) takes into account the need for establishing the extremely essential inter-relations between functionaries of various grades; (iii) provides guidelines for the production of health personnel on the basis of realistically assessed manpower requirements; (iv) seeks to resolve the existing sharp regional imbalances in their availability; and (v) ensures that personnel at all levels are socially motivated towards the rendering of community health services.

A. Rajasekaran, President National Board of Examination, New Delhi, in his convocation address in *University News*, June 5-11, 2006 observed that our present system of medical education was inherited as legacy of the British. Even though beneficial to our progress it has not fulfiled the aspirations and expectations of our people particularly rural poor. Starting from Bhore Committee (1946) there were several attempt at reorientation of medical curriculum to produce a basic doctor or community physicians. Reoreintation of Medical Education (ROME Programme) of WHO for Asian countries was aimed at developing Medical Education system responsive and relevant to the needs of our country by making necessary curriculum changes.

The medical students entering the medical college is not adequately briefed on compassion and care, and learns the communiation skills and moral values. Instead his first exposure is to a cadaver in the anatomy dissection hall. Here comes the need for a preparatory course. In the present under-graduate medical education the preclinical years, which was two years earlier, has been reduced to one year to learn anatomy, physiology, Biochemistry with too much of information squeezed into the curriculum.

AIIMS can do a lot in this education but failed to do till its golden jubilee. It is high time for AIIMS to demonstrate its leadership in giving right direction to medical and health education.

7. Researches Bear no Relevance to Practical Problems: Need Action Research

There has been a lack of co-operation and co-ordination among the institutions engaged in teaching and research. This resulted in disjointed, isolated and rank duplication of scientific research in several national laboratories resulting in waste of scarce resources. The Public Accounts Committee in its 40th Report of the 5th Lok Sabha emphasised the importance of collaboration and co-ordination among various agencies engaged in medical research with ICMR taking the lead and suggested that energetic steps may be taken to enlarge the scope of collaboration to avoid repetitive research.

Besides, over the years, for a variety of reasons the medical research programmes in the country could not follow the path of problem-oriented medical research in priority areas such as nutritional disorders, control of communicable diseases, operational research for providing health care to all, research in medical education, health manpower planning, utilisation of health personnel, research in indigenous system of medicine, etc. The Sixth Draft Plan (1978-83) was also critical of the research policy pursued so far. It was stated that:

"Medical research in the past had, by and large, failed to lay emphasis on problems of immediate practical importance. Efforts were mostly towards collection of disjointed and isolated research work by individuals/agencies in the country."

The Estimate Committee in its 102nd Report pointed out that "the purpose of medical research is to bring about results of practical utility in the fight against disease with the maximum expedition possible and that little purpose will be served unless the results of research can find immediate application in the field. It is unfortunate that resources and time and talent of the medical community of the country have not been meaningfully utilised over the years according to well thought out priorities."[11] Thus, there is a need of costing of research projects in terms of time and money likely to be required for their completion. The aim of the research should be to solve health problems of the social significance to the country.

The foreign sponsorship of research projects has not been examined properly before accepting the proposals, The Public Accounts Committee in their 167th and 200th Reports have been very critical of the research projects conducted in collaboration with foreign organisations, e.g. Genetic Control of Mosquitoes Unit Projects, the Bird Migration and Arbovirus studies, the ultra low volume spray experiments, the Pantnagar Microbial Pesticides project and some of the research projects undertaken in West Bengal and Narangwal in collaboration with the John Hopkins University. The Committees are not unwilling to concede the importance of research efforts, the projects examined revealed a rather casual attitude and indifference on the part of the authorities concerned towards foreign supported research in India. The Committee reiterated the imperative need for the utmost care, caution and critical scrutiny before approving foreign sponsorship of research projects undertaken in India, particularly when such projects have military or quasi-military implications of an almost incalculable character. Such researches must be got conducted by the Indian scientists. If the foreign collaboration is indispensable, research ventures should ensure the following:

(a) that such ventures are not only of potential value for the country but are of immediate productive utility;
(b) that the objectives of the projects are clearly spelt out and the research plans are notified in advance so as to avoid any ambiguity;
(c) that the collaborating Indian agency or institution has personnel with the requisite qualification and equipment to concurrently evaluate and monitor the progress of the research;
(d) that the technical and administrative control of the projects and determination of policies vest only with the Indian agencies and personnel concerned;
(e) that all data and materials collected are shared with the Indian collaborators;
(f) that any kind of secrecy in the conduct of research is eschewed and that the results of the research are made public; and
(g) that all research is conducted in accordance not only with the country's own environmental standards but the international environmental standards as well. In the new millennium, research must also be encouraged in the areas.[12]

AIIMS can take up such research which can solve the heath problems of the country.

8. Good Relationship between Minister and Experts

AIIMS is a complex organisation which requires good governance to operate. There is shortage of staff, lack of facilities for patients, overcrowded. There is a need of good governance which can manage the problems of a complex organisation like AIIMS.

Since the minister occupies the top position in politico-administrative hierarchy. It is essential that he should have full legal and constitutional authority to administer with good governance the affairs of his department. Theoretically it is feasible but in practice, he cannot achieve much whether it is policy-making or implementation or evaluation unless he gets due co-operation, help, participation, involvement of the personnel of his department. The volume of work with the Council of Ministers at the Union and the state levels is so large and the problems so complicated that it is impossible for any number of ministers to deal with all the matters themselves. The civil servants provide all the information and analysis for the guidance of the ministers and the cabinet. The channel through which a minister must operate is the secretariat. The secretariat acts as an institutionalized memory to enable the government to examine the feasibility of the proposed policy.

Sir Warren Fisher, in a memorandum to the Tomlin Commission (U.K.) defined the duties of the civil servant *vis-a-vis* the minister as follows:

Determination of policy is the function of a minister and once a policy is determined it is the unquestioned and unquestionable business of the civil servant to strive to carry out that policy with precisely the same energy and precisely the same goodwill whether he agreed with it or not. This is axiomatic and will never be in dispute. At the same time it is the traditional duty of civil servants while decisions are being formulated, to make available to their political chief all the information and experience at their disposal, and to do this without fear or favour, irrespective of whether, the advice thus tendered by accord or not with the minister's initial view. The presentation to the minister of relevant fact, the ascertainment and marshalling of which may often call into play the whole organization of a department, demands of the civil servant the greatest care. The presentation of inferences from the facts equally demand from him all the wisdom and all the detachment he can command.

The preservation of integrity, fearlessness, and independence of Thought and utterance in their private communion with ministers of the experienced officials selected to fill the top posts in the service is an essential principle in enlightened government, as whether or not ministers accept the advice frankly placed at their disposal, and acceptance or rejection of such advice is exclusively a matter for their judgement. It enables them to be assured that their decisions are reached only after the relevant facts and the various considerations have, so far as the machinery of government can secure been definitely brought before their minds.

In the last three years, more than half a dozen senior faculty members have left AIIMS. Last summer, three senior, high-profile doctors associated with AIIMS for nearly three decades, left. They left because they were disillusioned with the system.

9. Faculty in AIIMS may Follow Code of Ethics to Maintain the Dignity and Prestige of the Institution

The document prepared by Deptt. of Administrative Reforms and public grievances has chalked out a Code of Ethics which need implementation. The objective of Code is to prescribe standards of integrity and conduct that are to apply in the public services. The principles stated below underlie and supplement the rules and laws to regulate the public and private conduct of various public services.

Selflessness: Holders of public office should take decisions solely in terms of the *Public interest*. They should not do so in order to gain financial or other material benefits for themselves, their family, or their friends.

Integrity: Holders of public office should not place themselves under any financial or other obligation to outside individuals or organisations that might influence them in the performance of their official duties.

Objective: In carrying out public business, including making public appointments, awarding contracts, or recommending individuals for rewards and benefits, holders of public office should make choice on merit.

Accountability: Holders of public office are accountable for their decisions and actions to the public and must submit themselves to whatever scrutiny is appropriate to their office.

Openness: Holders of public office should be as open as possible about all the decisions and actions that they take. They should give reasons for their decisions and restrict information only when the wider public interest clearly demands.

Honesty: Holders of public office have a duty to declare any private interest relating to their public duties and to take steps to resolve any conflicts arising in a way that protects is the public interest.

Leadership: Holders of public office should promote and support these principles by leadership and example.

These principles apply to all aspects of public life. The Committee has set them out here for the benefits of all who serve the public in any way.

10. Time Management

Tertiary hospital like AIIMS must concentrate their time on vital issues. Time is not thought of as a source. However, it is the most important and crucial factor as time is inelastic and non-renewable. An event cannot take place unless there is a time for it. Time and tide wait for none. We may keep in mind that time is neutral, i.e. it is neither good not bad by itself. Therefore, to blame the time for any inaptitude for failure will be quite unfair.

11. Lack of Effective Inter-personal Relations—Need of Harmonious Relationships

Manager of today need to be trained in understanding the inter-personal relationship and their management to insulate the organization from internal behavioural disturbances. There are three inter-personal needs, (i) inclusion—need for interaction and association, (ii) control—the need for authority and power, and (iii) affection—the need for being loved and cared. Developing a successful inter-personal relation, conducive to achievement of organizational goals, is a challenging task and a slow process. IT requires a deep psychological understanding of oneself as well as of others, with whom one comes in contact in various organizational capacities.

12. Researchers have No Impact on Hospitals

AIIMS must develop modules which can be used for practicing doctors through video conferencing so that good medical education as well as continuous medical education can be spread among doctors so that people can be benefited of modern medicine at an affordable cost. There is not doubt about the excellence of AIIMS in academic achievement. However, AIIMS failed in its mandate of making medical education suitable for rural and poor people in the country. The leadership role of AIIMS was not put into practice.

13. Recruitment of Medical Personnel, not based on Merit

The success of any institute depends on its highly talented medical personnel. To quote *The Telegraph,* dated 22 Dec. 2007 (Report covered by Charu Sudan Kastrui) clearly observed that The All India Institute of Medical Sciences (AIIIMS) used unfair practices "designed to regularize" in-house teachers to fill posts for an entire decade, a health ministry inquiry has found.

The finding suggests several candidates from outside the campus were deprived of a chance to work in India's premier medical institute.

If the ministry decides to risk charges of witch-hunt and a possible backlash, upto 70 faculty members who were promoted between 1993 and 2003 could be demoted. The AIIMS authority, called the Institute Body, accepted the inquiry report yesterday.

Government rules and court orders were flouted in appointing teachers at the institute from 1993 to 2003 under two different directors, the committee has found.

Standard government rules require institutes to publicly advertise for vacant posts, and treat outside applications on a par with those from their own teachers seeking promotions.

From 1993 to 2002, AIIMS did not advertise outside the campus for posts, instead promoting *ad hoc* appointees to full-time jobs as teachers.

During this period, 152 out of 219 *ad hoc* posts were filled "in an arbitrary manner", the committee said in its report, a copy of which is with *The Telegraph*.

"It is sad to see the manner in which the rules were flouted by successive administrations to secure a coterie that would back them under all circumstances, "a senior official on the five-member inquiry team said."

In 2003, advertisements were issued in newspapers for 170 associate professors at the institute. In all 762 people cleared the preliminary selection criteria and were called for interview. These included 151 assistant professors (a grade lower than associate professors) and 611 applicants from outside the AIIMS.

Among the 611 outside candidates were 209 reserved category candidates, the report says. But in the final selection, only 19 per cent of the seats went to applicants from outside the AIIMS, despite being "equally suitable candidates", the committee has said. "The committee concluded that the selection process lacked fairness and was designed primarily to regularize the existing *ad hoc* assistant professors in large numbers", the report said.

Seventy of those selected between 1993 and 2003 were found to have poorer credentials than many other applicants who were not picked, the committee has said. But the ministry is treading with caution on the 70for fear that it may be accused of vindictiveness—a charge leveled by an associate professor who was promoted from an *ad hoc* post in 2003.

"This is vindictiveness at its peak . . . nothing else. The health ministry is not satisfied with removing (former director), P. Venugopal, they want to remove anyone else who can challenge them", the doctor from the pathology department said.

Several of the 70 faculty members are said to be close to Venugopal, who was expelled recently as director after a turf war with health minister Anbumani Ramadoss. Although the controversial selections were made in the period just before Venugopal was appointed director, cases against the appointments were filed soon after he took over. The panel was set-up in January.

This is highly serious as it encourages in house breading and merit becomes a secondary consideration. It becomes a closed door entry, suicidal to the growth and development of an institution of National Importance.

CONCLUSION

AIIMS is doing excellent work in medicine. Its students are spread throughout the world and occupying eminent positions. In India AIIMS has contributed in making available medical faculty, eminent doctors and other paramedical staff. Even taking the name of AIIMS brings before a person an idea of excellent institution. However, AIIMS must see that this institution must benefit the common man and not remain only in ivory towers. AIIMS must meet the needs of common man at a cost which he can afford.

Notes and References

1. Tripti Nath in the *The Tribune*, Oct. 7, 2007, Spectrum "AIIMS: Ailing Institute."
2. *The Tribune*, Chandigarh, Thursday, 28th November 2007, p. 2.
3. *The Tribune*, Chandigarh, Friday, November 30th 2007, p. 10.
4. *Hindustan Times*, Chandigarh, Friday, November 30, 2007, p. 12.
5. *The Tribune*, Chandigarh, Monday, December 3, 2007, p. 10.
6. *The Economic Times*, Tuesday, 4 December, 2007, p. 2.
7. AIU, *University News*, March 13, 2000.
8. Lok Sabha Secretariat: 102nd Report, Estimates Committee, (Fifty Lok Sabha), p. 4.
9. Lok Sabha Secretariat, 102nd Report, Estimates Committees, Fifth Lok Sabha, p. 4.

10. Madhu S. Mishra, Health Policy and Management of Health Care delivery services in India—Issues and Challenge in Public Health in India: Five Decades, 50th Anniversary of India's Independence, pp. 27-28.
11. Lok Sabha Secreariate: Estimates Committee, 102nd Report, (5th Lok Sabha), New Delhi, 1975, pp. 92-94.
12. Lok Sabha Secretariat, Public Accounts Committee: Fifth Lok Sabha, 200th Report, 1976, New Delhi.

APPENDIX I

YEARLY STATISTICAL HEALTH BULLETIN

1.	Total patients admitted	80,140
	a. Adults and children	77,803
	b. Newborn infants	2,337
2.	Total number of patient care days in hospital (as per daily census)	415,931
	a. Adults and children	409,462
	b. Newborn infants	6,469
3.	Daily average number of patients	1,140
	a. Adults and children	1,122
	b. Newborn infants	18
4.	Average bed occupancy ratio (BOR)	83.2
	a. Adults and children	83.4
	b. Newborn infants	72.0
5.	Average length of stay (ALS)	5.2
	a. Adults and children	5.3
	b. Newborn infants	8.8
6.	Births in hospital	2,337
	a. Male babies	1,261
	b. Female babies	1,073
	c. Intersex	3
7.	Total deaths (including newborns)	2,908
	a. Death under 48 hours	768
	b. Death over 48 hours	2,140
	c. Gross death rate (%)	3.6
	d. Net death rate (%)	2.7

Source: 49th Annual Report, 2004-05 of AIIMS, New Delhi, p. 36

Appendix II

INPATIENT CRUDE MORTALITY STATISTICS

S. No.	Department	Admissions	Deaths			Death rate (%)	
			Total	Under 48 hours	Over 48 hours	Gross	Net
1.	Anaesthesiology	785	-	-	-	-	-
2.	Cardiology	7790	235	72	163	3.0	2.1
3.	Cardiothoracic and Vascular Surgery	3269	233	19	214	7.1	6.6
4.	Dental Surgery	209	-	-	-	-	-
5.	Dermatology	3738	8	1	7	0.2	0.2
6.	Endocrinology	474	5	2	3	1.1	0.6
7.	Gastroenterology	1868	240	49	191	12.8	10.5
8.	Gastrointenstinal surgery	701	38	2	36	5.45.2	9.
9.	General surgery	6325	180	46	134	2.8	2.1
10.	Haematology	5943	113	47	66	1.9	1.1
11.	IRCH (Private ward)	449	87	43	44	19.4	10.8
12.	Medicine	3519	575	180	395	16.3	11.8
13.	Nephrology	3394	147	46	101	4.3	3.0
14.	Neuro-anaesthesia	10	-	-	-	-	-
15.	Neurology	2514	211	30	181	8.4	7.3
16.	Neurosurgery	4322	405	103	302	9.4	7.2
17.	Newborn	2337	51	23	28	2.2	1.2
18.	Nuclear medicine	476	-	-	-	-	-
19.	Obstetrics and Gynaecology	9364	22	4	18	0.2	0.2
20.	Orthopaedics	4207	35	4	31	0.8	0.7
21.	Otorhinolaryngology	4546	17	7	10	0.4	0.2
22.	Paediatric surgery	2210	62	10	52	2.8	2.4
23.	Paediatrics	6187	189	63	126	3.1	2.1
24.	Physical Medicine and Rehabilitation	29	-	-	-	-	-
25.	Psychiatry	377	-	-	-	-	-
26.	Radiotherapy	188	36	15	21	19.1	12.1
27.	Urology	4909	19	2	17	0.4	0.3
	Total	80140	2908	768	2140	3.6	2.7

Source: *Ibid.*

APPENDIX III

ATTENDANCE IN OPDS AND SPECIALTY CLINICS

Department	*New Cases*	*Old Cases*	*Total*
1	*2*	*3*	*4*
ANAESTHESIA			
Specialty Clinics			
Pain	1,795	5,208	7,003
Pre-anaesthesia	7,045	1,349	8,394
DENTAL SURGERY			
General OPD	29,714	27,234	56,948
Specialty Clinics			
Combined cleft palate	81	346	427
Oral prophylaxis	2,112	7,456	9,568
Orthodontics	1.094	7,215	8,309
Prosthodontics-*cum*-maxillofacial prosthesis	174	2,569	4,743
Restorative-*cum*-endodontic	7,648	4,810	12,458
Trigeminal Neuralgia	128	402	530
DERMATOLOGY			
General OPD	32,907	26,517	59,424
Specialty Clinics			
Allergy	445	870	1,315
Dermatological surgery	305	665	970
Leprosy	336	1,742	2,078
Pigmentation	550	1,619	2,169
Sexually transmitted disease	1,039	1,730	2,769
ENDOCRINOLOGY	9,537	16,215	25,752
GASTROENTEROLOGY	17,925	26,161	44,086
HAEMATOLOGY	4,206	14,121	18,327
MEDICINE			
General OPD	67,000	63,389	130,389
Specialty Clinics			
Chest	1,836	4,011	5,847
Geriatric	186	813	999
Rheumatology	233	5,957	6,190
NEPHROLOGY	5,628	14,357	19,985
Renal Transplant	79	4,536	4,615
NUCLEAR MEDICINE	1,644	2,007	3,651
OBSETETRICS AND GYNAECOLOGY			
General OPD	32,749	45,511	78,260
Specialty Clinics			
Antenal	1,059	5,955	7,014
Endocrine gynaecology	154	207	361

(Contd.)

1	2	3	4
Family welfare	3,020	5,188	8,208
High-risk pregnancy	1,741	9,462	11,203
Postnatal	181	90	271
ORTHOPAEDICS			
General OPD	81,337	147,112	288,449
SPECIALTY CLINICS			
Club foot (CTEV)	248	1,164	1,412
Follow-up	-	6,703	6,703
Hand	801	1,080	1,881
Polio	73	31	104
Scoliosis	498	1,131	1,629
Tuberculosis	-	2	2
OTORHINOLARYNGOLOGY AND RUAS			
General OPD	5,305	32,227	77,532
Specialty Clinics			
Audiology	179	104	283
Hearing	675	871	1,546
Rhinology	118	58	176
Speech	1,340	851	2,191
Vertigo	109	107	216
Voice	461	573	1,034
PAEDIATRICS			
General OPD	33,493	32,208	65,701
Specialty Clinics			
Chest	478	3,256	3,734
Follow-up TB	235	1,235	1,470
Genetic and birth defects	1,287	936	2,223
High-risk neonatal	232	1,264	1,496
Neurology	1,760	4,418	6,178
Renal	492	3,265	3,757
Well baby	658	19	577
PAEDIATRIC SURGERY			
General OPD	7,486	10,624	18,110
Specialty Clinics			
Hydocephalus	31	334	365
Intersex	33	33	66
Urology	268	2476	2744
PHYSICAL MEDICINE AND REHABILITATION	12,698	9,570	22,268
PSYCHIATRY			
General OPD	1,227	-	1,227
Specialty Clinics			
Child guidance	428	205	633
Walk-in	12,783	22,999	35,782
RADIOTHERAPY			
General OPD	1,425	57,962	59,387

Specialty Clinics			
Radiotherapy in gynaecology	701	11,282	11,983
Radiotherapy in surgery	1,351	10,606	11,957
GENERAL SURGERY	34,408	24,042	58,450
UROLOGY	10,004	19,236	29,240
THERS			
Casualty	156,217	-	156,217
Employees Health Scheme	105,871	70,577	176,448
Marriage Counselling clinic	2,449	2,705	5,154
Nutrition	5,196	1,046	6,242
Total	756,806	790,024	1,546,830

Source: Ibid.

APPENDIX IV

REGION-WISE DISTRIBUTION OF INPATIENTS

Region	*Number of Patients*
Delhi	43,271
Uttar Pradesh	12,863
Haryana	9,058
Punjab	689
Rajasthan	1,548
Bihar	5,840
Other states	6,556
Other countries	315
Total	80,140

Source: Ibid.

APPENDIX V

DEPARTMENT-WISE DISTRIBUTION OF INPATIENTS (2004-2005)

S.No.	Departments/Sections	Numbers
1.	Anaesthesiology	785
2.	Dental Surgery	209
3.	Dermatology	3738
4.	Dr. B.R. Ambedkar IRCH	449
5.	Endocrinology	474
6.	Gastroenterology	1868
7.	Gastrointestinal surgery	701
8.	Haematology	5943
9.	Medicine	3519
10.	Neonatal	2337
11.	Nephrology	3394
12.	Nuclear Medicine	476
13.	Obstetrics and Gynaecology	9364
14.	Orthopaedics	4207
15.	Otorhinolaryngology	4546
16.	Paediatric Surgery	2210
17.	Paediatrics	6187
18.	Physical Medicine and Rehabilitation	29
19.	Psychiatry	377
20.	Radiotherapy	188
21.	Surgery	6325
22.	Urology	4909
	Sub-total (MAIN)	62235
23.	Cardiology	7790
24.	Cardiotheracic and Vascular Surgery	3269
25.	Neurology	2514
26.	Neurosurgery	4322
27.	Neuro-anaesthesia	10
	Sub-total (CNC)	17905
	Grand Total	80140

Source: Ibid.

Appendix VI

SURGICAL PROCEDURES

S.No.	Department	Major	Minor	Total
1.	Casualty	5	8106	8111
2.	Dental Surgery	1831	8633	10464
3.	Gastrointestinal Surgery	466	19	485
4.	Gynaecology	1756	5156	6912
5.	Obstetrics	1021	1488	2509
6.	Orthopaedics	2439	1559	3998
7.	Otorhinolaryngology	1603	21770	23373
8.	Paediatric Surgery	1308	3088	4396
9.	Surgery	3439	10182	13621
10.	Urology	1636	8269	9905
	Sub-total (MAIN)	15504	68270	83774
11.	Cardiothoracic and Vascular Surgery	3641	5	3646
12.	Neurosurgery	2920	498	3418
	Sub-total (CNC)	6561	503	7064
	GRAND TOTAL	22065	68773	90838

Source: *Ibid.*

11

Governance of Fortis Hospital, Mohali

Fortis Health Care Limited (FHL) is an enterprise from the promoters of Ranbaxy, India's largest pharmaceutical company and a global giant. With the first flagship venture of the *Group,* Fortis Hospital at Mohali in 2001 today the Forts network has grown to ten hospitals with a bed capacity of around 1600 beds establishing itself as one of India's leading advanced tertiary care Health Care Group.

Fortis, Mohali, is the region's leading multi-speciality hospital, with a super-speciality in Heart. The world-class environment is nurtured by an affiliation with one of the world's leading health delivery systems, Partners HealthCare System Inc. (PHS), USA. The affiliation facilitates FHLs access to: clinical protocols, quality assurance, criteria for accreditation in accordance with US hospital standards besides training material for staff and recommendations concerning critical medical equipment.

Fortis, Mohali's emergence as a premier super-speciality facility in North India has been underlined by the accomplishment of numerous high-end procedures such as: Cardiac Re-Modeling: Pediatric Arterial Switch operation, Aortic Aneurysms; Kidney Tumour removal to cite a few. With the addition of the Escorts Heart Institute and Research Centre, Fortis Health Care Limited today runs amongst the largest Cardiac Program in the world with over 6000 surgeries, 5000 Angioplasties and 14000 angiographies on an annual basis. The competencies of the two systems jointly will help in enhancing service delivery capability and set benchmarks for the way health care is delivered in India.

Fortis Health Care Ltd. is fast establishing a major presence within the National Capital Region of Delhi. In a span of one year the new 350-bed Fortis Hospital in Noida, has become India's leading tertiary care hospital in Orthopaedics and Neuro Sciences. This is possible because of our doctors—Dr. Ashok Rajgopal, one of India's most experienced Orthopedic Surgeons who performed 1000 Surgeries in the first year and

Dr. A.K. Singh, Director, Neuro Sciences who is credited to being amongst the first in performing many critical procedures. Fortis Hospital Noida also provides tertiary treatment in key specialities such as: Renal Sciences; Genitourinary diseases; gastrointestinal diseases as well as many other disciplines.

In just about five years since the first hospital, Fortis Hospital Limited is rated amongst top two in India in terms of: Cardiac Procedures. Total Knee Replacement, Total Hip Replacement and in Neuro Sciences. Besides cutting edge surgeries are performed in Cosmetology Opthalmology. Dental, ENT, Oncology, Minimal Invasive Surgery, Women and Child Health to name a few within the Group Hospitals.

What differentiates Fortis Health Care Limited is its strict adherence to best international clinical protocols in Patient Handling. Operation Theaters, ICU Management and Emergency Care. Our Doctors—mostly Western trained, caring nurses, technicians and hospital staff makes the patient feel at home away from home. In order to provide International Patients with the highest level of service quality from arrival to departure in India with seamless registration and discharge with an element of warmth, we have created the Fords International Patient Service Centre at New Delhi. With the burgeoning Fortis network, patients at any Fortis hospital become beneficiaries of an enriched wealth of interactive medical expertise and a reassuringly consistent quality of medical treatment-medical excellence that is enhanced through compassionate care the Fortis way.

Escorts Fords Heart Institute and Research Centre provides world class cardiac and heart treatment in the most affordable ways.

Escorts Heart Institute and Research Centre (ERIRC), was setup to bring to India the best cardiac care and infrastructure, training of cardiac surgeons and cardiologists and to conduct research as per International standards. It has completed over 20 years of journey in providing one of the highest standards of cardiac care in Asia.

Fortis' world-class environment is sustained through an association with one of the world's leading hospital systems. Partners Health Care System Inc. (PHS), USA and its founding members, Massachusetts General Hospital and Brigham and Women's Hospital, which are the leading teaching hospitals of the Harvard Medical School. A strong partnership that enables access to clinical protocols, quality assurance, and criteria for accreditation in accordance with international hospital standards besides training material for staff.

The Fortis team of expert doctors mostly western trained, is supported by highly skilled nursing professionals, technicians, and aided by state-of-the-art medical equipment at their command.

Fortis recognizes that international patients have special needs and requirements. To provide a highly specialized and dedicated service, Fortis has created the Fortis International Patient Service Centre at New Delhi, India. For you, this means a menu of seamless services that will make your treatment and trip hassle-free, i.e. from greeting you at the airport, to your registration and discharge, and even organizing the ground handling of any post-treatment travel.

The Fortis Hospital at Mohali in Punjab with a 209-bed capacity was the first facility of its kind in the region. Amongst other specialties, it runs the largest Cardiac Program in North-West India.

The hospital is a Super Specialty Cardiac Hospital. Here cardiologists, heart surgeons, nurses and other health care professions provide the latest treatment and the best care for all forms of heart disease.

The hospital was the first facility set-up towards achieving the dream of the late Dr. Parvinder Singh, Chairman and Managing Director of Ranbaxy Laboratories Ltd. Set on a sprawling 8.22 acres, it is the largest Cardiac Care Hospital in the region. The hospital has been designed and equipped with the latest technology, Information Technology systems, a telemedicine programme and carefully selected doctors, nurses and support staff.

Bringing breakthrough technologies to the operating room, the hospital is setting the highest International standards in as many as 26 Medical specialities. All our efforts are geared to giving patients the highest degree of skill, world-class cardiac care and comfort.

The hospital, which was awarded the Best Design Award by the American Institute of Architecture in 1999, has the following facilities:

A Multi-specialty Medical Centre with day care facilities.
Outpatient care to fulfil the local demands.
NABL certified path lab.
State of art blood bank.
State of Art Operation Theatres with laminar flow with shadow less lighting.
A 24 hours Emergency Ambulance Service.
A dedicated Emergency and Trauma Centre
Mohali's only 24 hours Chemist Shop
Free home collection of Pathology Samples.

FORTIS HOSPITAL, MOHALI

A Commitment of Excellence to Patients and Community

Accredited by the JCI and NABH, Fortis Hospital, Mohali is constantly striving to be as patient-centric and attendant-friendly as possible. Eminent and proficient doctors and a highly efficient nursing faculty of the hospital work painstakingly towards ensuring safety and effectiveness of medical treatment, taking into account individual disparities in health conditions. The hospital aims at satisfying patients, family and community while studiously respecting patients' rights and educating them about their responsibilities in receiving the best out of our health care facility. It is this partnership between patient and the hospital that we cherish the most.

Fortis Health Care was founded in 1996 by the late Dr. Parvinder Singh, the architect of major pharmaceutical company, Ranbaxy.

The mission of Fortis is—

"To create a world class integrated health care delivery system in India, entailing the finest medical skills combined with compassionate patient care."

The hallmark of Fortis hospitals, distinguishing them from their contemporaries, is the element of 'patient centricity' in hospital designs, services, programs and most significantly, in the caring approach of its medical and non-medical people. This is also very well depicted by the Fortis logo—with two green hands nurturing and healing the enclosed human figure with a vibrant dynamism shown by the red dot at the top.

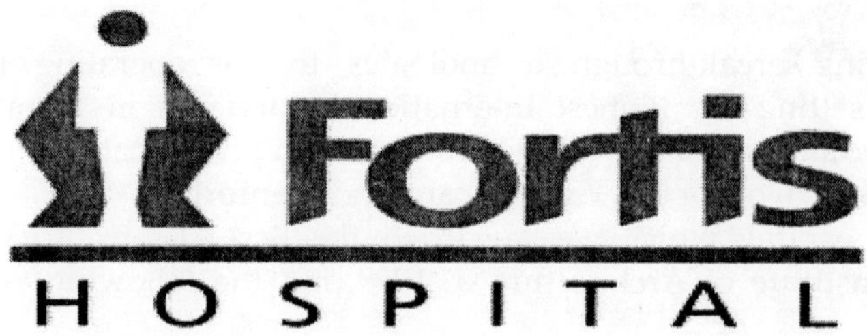

A set of VIRTUOUS Values form the ethos of the company, and are observed like a religion (Vision; Integrity; Respect; Trust; Understanding; Own; Uphold and Share).

Fortis Health Care Limited, which acquired Escorts Heart Institute and Research Centre Limited in September 2005, currently has a network of 14 hospitals and 8 satellite/heart command centres, including one heart command centre in Afghanistan. These specialty hospitals, which have been designed to provide high quality health care to the people of India through a hub and spoke model, include super-specialty centres providing tertiary and quarternary health care to patients in the field of Cardiac Surgery and Cardiology, Orthopedics and Joint Replacement, Neurosciences, Oncology, Nephrology, Gastroenterology, Gynecology and Obstetrics, Neonatology, Pediatrics and other general specialties.

As the flagship hospital of the company, Fortis Hospital, Mohali was inaugurated on June 28, 2001, and has recently completed 7 years of rapid expansion and growth. The commitment levels of all those who have brought it to this point have been fierce and uncompromising. Working relentlessly towards patients' satisfaction, the top brass is passionately involved in each step of qualitative improvement, adding new disciplines, dimensions and domains into the fabric of health care, with 'quality' and 'satisfaction' most emphatically the keywords. It is the CEO and MD of

Fortis Health Care Limited, Mr. Shivinder M. Singh, and his carefully handpicked team of administrators, along with a top-notch medical faculty that make the organization vibrant, dynamic and upwardly mobile.

Built on a sprawling 8.22 acres of land, Fortis Hospital, Mohali is the veritable torch bearer of super-specialty centres across the country. The hospital boasts of being awarded the Best Design Award by the prestigious American Institute of Architecture in 1999, and has unlimited scope for vertical expansion while retaining the carefully architected zones. While a compelling 200 founder employees continue to faithfully steer the large, organized team to new heights, many new departments have been introduced and policies created to ensure a continuous, healthy growth.

Initially set-up as 'Super-specialty in Heart' (Cardio Thoracic and Vascular Surgery, Invasive and Non-invasive Cardiology), Fortis Hospital, Mohali has not only found a place amongst India's most advanced cardiac hospitals, but is now also a well recognized multi-specialty facility (Anesthesiology, Cosmetic, Plastic and Reconstructive Surgery, Dentistry, Dermatology, Dietetics and Nutrition, Emergency Medicine, Endocrinology, ENT, Gastroenterology, General Surgery, Gynecology and Obstetrics, Hematology, Internal Medicine, Interventional Radiology, Lab Medicine, Medical Oncology, Minimal Access Surgery, Nephrology, Neurology, Neurosurgery, Nuclear Medicine, Ophthalmology, Orthopedics and Joint Replacement, Pediatrics, Physiotherapy, Psychiatry, Pulmonology, Radiology and Imaging, Rheumatology, Transfusion Medicine, Urology and Vascular Surgery) with accomplishments in numerous high-end procedures.

More than 100,000 patients avail the services in OPDs of the hospital each year. With 1200 cardiac surgeries, 1500 angioplasties, 600 other high end cath procedures, 500 joint replacement surgeries and 4500 other surgical procedures, the hospital has attained a numero UNO status in this region in a short span of 7 years.

JCI (Joint Commission International) Accreditation

The Gold Seal of the JCI accreditation is considered as the gold standard and the highest form of recognition in global health care. Fortis Hospital, Mohali received accreditation in August 2007, from the US-based Commission, which focuses on areas that directly impact patient care. The areas under their scanner include assessment of patients, utmost care of patients, patient and family rights, strict infection control for safety of patients, patients' education and documentation.

NABH (National Accreditation Board of Hospitals) Accreditation

In July 2008, within a year of getting the prestigious JCI accreditation, the Hospital was successful in acquiring the NABH accreditation, which is the most stringent form national accreditation for hospitals. For receiving these accreditations, approximately 600 standards were met with another 350 odd were complied with to achieve best practices in health care business! These included patients' safety, rights, facilities, physicians' credentials, besides formulating and adhering to policies and procedures of the organization.

The Tracer Methodology

Fortis Hospital, Mohali is the first and only hospital to have received the Joint Commission International, USA, as well as the NABH accreditations. Fortis Hospital, Mohali uses the "tracer methodology" to ensure that the patient is extended the highest quality of medical services required for his ailment. This methodology is an evaluation method which "traces" a single patient's experiences within the health care organization including the medical, nursing, hospitality, confidentiality, safety and several other aspects that lead to a comfortable and professional experience at the hospital.

Preventive Care through Lifestyle Medicine

At Fortis, we work on the premise that 'prevention is better than cure'. To ensure good health and well-being, the hospital offers several Preventive Health-check Packages to promote early detection and prevention of diseases and stress management. To this end, a Department of Lifestyle Medicine, under the banner of Clinic Rejuvé has been launched, which offers comprehensive programs to beat the stress and strain of urban existence.

MEDICAL FACILITIES

OPD facilities are available from 8 am to 8 pm. The hospital has 215 beds with patients having a choice of different categories of rooms. Besides well-appointed wards (4 to 10 beds each), double rooms (twin-sharing) and single rooms, there is luxury accommodation available as deluxe rooms, suites and presidential suites.

Critical Care Units have a patient-to-nurse ratio of 1:1. In all there are 97 critical care beds in 5 ICUs such as the Coronary Care Unit, Medical Intensive Care Unit, Cardiac Surgical ICU and Specialty Surgical ICUs, along with the General ICUs, managed by highly trained intensivists for life-saving measures. These units are located on the same floor as the OTs and Cath Labs for quick and efficient movement of the patient after surgery or in an emergency.

Cardiac Cath Labs to perform Coronary/peripheral/renal/carotid Angiography and Angioplasty, Pacemaker Implantation, Electro Physiology studies and Radio frequency Ablation, Ventricular/Arterial Septal Defect/ Patent Ductus Arteriosus Device Closure, IIVC Filter and Automatic Implantable Cardioverter Defibrillator, Balloon Mitral/Aortic/Pulmonary Valvuloplasty.

Non-Invasive Cardiology Lab provides Echocardiography, Stress Echo, TEE, Stress Test, Holter monitoring besides routine ECG.

Cardiac Operation Theaters equipped with high precision gadgets, new generation heart-lung machines, intra-aortic balloon pumps, touch screen flat panel monitors, advanced ventilators, cell savers and international laminar flow to ensure sterility and prevent infection during surgery and are directly connected with CSSD.

Emergency Care

Initially examined in the Triage area, the patients are transferred to observation room after basic evaluation. In life-threatening situations, the patient is shifted to the Code Blue room where facilities for cardiopulmonary resuscitation like defibrillation endotracheal intubation, etc. are available. Code Blue is an Emergency call for an incident where a patient in the hospital requires immediate attention for cardiopulmonary resuscitation. The call is made on a public address system for the entire Code Blue team to rush to the site where the patient has collapsed.

Ambulances

Four fully equipped rescue and intensive care ambulances with defibrillators, portable ventilators, portable monitors and even IABP with emergency pharmacy and trained staff.

Day Care Oncology

This for single and multi-drug infusion chemotherapy has been introduced, which is a unique facility offering advantage to patients who require short-term admission.

Dialysis

The hospital has an ultra-modern dialysis centre, equipped with latest machines with the facility of NIBP monitoring during the procedure, in-built alarms, plasmapherisis module, etc. Exclusive machines are allocated to HbsAg/HIV/HCV positive patients.

Endoscopy for advanced upper and lower GI and for ERCP.

Radiology Department offers imaging services such as 64 Slice CT Scan, MRI, Ultrasound, X-ray and Mammography.

Nuclear Medicine

Pathology Lab is staffed with highly skilled technicians and equipped with digital analyzers. This NABL accredited Laboratory offers diagnostic facilities with accuracy and ethical standards for the detection of a disease so as to help the clinicians prescribe effective, timely treatment and offers services round the clock for inpatients as well as outdoor patients. Facility for home collection of samples is also available.

The lab has complete automation in Biochemistry, Hematology, Coagulation, Serology, and Microbiology.

Lithotripsy and Urology Lab provides high precision uro-dynamics assessment of patients in order to give an objective measurement to support clinical assessment. Uro-dynamics is an essential part of the diagnostic armamentarium of the urologist, gynecologist, pediatricians and geriatricians. The investigations available include Uroflowmetry, Cyclometry and Urethral Pressure Profile (UPP) besides treatment of kidney stones.

Pulmonary Lab provides precise and reliable methods for understanding numerous facets of respiratory diseases.

Neurophysiology Lab offers Electroencephalography, Nerve Conduction Studies, Electromyography and Visual Evoked Potential.

Blood Bank is equipped with advanced techniques for processing/ screening of blood and its components. All mandatory screening for the transfusion transmissible diseases like HIV 1 and HIV 2, HBV, HCV, Syphilis and Malarial parasite are done with the more sensitive specific ELISA method rather than using the cheaper rapid methods which have low sensitivity. Committed to quality, the Blood Bank also performs Hepatitis B Core Antibody and also the Malaria Antigen Test to ensure the highest level of safe blood.

Rehabilitation and Physiotherapy facilitates quick management of patients. Qualified physiotherapists work to provide treatment for various musculoskeletal, cardiothoracic, neurological, orthopedic, pediatric, occupational diseases and also deal with ergonomics, and care of elderly. Equipped with the latest electro-therapeutic equipment, exercise unit and gymnasium facilities; the department caters to both inpatients as well as outdoor patients, along with domiciliary physiotherapy services.

Clinical Nutrition and Dietetics provide diet consults to all inpatients and outpatients. Specific and individualized counseling on the basis of clinical parameters, doctors' prescriptions and diagnostics is mandatory for all inpatients with diet planning and monitoring.

Fortis Paalna is an exclusive and contemporary Obstetrics department with labour-delivery suites.

Pain Clinic deals with management of chronic pain disorders.

Fortis City Centre is a satellite extension of the hospital in the heart of Chandigarh with OPD, Preventive Health Check, Dental and Ophthalmology facilities.

Health programmes such as Yoga, Aerobics, Lamaze, and Gymnasium are also offered to the community for holistic healing

OTHER FACILITES

The hospital has a huge array of support facilities available for the patients and their attendants.

Fortis Inn is special rehabilitation centre, located on the campus, which not only provides step-down care for out-station patients but is also a boon for attendants of the patients traveling from far and wide. The Inn has 30 well furnished and centrally air conditioned rooms with all amenities and a 24-hour café offering multi-cuisine meals at affordable prices.

Other facilities include Café Coffee Day, Hot Shoppe/Nestle Coffee Bar, Chemist Shop,

Gazebo, Business Center, Bank and ATMs, Prayer Room, Kids Corner and Book Café.

Patient Welfare Department

Patient satisfaction and feedback through a structured Patient Welfare Program is an integral and unique part of Health Care Delivery System at Fortis Hospital, Mohali.

The Welfare Officers act as a link between the patient and the hospital. They are patients' advocates and constantly strive to provide solutions to personal problems, thus improving the overall quality of care provided. The Welfare Officers also keep in touch with discharged patients to strengthen the hospital-patient bond. The patients are inducted to the 'Friends of Fortis' program where they informally meet their doctors/ specialists.

Corporate Social Responsibility

Since the inception of the hospital there has been a very intense and committed effort to cater to all sections of society—including the weaker sections.

The main objective of Fortis Outreach Programs is to increase awareness about preventable diseases like cardiac diseases, diabetes, cancer, osteoporosis and hepatitis, etc. amongst people of the region. The programs are carried out with the active participation of the government, NGOs and local bodies. Some of the popular outreach initiatives are:

- ACTFAST: For HIV/AIDS awareness
- CHETNA: For extending life saving medicine to the underprivileged girl child
- CHIRANJEEVI: For the health care of school children
- SAHAAYAK: Support group for Dialysis patients
- SAARTHAK: Support group for Cancer patients
- CME (Continuing Medical Education) Program
- OUTREACH OPDs: Free OPD by specialists in remote areas of the region
- FORTIS GOLDEN AGE CLUB: Special facilities/discounts for senior citizens
- FRIENDS OF FORTIS: For ex-patients of Fortis
- TELEMEDICINE: connecting with remote areas through telephone and TV
- RURAL OUTREACH: Educational programs for the rural populace
- FORTIS-ROTARY HEARTLINE: Cardiac surgeries for underprivileged children
- HAMAARI BETI: A campaign against female foeticide and infanticide

Against this backdrop, the company has established:

- Fortis Health Care Charitable Trust (FCT)
- Fortis Health Care Charitable Foundation (FCF)

Revival/upgradation of community hospitals

Another area that Fortis Hospitals have seriously looked into is upgrading and reviving community hospitals so that quality health care is extended and distributed to all parts of the country. Some examples of these are Sanjay Gandhi Hospital (SGH), Amethi, and Khushi Neemrana. A recent report in the *Economic Times* (Chandigarh edition, July 25, 2008) states that Fortis Health Care has offered to invest Rs. 3,471 crore in the Health Care Sector of Punjab, for PPP-based models, which will give a tremendous boost to the ailing and incapacitated health care centres of the state.

Fortis Health Care was established with the very clear aim of achieving excellence in health care that is worthy of global recognition. Starting with our Hospital Information System, to our human resource, to our Infection Control measures, to the bed-to-floor space, and down to the patient-nurse ratio, Fortis painstakingly maintains international standards.

STATE-OF-THE ART CATH LAB INAUGURATED BY SARDAR SUKHBIR SINGH BADAL, SEPTEMBER 5

Impressed by the facilities at Fortis Hospital, Mohali during his visit to the hospital on the inauguration of the Cath lab at Fortis, Sardar Sukhbir Singh Badal commented "Health Care is a priority area for Punjab and the State Government is more than willing to facilitate the setting up of such advanced hospitals like Fortis."

Speaking on the occasion, Mr. Shivinder Mohan Singh, CEO and MD of Fortis Health Care Limited, stated, "At Fortis, we continuously make fresh investments in the latest technologies. This is in keeping with our mission of creating a world-class integrated health care delivery system, entailing the finest medical skills combined with compassionate patient care. Our objective is to ensure that Fortis always remains a centre of excellence and the new Cath Lab is a big leap in this direction."

MANAGEMENT OF ACUTE HEART ATTACK—PRIMARY ANGIOPLASTY THE TREATMENT OF CHOICE

—Dr. G.S. Kaira

The management goal of acute myocardial infarction (Heart Attack) is prompt revascularization. Recent years have seen improvements in both pharmacological and mechanical methods of revascularization of the infarct related arteries.

Percutaneous Transluminal Toronary Angioplasty (PTCA) involves passing a tiny, deflated balloon through the arterial system usually through an artery in the leg (Transfemoral) or in the wrist (Transradial) to the narrowed coronary artery. The balloon is then inflated, causing the walls of the balloon to dilate (expand) the narrowed artery, thereby restoring blood flow to the heart muscle in the event of Heart attack. A stent (an expandable tube usually made of wire mesh) is often placed to prevent the narrowing from recurring and restoring the blood flow in the choking artery.

Benefits

Angioplasty can effectively restore blood flow to the arteries of heart in over 90 percent of patients, relieve angina and improve a person's ability to exercise. Since angioplasty does not require surgery, complications are relatively infrequent and hospital stay and convalescence are usually brief. In most cases, patients are able to walk on the day following the angioplasty and can resume their normal activities, including returning to work, within a week, at the doctor's discretion.

Severity of angina

People who have severe angina tend to derive more benefit from interventional treatment than from medical treatment.

Presence of advanced heart disease

Coronary heart disease may lead to poor pumping function of the left ventricle, (the heart chamber that pumps blood around the body), called low EF and it may even lead to a serious condition called congestive heart failure. People with these advanced types of heart disease may benefit more from interventional treatment primarily bypass surgery, than from medical treatment. In fact, interventional treatment may even reverse abnormal function of the left ventricle in some cases.

Patients with one narrowed coronary artery are often advised to select medical treatment, unless this treatment fails to control angina; if angina persists with medical treatment, angioplasty is often recommended.

PRIMARY STENTING IN ACUTE MYOCARDIAL INFARCTION

In acute myocardial infarction, successful restoration of the blood flow in the affected artery by primary angioplasty, can result in preservation of left ventricular function. Direct stenting, without predilation, reduces procedural time, radiation exposure, and costs. Inpatients with an acute myocardial infarction, direct stenting may also reduce embolization of plaque constituents, lowering the incidence of the no reflow phenomenon, thereby increasing myocardial perfusion and salvage. Although primary stenting improves the short-term outcome of patients, there is growing evidence that the main benefit of stenting is freedom from long-term recurrence of restenosis and myocardial infarction. Primary stenting is an effective therapy for even patients with an acute myocardial infarction who have a left main coronary artery stenosis, particularly when associated with cardiogenic shock.

CRITICAL CARE UNITS AT FORTIS HOSPITAL, MOHALI

The Intensive Care Units at FHM are managed by experts in critical care, with a patient-to-nurse ratio of 1:1 (for ventilator patients) and 1:2 for step down. FHM has the following CCU's:

- Surgical Intensive Care Unit (SICU)
- Coronary Care Unit (CCU)
- Medical Intensive Care Unit (MICU)
- Speciality Intensive Care Unit (SPICU I and SPICU II) Intensive care units have been planned on the same floor where the operation theatres and cath labs are also located. There is an inside corridor from the Cath Lab to Cardiac OT for shifting patients in emergency without any delay.

The process flow at CCU should incorporate the following parameters for a successful process. . .

- Transfer in:
- Blood Bank
- Investigations (lab, bedside and CT)
- Pharmacy
- Cross-referral
- Transferout
- Manning
- Performance Management.

FHM specializes in the following manner in the Critical Care Unit processes:

- Bed requests are sent the previous day when the angioplasties are slotted.
- Blood compatibility is checked thoroughly and expiry date of blood is checked before transfusion by counter-checks.
- Lab GDA collects routine samples from CCU at specified times during the day and night and emergency samples are sent through the CCU GDA.
- Stat indents are colored differently so that the pharmacists can see it and keep the drugs ready immediately for the GDA.
- Automatic SMS is generated to cross-referral consultants with patient details once cross-referral request is entered on the system.

- Beds are booked a day in advance and communicated to the bed manager so that CCU beds are not blocked by patients over staying due to lack of availability of ward beds. Discharge summary for CCU stay is prepared by the MO and completed discharge summary is handed over during transfer of patient to the ward. Direct discharges are carried only if the situation demands.
- Lastly, the manning and performance management is carried out for a smooth and flawless process flow.

Equipment

All the ICUs at Fortis Hospital are equipped with the most modern and highly specialized equipment. Some of this equipment, which forms an integral part of the patient care, and sets Fortis Hospital, Mohali a class apart, are:

Ventilators

The newer generation critical and life saving machines are patient and user-friendly with alarms and set-up buttons simplified. We, at Fortis Health Care, have opted for the Seimens 300A which is the latest ventilator on the market. It not only is able to sense whether the patient is breathing spontaneously but also allows him to do so if this is adequate. The same ventilator can be used for adults, paediatrics and neo-natals.

Monitors

We have opted for the Agilent wide touch screen monitors, which are able to provide at least 3 pressure traces along with other parameters such as heart rate, respiration, temperature, ABP, etc. This is also networked into a central nursing workstation so that all the parameters of patients are seen on one screen making access easier. All these monitors are networked through a central server and interfaced with HIS. The doctors can view these parameters sitting in their chambers.

ICU Beds (HILROM)

Some of the special features about these beds are that, they are electrically operated through remote switches can be tilted up and down or sideways. Provides ease in the movement of the patient from Cardiac OT to SICU and *vice versa*. Provision has been made for keeping monitors, oxygen cylinders, infusion pumps and syringe pumps, without affecting the patient comfort.

Mattress (Ripple mattress)

Helps in reducing the incidences of bed-sores to the patients when he may be lying down in the same position for days altogether.

SICU Pendants

These imported pendants from Drager (Germany) are installed next to the patient bed, which can rotate upto 270 deg, providing medical supplies e.g. oxygen, compressed air, vacuum, electrical outlets (UPS and non-UPS). This can house monitors, infusion pumps, IABP, BIBAP (type of ventilator), etc. This provides effective space utilization and ease of operation.

Bed Head Panel

Bed head panels have been installed in CCU, MICU. They are used for supplying services like oxygen, compressed air, vacuum, electrical outlets (UPS and non-UPS), nurse call system, data and voice outlets in patient rooms.

Intra Aortic Balloon Pump (IABP)

This critical and life saving device is used to increase the blood pressure of the patient whenever it falls down below certain desired limits. Apart from SICU, CCU and MICU, this equipment is also used in OTs, Cath lab and ER.

Infusion/Syringe Pumps

Used for delivering accurate dosage of medicine to critical patients at a particular rate.

Critical Care Stat Lab

Houses the facilities for immediate testing of blood gases, electrolytes for critical patients and is located within the ICU.

A NEW TREATMENT OPTION FOR HEART FAILURE

—Dr. H.K. Bali

Heart failure prevalence has been increasing and it has acquired an epidemic proportion. Worldwide, more patients get admitted to hospitals with heart failure than with any other disease including heart attack and cancers. Two major factors have contributed to this changed scenario; one is increasing longevity and the other is better and longer survival after various types of heart diseases. With the widespread availability of thrombolytic drugs and primary angioplasty, more and more patients are surviving after a heart attack. Similarly, survival after valvular surgery, bypass surgery and other cardiac surgeries has improved remarkably. Many of these survivors develop left ventricular dysfunction and heart failure over a period of time.

These patients present with symptoms of progressively increasing breathlessness, nocturnal dyspnea, pedal edema and congestive hepatomegaly. Their quality of life is adversally affected and they require repeated hospitalization for control of symptoms of heartfailure. They are at a very high risk of sudden cardiac death due to high grade ventricular arrhythmias and also for embolisms both in the pulmonary and systemic circulations.

Till a couple of decades back, very few treatment options were available for them and most of the available drugs could provide only symptomatic relief. These drugs had no effect on survival and very little, if any, effect on quality of life. Since 1988, few groups of drugs have become available which in addition to symptom relief also have been shown to improve survival in large multicenteric placebo controlled trials. ACE inhibitors and beta blockers are the two groups of drugs which have been shown to have these effects.

Unfortunately despite the availability of these drugs and a number of newer drugs, these patients continue to have a very high mortality and repeated admissions for heart failure worsening putting enormous burden on exchequer and health care resources. A large number of these patients are ultimately candidates for heart transplant. Unfortunately there are logistic limitations for widespread availability of heart transplantation as enough donor hearts are not available.

In the last few years, cardiac resynchronization therapy has become available to many of these highly symptomatic patients. It involves implantation of a permanent pacemaker with three leads. In addition to the conventional dual chamber pacemaker, a third lead is placed in the coronary sinus tributary to stimulate the posteriolateral left ventricular wall.

This biventricular pacemaker restores the atrioventricular and interventricular synchrony and therefore improves cardiac function.

This device is implanted in inpatients with severe heart failure (NYHA III and IV), severe left ventricular dysfunction and having certain ECG criterion (LBBB pattern with QRS > 0.012 sec) and echocardiographic criterion (EF< 35% and MR). A large number of these patients meeting this criterion improve after cardiac resynchronization therapy, making this therapy the most rapidly increasing therapy in heart care worldwide. Some of these patients improve instantaneously, while others improve over a period of few weeks to few months. A large majority of these patients improve at least one functional class while a minority a show a more robust response. Effort tolerance is improved, frequency of hospital admissions is reduced and quality of life is improved. Few recent trials have also shown a positive effect on survival. As these patients have severe left ventricular dysfunction, most of these patients are given a combination of biventricular pacemaker and implantable defibrillators (Combo device). A minority of patients despite fulfiling the clinical, ECG and echocardiographic criterion do not benefit from this therapy. In large trials such patients constitute around 15% of patients. Efforts to identify such "non-responders" prior to implantation are aggressively being looked.

Experience with this treatment has been very gratifying the world over and thousands of patients have been given "CRT" with excellent response. In India also the number of procedures is increasing remarkably. Although, there is a definite learning curve, the implantation procedure is quite simple thereafter.

We have implanted quite a few of these biventricular pacemakers including few: Combo devices and the patient response have been very satisfying. Although price is a limiting factor, considering the excellent response, this treatment should be offered to all patients with severe heart failure who fulfil the clinical, ECG and the echocardiographic criterion.

"Dr. Bali has extensive experience of performing both elective and emergency coronary interventions and has been responsible for introducing primary angioplasty for patients of acute myocardloal infarction in this region. This includes interventions inpatients with stable coronary artery disease, acute coronary syndrome, acute myocardial infarction, cardiogenic shock and patients with severe left ventricular dysfunction. He has pioneering original work in heart failure pathophysiology and management. He was part of the team which described a new syndrome of "heart failure at very high altitude" for the first time in world literature. Dr. Bali has the largest experience, worldwide, in angioplasty/stenting in Takayasu arteritis (pulseless disease) and this work has been widely reported in International literature."

WORLD HEART DAY CELEBRATIONS AT FORTIS (SEPTEMBER 28 TO OCTOBER I)

- **Launch of Sahyog (Sept. 28)**—Announcement of extremely subsidized cardiac surgery package for underprivileged rural section.
- **Walkathon (Sept. 28)**—Walk for Heart by Dr. H.K. Bali in association with *Times of India* at Sukhna Lake. Mr. Ashish Bhatia and Dr. Ashok Chordiya graced the event.
- World Heart Mela **(Sept. 29, 30)**—Fortis organised Health mela by putting up various stalls in the OPD and IPD.
- **Friends of Fortis (Oct. 1)**—Dr. T.S. Mahant addressed the audiences regarding the value of laughter for a healthy heart. The talk was followed by an entertaining evening with comedy King, Bhagwant Maan.

Luteum conducted to celebrate World Heart Day

- **Dr. RK Jaswal** delivered a lecture on 'Prevent Heart Diseases and Lifestyle Management' at Panjab and Haryana High Court, September 26.
- Lectures of **Dr. G.S. Kaira** and **Dr. Ambuj Choudhary**, with Sadbhavna Heart Foundation, were conducted at Patiala on September 27.
- **Dr. A.S. Bawa** was invited to speak on 'Newer Modalities in ED' at a program in IMA on September 27.
- **Dr. Arun Kochar** was invited to speak on 'Stress and heart disease' at Chitakara School of Mass Communication, Chandigarh on September 30.

HEALING HEART THROUGH WRIST

—Dr. R.K. Jaswal

Dr. R.K. Jaswal, Additional Director in Cardiology at Fortis Hospital, Mohali, is now performing tranradial interventions with 0% complications till date. His vast experience in this field has given him the honor of being the faculty member of TCT (Trans Catheter Techniques)—Asia Pacific Seoul, South Korea. Here is an account of what transradial (wrist) procedures mean and why they are gaining popularity.

Angiographies are, in today's fast-paced and stress-laden lives, a quick and safe means of deciphering if your heart is functioning to its optimum. Often angiographies show obstructions in arteries that are almost simultaneously treated by angioplasties, which in a layman's words is ballooning and stenting of the artery, so that the obstruction is removed.

It is a myth that angiographies and angioplasties are "dangerous." With the advancement in expertise and technology, only one of 1000 persons suffers a complication during an angiography and one in 100 during an angioplasty, which would be the ratio in any other invasive procedure too. The message is that DO NOT have apprehensions regarding getting an angiography done, and also do not compromise on the quality of medical expertise or facility that you opt for!

For a long time, coronary angiography and angioplasty procedures have been performed through the thigh (transfemoral approach). Today, transradial access for coronary procedures is preferred by the patients, and complex angioplasties are being performed through the radial approach.

Some of the significant advantages of the transradial approach over the conventional approach (via thigh artery) are:

- Although more difficult for the interventionalist to perform, it is pertinent to note that this new approach is less complex and very comfortable for the patient.
- Transradial approach allows the patient to be mobile immediately after the procedure while in the conventional approach the patient has to lie down flat on the bed for at least 6-8 hours after angiography and 12-18 hours after coronary ballooning and stenting.
- The conventional approach is associated with several problems due to prolonged immobilization, such as:
  - Backache
  - Urinary retention
  - Patients of bronchial asthma and heart failure find it extremely uncomfortable to lie in bed for extended durations.

All these problems are virtually absent in the transradial approach.

- Femoral artery used as the access site in the conventional angiography. Angioplasty lies deep and is not easily compressible. Therefore the chances for major hematoma requiring blood transfusions and residual femoral artery detects requiring surgical correction are as high as 2-8% in the transfemoral approach. These complications are nearly 0% in transradial procedures.
- Thigh vein and nerve that accompany the thigh artery, which is the access site in the conventional procedures, are liable for damage in conventional angioplasties. However, the risk and complications of damage to these is virtually absent in the transradial approach.
- Needless to say, patients world over overwhelmingly prefer it. In a survey in the U.K. all except 2% patients prefer only transradial approach to the conventional Transfemoral approach.

Transradial Interventions have fewer complications but are technically more difficult to perform. The level of complexity for the surgeon makes the procedure exceptional and rare. But not anymore! A growing number of patients are opting for this procedure. This relatively new technique promises lower morbidity and improves patient satisfaction. Its effects on quality of life after the procedure, patient preference, and cost are gradually beginning to delineate that the popularity of this procedure is on the rise.

CONCLUSIONS

- Among patients undergoing diagnostic cardiac catheterization, transradial access leads to improved quality of life after the procedure, is strongly preferred by patients, and reduces hospital costs.
- The transradial approach to coronary interventions is both feasible and safe inpatients with acute myocardial infarction. This option may be most appealing inpatients at high risk for developing vascular complications of arterial access.
- That is the reason that transradial access is the safest and most comfortable for patients who undergo urgent ballooning and stenting as life saving procedures following a heart attack (primary angioplasty).

COMING SOON: RADIAL LOUNGE AT FORTIS HOSPITAL, MOHALI

FORTIS CELEBRATES 2ND ANNIVERSARY OF CHETNA ON INTERNATIONAL GIRL CHILD DAY, SEPTEMBER 24

Chetna is a unique initiative of Fortis aimed at providing the underprivileged girl child an equal opportunity to health care, promising her a healthier and brighter tomorrow. Right from its inception, Fortis has been sensitive to the needs of all sections of society including the weaker sections—and has always come forward to assist them."

Health Check Camp at Bal Sadan Association (orphanage) for the underprivileged girl child, September 24

A special health camp was also held at Bal Sadan Association, Panchkula, an orphanage for girl children. Ageneral health check-up of all 45 girl children was conducted at the orphanage by a team of Fortis doctors and paramedical staff. Five needy girls were given Chetna cards which will entitle them to free consultations at Fortis Hospital for one year.

Baby Shruti given a new lease of life on 2nd anniversary of Chetna

A free cardiac surgery was conducted on *6 year old Shruti,* an underprivileged girl child. Shruti had Congenital Heart Disease and an Atrial Septal Defect Closure procedure was successfully conducted on her by **Dr. T.S. Mahant.**

Dr. Ashok V. Chordiya commented: "being of assistance to associations like the Baal Sadan or young children like Shruti brings a new meaning into the lives of all of us at Fortis. We are very happy that we are able to make a contribution in helping their lives become better."

STATE-OF-THE-ART SPECIALISED DENTAL CLINICS INAUGURATED AT FORTIS: JULY 15

Two state-of-the-art specialized Dental Clinics were inaugurated at the Fortis City Centre, Sector 9, Chandigarh and Fortis Hospital, Mohali, ushering in a new era of Specialty Dentistry to the city. The multi-specialty Fortis Dental Centres have been set-up in partnership with a renowned chain of Dental Clinics—Axiss Dental. Mr. H.S. Mattewal, Advocate General, Punjab inaugurated the Dental Centre. Speaking on the occasion, Mr. Shivinder Mohan Singh, CEO and MD of Fortis Health Care Limited, said, "Chandigarh needed a specialized Dental Clinic which would provide all dental modalities as well as diverse dental specialties under one roof. As health care providers it was our duty to bring this facility to the city."

The Dental Centres are the first of their kind in the city and senior specialists from Delhi will be visiting them regularly. The Centres are equipped with cutting edge technology and shall offer specialties such as

Endodontics, Orthodontics, Prosthodontics, Periodontics, Oral and Maxillofacial Surgery, Pedodontics, Implantology, etc.

TEAM MOHALI (ORTHOPEDICS) DOES IT AGAIN!

The ORTHOPEDICS Team at FHM can boast of recording a remarkable 130 joints performed in September (Knees 122/Hips 8). This has also established a personal landmark for Dr. Manuj Wadhwa he has performed 131 joints in this month (116 at Mohali and 15 at Amritsar). With the hard work, team spirit and determination that each Fortisian has shown through the Orthopaedic Camp, FHM will continue to arrive at new milestones in other specialties as well.

12

Secondary Health Care Administration in Thailand#

Before we discuss the hospital administration, let us mention briefly the structure and role of Ministry of Public Health in Thailand. The country's administrative structure consists of Bangkok Metropolis area, 73 provinces and 163 municipalities. The Bangkok Metropolis is headed by a governor and his four deputies. Each province is headed by a governor who is appointed by the Ministry of interior. Each Municipality is headed by a mayor who is elected by Municipal Council.[1]

The typical province has a population of about 500,000 and the smallest well over 10,000. Each province is composed of about 3-20 districts (amphoes) depending on population and area. There are 628 district (amphoes) and 82 smaller districts (gingamphoes). Each district is administered by district officer (nai Amphoe), a civil servant appointed by the Interior Ministry who is responsible to the Provincial Governor. Each sub-district is under the supervision of a deputy district officer responsible to the district officer.

There are 5,608 communes (tambons) and 56,286 villages (mubans). Majority of the communes and villages are not legally recognized as part of the administrative system of the country. A commune consists of a group of villages. The tambon head official acts as registrar and as intermediary between the district officer and the village headman. The village is the smallest unit consisting of a cluster of 50 households, having about 200 inhabitants, and is headed by a village headman (puyaiban) elected by the inhabitants of the village.

This is a piece of doctoral Research by Krienkerai Klnoboul, first Secretary, Thais Embassy, Under the guidance of the Author who visited Thailand alongwith the students.

The functions of the various Ministries in Thailand are very similar to those of the major sub-division of the executive branch of any modern government. The general pattern of organization at the ministry level is relatively standardized and long established. The head of each Ministry is its political chief—the Minister—who is responsible to the Cabinet for the proper functioning's of his Ministry and its subordinate Departments. The minister may be assisted by one deputy or assistant Minister or more holding a political appointment. Each Minister has attached to him one political secretary or more whose appointment and removal is effected by the Cabinet. In each Ministry, the Secretary, his assistants and staff, form the Office of the Secretary to the Minister.

MINISTRY OF PUBLIC HEALTH

The principal governmental agency but by no means the only one responsible for health services is the Ministry of Public Health.[2] The Ministry of Public Health (MOPH) has undergone several re-organizations since its founding and at present (2000) its responsibilities at the central level are divided among six departments or offices:

1. Office of the Under-Secretary of State for Public Health.
2. Department of Medical Services.
3. Department of Communicable Disease Control.
4. Department of Health.
5. Department of Medical Sciences.
6. Office of Food and Drugs Committees.

The six Departments of Offices of the Central MOPH further organized into 'divisions' with a wide variety of functions.

1. Office of the Under-Secretary of State for Public Health

The office of the Under-Secretary of State, besides its administrative functions and correlation of the work of the various departments, exercises its duties through the Divisions of Medical Registration, International Health, Food and Drug Control, Nursing and also through the Medical Council, the Committee for the Control of Drugs, the Committee for Food Quality Control, the Committee for TB Control, the Committee for V.D. Control, the Filariasis Contol Board, the Primary Health Care Board, and Office of National Advisory Board for Disease Prevention and Control. Latest additions to this Board are the Division of Malaria Eradication, the Division of Filaria, the Division of Vital Statistics and the Health Planning Division.

2. Department of Medical Services

The Department is responsible essentially for the management or supervision of large governmental hospitals. These include, for example, the mental hospitals operated directly by the Central Ministry and the large general hospitals at the provincial level. The National Cancer Institute and the Institute of Pathology, which engage themselves in both patient care and research, are also under this Department. It should be noted, however, that they are numerous smaller district hospitals of the MOPH that are not under the supervision of this Department. Furthermore, there are several hospitals under other ministries of the Government, and also an expanding number of purely private hospitals (both non-profit and for-profit) which are not supervised by the Department of Medical Services.

3. Department of Communicable Disease Control

This Department is responsible for nation-wide campaigns against several selected communicable diseases of relatively high prevalence in Thailand. These include malaria, tuberculosis, filariasis, venereal disease and leprosy. The operation of these disease control programmes are mainly through a "vertical" flow of authority from the Central Government out to the provinces and municipalities. Although, there has been, in recent years, a movement to decentralize health programmes and enlarge the "horizontal" scope of authority at the provincial level, these communicable disease control programmes are still managed essentially from the top of the pyramidal structure of the IMOPH.

4. Department of Health

This Department is responsible for supervision of most of the other preventively-oriented programmes of the Ministry. These include such fields as nutrition, family health, dental health services and environmental sanitation. Highly important has been the delegation to this Department of responsibility for several special innovative programmes in "primary health care." Moreover, since most of the family (maternal and child health and also family planning) health services are delivered through a nation-wide network of facilities for ambulatory service health centres, mid-wifery centres, and also 'medical and health centres' the standards for operation of these facilities are promulgated and supervised by the Department. Most of the medical and health centres are at the district level and contain a small number of beds (10 to 30) for minor illness or emergency cases. These centres have recently come to be designated as "district hospitals." Inspite of the functions of these small hospitals being mainly curative rather than preventive, their technical supervision has remained with the Department of Health.

5. Department of Medical Sciences

This Department has as its main objectives for promotion of research in medical sciences and the provision of modern diagnostic procedures in the treatment of prevention of diseases. It is also responsible for the management of a variety of technical services which are performed mainly at the Central Government level. These include, for example, a Radiation

Protection Service Division, an Entomology Division and a Virus Research Institute. The National Health Laboratories Project Division is exceptional in attempting to organize a network of clinical laboratory services throughout the country, as well as operating a major central laboratory in Bangkok.

6. Office of Food and Drugs Committees

Office of Food and Drugs Committee, the newest of the major administrative entities of the MOPH, has responsibility for protecting the population against hazards in the consumption of food or drugs or the use of the cosmetics. As we shall see, the use of drugs in Thailand both those that are medically prescribed and those purchased directly over the counter by patients—absorbs a substantial share of all expenditures for health purposes in the nation. The establishment of this Department signifies an effort by the MOPH to introduce greater controls over this important health problem. Tackling the problems of substances' abuse (drug addiction) is only part of this larger pharmaceutical problem.[3]

Under the general surveillance of the latter Department but operating as a semi-autonomous government enterprise, is the Governmental Pharmaceutical Organization (GPO). This public entity was started in 1939, originally under the Ministry of Economics to prepare drugs for use in governmental facilities and to save on foreign exchange. In 1942, when the MOPH was formed, it was transferred there and eventually combined with the Division of Medical Depot of the Department of Medical Sciences. Currently, the GPO produces 384 items which, it is estimated, constitute nearly half of the drugs and vaccines distributed to governmental hospitals and health centres.

Since 1950, the activities of the above Departments have been expanded by the assistance of and co-operation with the following international and foreign organizations: the World Health Organization, the United Nations Childern's Fund, the United States Agency for International Development, the Rockefeller Foundation, the China Medical Board of New York and several governments under the Technical Co-operation Scheme of the Colombo Plan. The projects which have benefited by the international and foreign aids are malaria eradication, yaws control, tuberculosis control, maternal and child health including family health, community health development and village sanitation, environmental health, vital health statistics, medical education, trachoma, leprosy control, health education of the public, nursing and mid-wifery education, nutrition promotion and training of personnel.

Field Administration: Local Health Administration

Traditionally, the numerous functions of the MOPH just summarized were carried out under higher centralized authority, but in recent years, stress has been put on the delegation of responsibilities peripherally towards the local level.[4]

Each of the 73 Provinces has an Office of the Provincial

Ministry of Health's Service Institution at Provincial Level			
Regional:	9 region	Regional Hospital	(14 hosp.)
Provincial:	73 provinces	Provincial and district hospital	(73 hosp.)
District:	628 Amphone	Medical and health	(323 district centre hosp.)
Tambom:	5608 Tambom	Health Centre	(4204 centres)
Big Village		Mid-wifery centre	(2271 centres
Villages:	56,282	Village Health post	

Field Offices

The Ministry of Health has field offices spread throughout the country. There are 14 Regional Hospitals, 73 Provincial Hospitals, 323 District Hospitals, 4,204 Health Centres, 2,271 Mid-wifery Centres and Village Health posts.

Chief Medical Officer

The PCMO is a public health physician, who is responsible for supervision of both preventive and curative functions of the MOPH throughout his province. Thus, he oversees the Provincial General Hospital of which there is at least one in each province and sometimes two, making a total of 88. These hospitals vary in size from 60 to as much as 800 beds. The PCMO is also responsible for the technical supervision of the work of the District Health Offices in the province. These Offices are headed by a District Health Officer (not a physician), who is typically a sanitarian with additional training in general public health administration.[5]

Within some, but not all of the districts, there are District Hospitals of 10 to 30 beds, staffed by at least one physician along with nurses and other health personnel. Also, within some but not all of the sub-districts or communes (tambons) there are health centres staffed by nursing and other allied health personnel (but not physicians). In some but not all of the villages, especially the larger ones. There are mid-wifery stations, staffed simply by a trained auxiliary midwife. The last two types of health facilities come under the general supervision of the District Health Officer, but the District Hospitals, being staffed with physicians are more particularly the direct technical and administrative concern of the PCMO.[6]

The PCMO is appointed by the central Under-Secretary of State for Public Health, and is technically responsible to him. He may be advised and assisted also, however, on various technical problems by specialists from the several other departments of the central MOPH. For example, on problems of administrative area, the PCMO is administratively responsible to the Governor of his province, who is appointed by the Department of

Local Administration of the Ministry of Interior. Provincial Governors are important officials in Thailand, and it is evident that PCMO must exercise great discretion in combining his technical responsibilities to the central MOPH with his administrative responsibilities to the Provincial Governor.

In the same way, the District Health Officer, while technically responsible to the PCMO is administratively responsible to the generalized District Officer. The latter official, like the Provincial Governor is part of the network of authority of the Ministry of Interior. The most recent development in the network of local health services under the MOPH is the "programme of training and activity" of "village health volunteers" (VHV) and "health communicators" (HC) in selected villages throughout the nation. Starting with the movement to limit population growth by encouraging family planning (FP), this programme has broadened to encompass the provision of general primary health care. These village people are part-time health workers who depend for their livelihood on some other occupation. They are not considered part of the bureaucratic structure of the MOPH or any other Government agency.

Thus, it is evident that MOPH, both centrally and at the several peripheral levels, has a very wide range of functions. They embrace both preventive and curative services, and they involve liaison with various officials of provincial and local Government within the nation-wide network of the Ministry of Interior. Even so, as we shall see, there are numerous health activities under the private sector. On the whole, the scope of MOPH authority does not extend to these other activities; when it does the relationship is quite indirect. The Ministry of Public Health must ensure cooperation and co-ordination among allied agencies to achieve good results. It needs to develop an effective information system network to involve all allied agencies.

HOSPITAL ADMINISTRATION

Since many health problems require a level of medical treatment and personal care that extends beyond the range of services normally available in the patient's home or in the physician's office, modern society has developed formal institutions for patient care intended to help meet the more complex health needs of its members. The hospital, the major social institution for the delivery of health care in the modern world, offers considerable advantages to both patient and society. From the standpoint of individual, the sick or injured person has access to centralized medical knowledge and technology so as to render treatment much more thorough and efficient. From the standpoint of society, hospitalization both protects the family from many of the disruptive effects of caring for the ill in the home and operates as a means of guiding the sick and injured into medically supervised institutions where their problems are less disruptive for society as a whole.[7]

Today, a hospital is a place for the definition and treatment of human ills and restoration of health and well-being of those temporarily deprived of these. A large number of professionally and technically skilled people apply their knowledge and skill with the help of complicated equipment and appliances to produce quality care for patient. The excellence of the product—the *raison d'etre* for a hospital, therefore, depends on how well the human and material resources are applied to promote patient care.

Functions

(a) Patient Care

The first and foremost function of a hospital is to give care to the sick and injured and restore the health of diseased persons. Ethically, his care should be given to all without discrimination of social, economic or racial nature. However, the hospitals as national investment in people's health and as centres for scientific practice of medicine, must do many more things than 'produce' medical care. To quote Perry: "The success with which a hospital contributes towards meeting the patients' needs can be measured by the fullness of the life he is able to lead on leaving it."[8]

(b) Training

Education and training of doctors and nurses have traditionally been carried out in hospitals. It is a workshop wherein the student learns by seeing what his superiors and peers do. Radiology, laboratory, radiotherapy, highly advanced surgical techniques demand a variety of skills and knowledge, all of which cannot be mastered by the doctor specialists. These activities have created the need for a large number of skilled technicians who are today the vital support to the specialist whether he is the surgeon, physician, diagnostician or therapeutist.

These people are indispensable for the all-round excellence of all specialist work. To develop these technical skills, a programme should be organized by the hospital under the direction of people who have the required experience, knowledge and attitude to teach others. The purpose of in-service education and training programme is to develop such knowledge and skills in all categories of paramedical personnel as are required to make them fit for the job they hold and keep them attuned to the growing needs of their jobs.

(c) Medical Research

The third important function of hospital is to give support to medical research. A good hospital, where the quality of professional work is excellent, is an ideal ground for medical research. As a matter of fact, excellent professional care of patients largely result from the fruits of research into new problems. An attitude of enquiry and investigation should permeate through the day-to-day care of patients. The hospital can develop facilities for research with comparative ease and speed if the staff and administration are properly motivated. True, elaborate research is expensive. There, nevertheless, remain clinical investigations of applied nature that call for little capital investment. Responsibility for creation of new knowledge is that of any enlightened profession. It is in a hospital that opportunities exist, if not abound, for organized as well as individual initiative for research.

(d) Health Education

The fourth and final object is to support and assist all activities carried out by various public health and voluntary agencies to prevent disease and promote positive health attitudes in the community through health education. Health education, immunization, social and economic rehabilitation are some of the many activities for which the hospital may provide assistance in terms of physical facilities and advisory services to staff. As a matter of fact, in the western countries, this aspect of the hospital as a community health centre is being emphasized more and more. Many ways are being devised to integrate the hospital with the activities of community health agencies.

Administration of such a complex organization requires blending of technical and administrative competence in the right quantity, at the right time, at the right place, by the right man and in the right way or process. Each hospital is a distinct entity and as such each has to be tailored to the specific aims to be accomplished, the specific tasks to be performed, the volume of services to be rendered and the type of the community to be served. The basic purpose of the hospital is "better patient care" and return the patient back to the community as a productive unit of that community. Hospital administration is an activity to secure better output through optimum utilization of inputs. It is not so easy, as it might seem, to determine the number of hospitals and the number of beds within them, in Thailand. Various reports from different agencies tabulate the hospital resources of the specific agency but an overall tabulation of hospital bed resources, of multiple sponsorships, is not currently available.

In Thailand, there were 491 hospitals and other establishments for inpatient care, with a total of 45,393 beds.[9] Thailand had 60,590 hospital beds or 1.41 beds per 100 population.[10] This may be compared with Malaysia (Thailand's neighbour to the South), which in 1993 had a ratio of 2.63 hospital beds per 100U population. The problem is to determine the classification of these hospital resources by:

(a) type of hospital, i.e., general or for various special purposes, and
(b) sponsoring or the ownership of the facility.

(a) Types of Hospitals

The most detailed categorization of hospitals, by type, is reported in a Ministry of Public Health Publication Institutions containing beds were classified into four types as on the next page.[11]

In later years, the health centres with beds (also known as first-class

Type of Facility	*Number*	*Number of Beds*
Hospitals	279	52,005
Health Centres (most with beds)	329	193
Maternal and Child Health Centres	5	575
Midwifery Centres	48	402
Total	661	56,175

health centres) were redesignated as "district hospitals", those without beds (formerly called second-class health centres) were simply considered as "health centres." Accordingly, the facilities that are now designated as district hospitals of the Ministry of Public Health numbered 329 and had 3,168 beds, or an average of slightly less than 10 beds each.

Type of Bed Service	*Institutions*	*Beds*
General Hospitals	248	39,722
District Hospitals	329	3,169
All General Facilities	577	42,891
Specialized Hospitals	31	12,283
Maternal and Child Health Centres	5	575
Midwifery Centres	48	402
All specialized Facilities	84	13,260
All Types of Facilities	661	56,151

Focusing on the hospitals in the above tabulation, those considered "general hospitals", i.e., serving all types of patients, numbered 248, with 39,722 beds. This meant a ratio of general hospital beds of 0.9 per 1000 population. Hospitals for specialized conditions numbered 31, with 12,283 beds. In addition, all the beds in district hospitals (previously first-class health centres) are "general." Correspondingly all the beds in "maternal and child health centres", "midwifery centres" may be considered as "specialized." Thus, breakdown of the above listing of institutions, by type of health service, comes out as follows:

The discrepancy of 24 beds (56,176 minus 56,151) between the two tabulations is explained by the omission from the second tabulation of "second-class health centres", a few of which contained a total of 24 beds. Specialized hospitals are of several sub-types which may be identified as on the next page.

Thus, in summary, of all facilities with inpatient beds in Thailand, 84 with 13,260 beds or about 13 per cent of the facilities and about 24 per cent of the beds are in specialized facilities. The majority of these beds are in facilities related to mental disorder-17 institutions with 8,503 beds. Another

Type of Specified Hospitals	*Number*	*Beds*
Mental Disease	14	7,483
Mental Deficiency	2	520
Narcotic Addiction	1	500
Leprosy	2,320	
Tuberculosis and Chest Diseases	2	584
Tropical Diseases	1	100
Infectious Diseases	1	230
Eye Diseases	4	46
Maternity	1	50
Pediatrics	1	450
All Specialized Hospitals	31	12,283

2320 beds are for leprosy patients from though most people with this disease have relatively mild cases that are hospitalized. The remaining beds are in facilities for various diseases of demographic groups, mainly mothers and children.

From the viewpoint of the number of different patients served, the general hospital with 76 per cent of the beds are most important. The great majority of these are under the Ministry of Public Health at the provincial and district levels. In contrast to the specialized hospitals, the average length of stay of patients is relatively short. In 1975, it was only 5.9 days in all provincial hospitals (that is, at the provincial level, not district hospitals) and 10.3 days in the Bangkok City hospitals (but not counting the large medical school teaching facilities).[12] Thus, there is relatively rapid turnover in the use of general hospital beds. In most of the specialized hospitals, the average patient stays for several months or years.

(b) Hospital Sponsorship

Highly relevant to hospital planning, as well as to the whole distribution of health services, is the sponsorship of hospitals. Institutions under governmental control, particularly the Ministry of Public Health, are more readily subject to planning in relation to general population needs. Sponsorship is important mainly with regard to general hospitals. Of specialized hospital beds, only a handful—hardly 5 per cent are not governmental in sponsorship.[13]

Some of these figures requires explanation. The Ministry of Public Health data do not count beds in district hospitals which were identified as "first-class health centres" if these 3,193 beds are added the MOPH total becomes 26,456 beds. The other Ministries include the large teaching hospitals in Bangkok (Sirirat Ramathibodi, and Chulalongkorn Hospitals) under the State University Office as well as hospitals under the Ministries of Defence, Communications, Interior and other branches of Government.

Sponsorship	*General Hospitals*	*Number of Beds*
Ministry of Public Health	87	23,262
Other Ministries	63	11,463
State Enterprises	13	574
Municipalities	6	1,243
Private	79	3,180
All General Hospitals	248	39,722

The 13 hospitals of state enterprise include those of the railway system, the tobacco monopoly and other organizations.

It should not be inferred that care in Government hospitals is without cost to the patient. For drugs, laboratory and X-ray examinations, and various supplies, the vast majority of patients using public hospitals must pay. The very poor are theoretically exempted, but in practice few qualify for this completely free hospital care in public general hospitals.

Health Centres

Before 1975, these were classified as follows:

Class I: Medical and Health Centres
Class II: Health Centres
Class III: Midwifery Centres

Class I facilities typically had a few beds for accidents, maternity, or other conditions pending referral to a hospital; at least one doctor was on the staff. Class II units had no beds and were staffed entirely by auxiliary health personnel. Class III units were staffed solely by midwives (not nurse midwives) and sometimes also with an assistant sanitarian.

Since about 1975, there has been a gradual upgrading in the status of these types of units, and a fourth echelon of primary health care has been added. Class I "medical and health centres" are now designated as district hospitals with 10 to 30 beds, it has been easier to have them staffed with a doctor, since the mandatory 2-year period of rural services has been required of all new medical graduates.

The Class II health centres, now simply designated as health centres, have increased in number and in staffing. Many of them are now staffed with middle-level, personnel-nurse practitioners or wechakorn and their allotment of drugs and supplies has been increased.

The Class III units or midwifery centres have also been increased in number, and the scope of functions of the midwives has been broadened to encompass general family health (including family planning) and some basic primary health care for first aid to patients with minor illness or injury. The time of rural midwives is now devoted more than half to services other than attendance at child births and maternity care.

Finally, in a number of demonstration projects, a fourth echelon of "village health post" has been established where very briefly trained health volunteers—backed up by health communicators—offer basic primary care closer to village dwellers than any of three previous levels of health centres. This level of peripheral primary care facility has not required new construction, since the services are rendered directly in the home of the volunteer or, if he is a shopkeeper, in the store. Whether this type of facility will be spread throughout the country depends on evaluation of its effects in the selected demonstration area, especially that in Lampang Province. Unfortunately there is a serious problem of underutilization of all four levels of health centres in relation to the health needs of the population theoretically served.

Deficiencies in Coverage

Health planning in Thailand has for several years contemplated coverage of the population with the several types of hospitals and health centres described above, according to certain designated ratios. These have, as a minimum, simply corresponded to the structure of the political sub-divisions of the nation: provinces, districts, communes and villages. Although these constitute very rough guidelines, since each of these geo-political areas have different total populations, it is helpful to examine the coverage of the nation at present along these lines. The established facilities were as follows:[14]

Types of Facility	*Facilities Established*	*Percentage Coverage*
Provincial Hospitals	89	100 plus
District Hospitals	317	56.6
Health Centres	4,047	73.0
Midwifery Stations	1900	3.9

As indicated above, the provinces are relatively abundantly served by provincial hospitals in the capital cities, and in several provinces, there are two such hospitals. Many of these are old structures, which require renovation, but it is clear that the needs are more urgent at the more peripheral areas, close to Thailand's large rural population.

The coverage of 55.6 per cent indicated for districts, with district hospitals, is somewhat of an exaggeration, if one considers the adequacy of staffing. Of the 317 district hospitals, 62 are not yet stationed to the minimal standard. If the coverage is adjusted to take account of staffing, district hospitals would number 255 and the coverage would decline to 48.2 per cent. The great majority of these district hospitals (165 of them) have 12 beds, and nearly all the remainders have 30 beds.

Progress has been particularly rapid at the commune (tambon) level. The coverage at this level with health centres was reported as 57 per cent and it has now risen to 73 per cent. On the other hand, the coverage level of only 3.7 per cent for midwifery stations would seem to be based on an unreasonable criterion. Since the average village has only 500 to 600 population, one should not expect a midwifery station in every village; a cluster of two or three villages aggregating to about 2,000 population would actually be more consistent with planning objectives. On this basis, the coverage now achieved would be between 8 to 12 per cent.

With respect to the fourth level of "village health posts" for primary care, staffed by health volunteers, the objective is indeed to cover every village in the nation. Unfortunately, different sources in the Government report different number of facilities actually in place and in operation. The data is given above were obtained, as indicated, at the Thai Ministry of Public Health but they differ from figures reported in publications from other sources.[15]

Administrative Set-up

All hospitals—both general and specialized—under government sponsorship are administered or supervised by a physician who is assisted by various managerial and nursing personnel. The numbers and backgrounds of those associated vary, of course, with the hospital size (number of beds). The Hospital Director or "Chief Executive Officer" of the hospital is appointed by the Central Government authority responsible for the hospital. Thus, in Ministry of Public Health hospitals, both at provincial and district levels, this would be the Minister, ordinarily on recommendation of the Director of the Department of Medical Services. In hospitals under other Government agencies, such as the State University Bureau (which controls the large teaching hospitals in Bangkok) or those serving various state enterprises, the Hospital Director is appointed by the top official of that agency.

Most of the other supervisory personnel in each hospital are also appointed by the central authority, on the recommendation of the Hospital Director. Appointment cannot be finalized, however, until the Civil Service Commission has determined that the individual meets the requirement officially listed for the position. In fact, for any technical position in a hospital, such as a laboratory or X-ray technician, such review by the Civil Service Commission is required. In one case, in which one X-ray technician trained by a radiologist and considered very well qualified could not be appointed because she had not taken certain formal courses required in the rules of the Civil Service Commission.[16]

The entire staff of the public hospital is responsible ultimately to the Hospital Director, although this may be through an intermediary, such as the "Chief Nurse" or the "Secretary" (or business manager). The physicians on the hospital staff are always responsible directly to the Medical Director.

Staffing Patterns

In contrast to hospitals in the United States—although in common with hospitals in most developing countries—the physicians on all public hospital staffs are appointed to salaried position designated on an "organizational chart." Thus, the doctors are members of a "closed staff", and no physician who is not a member of this staff may admit a patient to a hospital bed, except, of course, in obvious emergencies. Thus, a patient may be referred to the hospital by a health centre doctor or a doctor in private practice, but after admission, the case is entirely the responsibility of a hospital doctor. After discharge, a report is supposed to be sent to any outside physician serving this patient, but such reports are evidently not always sent.

Probably the commonest practice of admission of a hospital patient is through "self-referral"—that is, the patient simply coming directly to the hospital outpatients department (OPD) on his own initiative. There, an OPD physician decides on whether admission to a bed is necessary. The case then becomes the responsibility of a hospital doctor, if it is a large hospital-such as at the provincial level or in Bangkok this doctor will be in one or another clinical departments (such as surgery, medicine, obstetrics, pediatrics or some other. For a private patient, that is, someone occupying a private or semi-private hospital room, the arrangements are different. Such a patient is admitted on the request of the hospital staff physician who has served this patient in his private practice. This physician, than takes care of the patient throughout his hospital stay. It should be explained that officially a government doctor may not charge for services rendered in a public hospital, even for patients in private rooms.

The usual custom, however, is for the physician to charge a certain fee for the services rendered in the private office or "clinic", when a patient is scheduled to be treated in the hospital with surgical or other procedures, the fee charged is simply calculated to cover the services rendered in the hospital as well. It need hardly be mentioned that these practices have developed in Thailand, as in certain other developing countries, because the official medical salaries for hospital work are so low (These salaries are standardized by the Civil Service Commission for all public hospitals, including those of state enterprises or the municipal hospitals of the Ministry of Interior, as well as in MOPH facilities). Earnings per hour in private practice are five to ten times higher.

In all MOPH hospitals, there are certain official standards for staffing, varying with the size and role of the institution. In the average Provincial General Hospital, for example, the standards call for one doctor to every 15 beds. For larger "regional hospitals" expected to serve several provinces for highly specialized services, the doctor to beds ratio is theoretically 1: 10. In practice, however, these standards are not yet being implemented; currently, the ratio of doctors in Provincial Hospitals generally is about 1:20 beds.[17]

Likewise, for nursing personnel, there are official standards, although they allow for flexibility in the proportions of professional nurses (with RN credentials) and auxiliary nurses. In Provincial Hospitals the standard calls for a ratio of five nursing personnel (of various level) to nine beds. This standard is currently attained, however, in only a small fraction of these hospitals.[18]

In District Hospitals, where the patients have less serious conditions, but at which it is expected that outpatients and preventive service will require a good deal of staff time, the personnel standards differ. For the typical District Hospital of 10 beds, there is required one doctor who takes clinical responsibility for all inpatients and outpatients, as well as being the Hospital Director. Other personnel in a 10 bedded District Hospital, according to official standards, should include:

Nurses:	8, of whom one has RN qualification.
Administrators:	3, of whom one is Secretary, plus 2 clerks.
Technician:	1, for laboratory tests.
Sanitation Control:	3, who also do communicable disease control.
Health Promotion:	4, including a health educator, public health nurse and others.
General Maintenance:	8, including a driver, a mechanic for repairs, etc.

For large 30-bedded District Hospitals, in addition to proportionately more doctors (3 or 4) and the above types of personnel, there should also be a pharmacist and a dentist. As in Provincial Hospitals, however, these various standards are seldom achieved at present. According to a high MOPH official, only about 10% District Hospitals currently meet these standards.[19]

In District Hospitals of 10 beds, these are typically set-up in two wards (for men and for women); there are not ordinarily any private beds. Provincial Hospitals have their public beds in wards of about 6-8 beds each, with between 5 and 15 per cent of the total beds reserved for private patients. The occupancy levels at these two types of hospitals are very different. District Hospitals typically are reported to have occupancies of under 59% although it would be more accurate to say under 25%. The explanation would not seem to be mysterious; on the relatively rare occasions when rural people feel sick enough to seek admission to a hospital (considered a fearful experience) they want to be treated in a hospital with various medical specialists and advanced equipment. Thus, they usually bypass the District Hospital and go directly to the Provincial Hospital, (it may turn out that the case is simple and could have been handled at the District Hospital, but it is simpler to give care than to send the patient back).

Assessment

(i) Provincial Hospitals, therefore, have very high occupancy levels as a rule—from 75 to over 100 per cent. Sometimes two patients must be put in one bed and extra beds crowded together in the wards or even the corridors, are common. It is also not uncommon to see the public wards terribly overcrowded, while the private rooms are half-empty. In view of this situation, the MOPH has attempted to build up the District Hospitals—especially since young doctors are now available to staff them under the mandatory public service law to reduce the pressures on Provincial Hospital. So far, the desired effect has not been participated perhaps if referral from a District Hospital or Health Centre becomes obligatory for acceptance in a Provincial Hospital (except of course in obvious emergencies), the occupancy problem, would be corrected.

(ii) The training of Hospital Secretaries for their administrative Responsibilities on budgeting, personnel, kitchen and laundry maintenance, house-keeping, etc., is surprisingly limited. It is done through a one or two-week course given by the MOPH in Bangkok. The Mahidol University Faculty of Public Health offers a course in "hospital administration" but this is limited to physicians or other professionals with a doctorate degree. Some reflection of this weakness in training may be the deficiencies in ordinary sanitary maintenance that characterize many Provincial Hospitals, by this may also be due largely to the relatively tight budgets on which he must depend, with inadequate nursing and house-keeping personnel.

(iii) Another comment about public hospitals in Thailand is called for the policy of making charges for drugs and diagnostic procedures to all but the very poorest patients. In practice, even though many patients have very low incomes nearly everyone pays something. Further indirect evidence of the deterrent effect of these costs is the very low rate of hospital utilization in Thailand as a whole. Based on 1973 data although published in 1997, the Thai population uses the general hospitals of the MOPH at the very low rate of 64 patient days per 1000 persons per year.[20] This may be compared with a rate of some 1800 days per 1000 persons per year in a developed country like Canada, but even to 500 days per 1000 in a developed country like Canada, but even to 500 days per 1000 in Government hospitals of neighbouring Malaysia.

(iv) A final aspect of the MOPH hospitals is their accessibility the population. A study of this was made, simply by relation Provincial Hospitals to the geographic centres of numerous political districts (Amphoe) whose population they served. The nation was analyzed in terms of its 5 official districts, plus 73 additional areas sometime considered "small district", making a total of 643 areas, these 358 were found to have "good" for reasonable access to a Provincial Hospital, meaning that the district contained a Provincial Hospital or was adjacent to a district population were within 50 kilometeres of it. In a second category were 111 districts not contiguous with a district, containing a provincial Hospital, but with a population mainly (but not: entirely) under 50 kilometers distance from it; these were termed "intermediate." Finally, these were 174, districts with "poor access" or "isolated" from a Provincial Hospital—being located where most of the population were over 50 kilometers away from such a hospital considering the many poor roads and inadequate public transportation, one can appreciate the difficulties faced by residents of these 174 districts in reaching Provincial Hospital.

Provincial Hospitals

Provincial hospitals, located in the capital town of every province in the country, by far account for the largest number of general hospital beds overall, as well as for hospitals within the control of the Ministry of Public Health. Ministry sources indicated there were 89 hospitals "labelled provincial hospitals" for the country's 72 provinces. Although a province normally only has one provincial hospital, indicated in the capital town, the excess number of provincial hospitals is a result of more than one general hospital being located in each of several larger provinces with dispersed populations. The average size of a provincial hospital remains about the same as in 1974, or slightly more than 250 beds per hospital. However, they range from as small as under 100 beds, to several hospitals now being expanded and upgraded as regional referral facilities with 600 to 700 beds, the size of the hospital varies roughly with the size of the provincial population it serves. The number of physicians varies with the size of the hospital, and MOPH standards suggest one doctor for every 15 beds in a provincial hospital, and one doctor for every 10 beds in the regional facilities. However, some of the smaller provincial hospitals in more isolated provinces have only four or five doctors in residence (range in 1978, 3-35 doctors/hospitals with an average of 10.5 doctors per hospital and the overall ratio throughout the country is about one physician for 20 beds.[21]

A CASE STUDY OF LAMPANG PROVINCIAL HOSPITAL

In 1942, a 25-bed hospital was built under the sponsorship of the Lamparg Municipality on a 20 acre plot. In 1950, the Department of Medical Services in the Ministry of Public Health took over responsibility for the hospital, purchasing adjacent land and adding new buildings and departments. The inpatient departments currently include: surgery, medicine, pediatrics and obstetrics-gynecology. The outpatients departments are obstetrics, gynecology and family planning, pediatrics (including well-baby immunization clinical), ear, eye, nose and throat minor (EENT); minor surgery (including orthopedics), and medicine. As in most provincial hospitals, some community health activities, such as family planning, well baby and immunization clinics, have been integrated into the outpatient departments.

Issues and Problems

(i) It is clear that although the budgets of both have increased each year, the operational resources available to the Provincial Health Office are small in comparison to those available for the Provincial Hospital. If capital funds were also added to these budget totals, the difference between the hospital and the Provincial Health Officer would be even greater. The difference between the two in resources available is emphatic when one considers that: the Provincial Health Office is responsible for seven district hospitals, about 70 district health centres, 35 midwifery centres, a variety of special purpose programme, and the primary health care volunteer network. The provincial hospital is a single facility.

(ii) As in all provinces of Thailand, the Director of the Provincial Hospital is nominally under the authority of the Provincial Health Officer. However, the Provincial Health Officer has little role in co-ordinating hospital activities and exercises no control over the Provincial Hospital's budget or administration, which flow through a separate line from the Ministry of Public Health. There has traditionally been no routine system of reporting hospital activities to the Provincial Health Office. These are a few factors which suggest a relative autonomy of operation of the Provincial Hospital within the provincial health care system.

(iii) In the near future, the Provincial Hospital's size may grow to 750 beds as it assumes regional hospital status. In recent years, as the hospital slowly increased bed capacity under its phased expansion plan, the inpatient load has not significantly increased. This is due, in general, to a much more slowly increasing hospital staff. As the new hospital units open in the near future, the problem of staffing will become extremely acute. It will most likely be some time before sufficient staff can be made available to, appropriately match the increased bed capacity. This suggests that there will be great pressure on current hospital staff to assume responsibility for the new capacity, and the increase in size and status of the hospital will undoubtedly open up new opportunities for advancement in the clinical departments. A major concern is that the already considerable pressure on the Community Health Department staff will become more pronounced as the department expands its role and that many of the very competent staff will be attracted to the new clinical positions available with more career potential.

(iv) Provincial Hospital and Provincial Health Office Administration still remain basically separated and uncoordinated. Informally, a number of staff within the provincial health headquarters were shifted to the Community Health Department in the hospital. However, administrative problems are encountered, the provincial health staff, who were never really under the authority of the Community one health Department Chief, shifted back to the Provincial Health Office.

(v) The Provincial Health Office is directly responsible for district hospitals, but there is no official link between the Provincial Hospital and the district hospitals technical support and resources could possibly be provided to district hospitals by the Community Health Department, but there is no official channel to institutionalize this. A further complication is that the district hospital itself is only responsible for the geographic area of the sub-district in which it is located, and is not responsible for health care in the full district. Health centres within the district and their staff fall under the responsibility of the non-physician District Health Officer. If a strong technical support and supervision network is to be established, a more appropriate arrangement might be the Community Health Department providing technical and administrative support to the district hospital, and the district hospital in turn providing some kind of support for wechakorn and other personnel in the sub-district health centres with overall co-ordination at the Provincial Health Office. This might also provide the means for rotating junior hospital staff into district hospitals or districts which do not have a physician at present, which would provide technical input to the district, as well as give experience and understanding to the hospital physicians in the needs of the rural health care.

Expanding Role of the Hospital

With the help of foreign aid and consultation, the hospital role was extended to the following:

(1) Temporary extension of the hospital outpatient department to district health centres.

(2) Establishing a Community Health Department in the hospital which eventually would have responsibility for direct support of rural health services.

Extended Outpatient Services

In the first phase hospital outpatient department services were extended to the district health centre in Hang Chat, the first district to which integrated services were introduced. Since the district health centre had no physician in residence, an immediate priority was to add one to the staff. The simplest approach to filling the position, and to initiating involvement of the hospital in rural health care, was to rotate provincial hospital physicians through the centre in Hang Chat at two-month intervals. The rotation programme continued for almost two years, providing services' during the clinic hours five days a week, until the new district hospital was completed and staffed by a permanently-assigned physician. During the period that provincial hospital physicians served in the Hang Chat health centre, the utilization of services there increased sharply in the years before physicians were rotated through Hang Chat, the average number of patients seen per month had been about 125. However, shortly after the physician rotations began, the monthly average more than doubled. Since the hospital physicians were only in transient assignments, their role was generally limited to providing medical care services and they did not have sufficient time or opportunity to lead the district health team. With the completion of the district hospital in Hang Chat, the permanently assigned physician assumed this responsibility.

Development of the Community Health Department

A community health department was proposes as a mechanism to effectively link the Provincial Hospital to the Provincial Health Office and rural health services. The hospitalized planner undertook the initial organization of the department, and became the department chief. An old building separate from the Provincial Hospital main buildings, was assigned to the Community Health Department.

The Community Health Department established in the Lampang Provincial Hospital was the first of its type in Thailand, although there were already a number of community health or community medicine departments in teaching hospitals associated with the medical schools. However, the function of community health departments in medical schools' has been primarily to train medical students and other health professionals. Each medical school faculty has generally chosen one rural district, served by a district hospital and outlying health centres, through which small groups of medical students have rotated for periods of upto six weeks. The field work in the rural district is occupied with class room lectures and is expected to prepare the newly trained physician for future work in rural areas.

Developing a community health department in a non-teaching provincial hospital was a complex talk. The objectives of such a department are somewhat different from those of a medical school department. The medical school normally selects small areas to be used as a field training site for students. The objective in Lampang, on the other hand, was to make the Community Health Department the centre for stimulating and co-ordinating health services in all rural districts, rather than in one selected area. Training is also an integral part of the department's role in linking the hospital with rural health centres. The Ministry of Public Health has recognized the need for community health departments in general hospitals and has planned to establish such departments in other provincial hospitals in Thailand. The Department of Community Health was initially headed by the Project's hospital planner, assisted by a public health nurse/ health educator, a social worker, an epidemiologist/statistician and secretary.

With a seriously limited number of available staff positions and resources at its disposal most of the early activities of the department were focused inside the hospital. These were:

(1) Organizing educational activities for the prenatal, well-baby postnatal and family planning clinics;
(2) Implementing educational activities and discharge counseling programmes in the various wards;
(3) Producing a variety of educational brochures and leaflets for distribution in the various outpatient clinics;
(4) Improving the public address system for broadcasting health messages periodically during the day;
(5) Improving environmental sanitation on the hospital premises; and
(6) Co-ordinating collective of hospital statistics and epidemiological reports normally sent to the Provincial Health Office.

While concentrating on activities inside the hospital during the initial period, the department's chief looked for opportunities to link the department with peripheral rural health services. In mid-1977, one such opportunity presented itself; the organization of a mobile vasectomy clinic. Under this programme which is a part of the National Family Planning; Project, teams were set-up within Provincial Health Offices in a number of provinces to provide vasectomies to village in rural locations. This was an ideal activity for the Community Health Department to expand rural services, as the chief of the department was a skilled surgeon specializing in urology. With assistance from the vasectomy training team of Ramathiborli Medical School, the first mobile clinic was organized in Hang Chat District in October 1977. The response was much greater than expected—ISO rural villagers had a vasectomy in the first two days of the clinic, confirming the acceptability of vasectomy in the rural areas. After the first clinic, the mobile team travelled to rural locations twice a month. A motivation team worked with local village leaders and health volunteers prior to the mobile team's visit.

The Family Health Division of the Ministry of Public Health provided a mini-bus for the mobile team as well as costs of supplies and per diam for participating staff. The mobile vasectomy team achieved important results during its first year of operation. Nearly one thousand vasectomies were performed compared with less than a hundred performed in the hospital in previous years.

The mobile clinic has filled a major gap in the generally successful National Family Planning Project. It seems apparent that many rural people are interested in having a vasectomy. But the Provincial Hospital where vasectomies have been most readily available, is not easily accessible to rural population, Bringing the service closer to their homes (the mobile clinics have been operated from rural health centres) has made it more convenient, and the high quality of service provided has reinforced acceptance among rural villagers. Chart 12.1 summarizes the current overall functions of the Community Health Department and plans for future additions. Chart 12.2 outlines the specific responsibilities of each unit within the Department.

Assessment of the Working of the Hospital

The assessment of the Hospital is based upon both primary and secondary data. Patient opinion survey was designed and 100 patients were interviewed, on random basis, for two weeks. Three questionnaires were designed to solicit the opinions of the employees in the hospital to ascertain their views on hospital functioning. The sample for questionnaires 1 and 2 included all the physicians (32); Dentists (2); Pharmacists (3); while Nurses (25); Nurse Aides (25) and Other Staff (SO) were selected on random basis. Besides, the record of the hospital was studied to analyze the functioning of the hospital.

The answers to the patients' opinion surveys have been analyzed in percentages and are given in Table 12.3. The analysis of the table indicates that the patients are satisfied by and large towards the services provided by the hospital as well as with the behaviour of the personnel working in the hospital. However, the following difficulties were mentioned by the patients and their relatives. We present here these and their probable solutions.

A. Problems of Outdoor Patients

(1) Though it is a fact that in the present decade of reforms communication with the District and Sub-divisional towns hits improved tremendously still there are remote and inaccessible areas from where patients find it difficult to come in time to get medical facilities at the outdoor. As such they have to wait for the next day for getting Medical facility unless the case is a serious one. This communication difficulty poses problems both for the patients and the staff of the hospitals.

(2) The facilities for investigation at the outdoor is very meager, as such the cases cannot be investigated properly.

(3) Even though the facilities exist, as the staff strength is very

meagre, the cases cannot be investigated and treated with greater speed and care.

(4) The supply of medicines falls short of the requirements because the budget provision for each hospital is fixed. Unless and until more budget provision for supply of medicines to different hospitals is made to cope with the rise of population and rush at the outdoor, most of the patients will have to go without

CHART 12.1

Current and Future Functions of the Community Health Department, Lampang Provincial Hospital, 1979

Community Health Department		
Hospital-based Services	•Community-based services	•Support for Peripheral Services
Immunizations	•Jail Health	•Medical referrals
Nutritions	•School Health	•Mobile clinics
•Health Education	•Community Information/ Education	•Special Services
•Communicable disease control and surveillance	•Mobile health services	•Technical Supervision
•Outpatient medical care	•Co-ordination of health activities in the Lampang municipality	•Technical supervision
•Outpatient medical care	•Co-ordination of health activities in the Lampang municipality	
•Environmental sanitation		
•Social Welfare		
•Drug addict care (outpatients)		
•Medical Care by radio or isolated areas		
•Malnourished children's ward		
•Ward for contagious diseases		
•Drug addiction ward		
•Geniatric services		

medicines. Sometimes, the most essential and cheap items of medicines are not supplied while costly and rarely used medicines are given.

B. Problems of Indoor Patients

(1) There is shortage of staff. As such the admitted cases cannot be looked after properly.
(2) Bed strength is meagre in comparison to the demands of admission cases—resulting in refusal of admission of genuine cases.
(3) Operation theaters are not upto the mark in most of the hospitals as they lack in equipments, trained O.T. staff, electrification, etc.

CHART 12.2

	Cost of trans-portation	*Cost of medicine of the relatives*	*Cost and expense*	*Total*
An outpatient	40	30	250	320
An inpatient	40	50/day	400	490/day

Note: The currency is in the Bahts.

General Problems

(1) Huge Cost of Transportation

It was found that villagers used up quite a lot of money in bringing themselves to be examined by the doctor, which was due to the difficulty in transportation and the expenses by the relatives who come along with the patients. The expense of one visit, in average, for a villager at about 11 kilometers away from the district hospital is:

Many villagers have faced troubles in transporting themselves to the district hospital and provincial hospital, especially during the night time. For the poor, the problems are much more serious as they have to manage their scarce money for food rather than medicines. It is suggested that the Government may help to set-up a village health fund from the villagers for supporting the volunteer in giving all services in primary health care to their members in the village. The fund needs to be controlled by a group of self-selected villagers called "Village Health Bank Committee."

(2) Lack of Functional Literacy

In the study, we also found that most of the poor patients did not want to see the doctor when they got ill, they would let the disease become complicated until they thought that they would die if no doctor was consulted. Usually it was too late for the patient to receive the proper treatment, and it would mean much larger amount of money in treating such a patient.

It is suggested that there is a need to co-ordinate health functions with other socio-economic factors. The first step in this context is to set-up a fund in the village and a programme for training of the health volunteer to make use of that fund in elevating the health status of the villagers.

(3) Absence of the Involvement of the Community

Most of the people contacted were of the view that the Health Administration never takes the people into confidence. To achieve its aim, a health team must be able to promote community participation, i.e., to help people to rely as much as possible on their own efforts and resources for their health needs. A health team must:

- understand and communicate with the community;
- encourage community participation in identifying problems and seeking solutions; and
- work in the community.

To establish good relations with the community a health worker or health team follows these steps:

(a) listen, learn and understand;
(b) talk, discuss and decide; and
(c) encourage, organize and participate.

(4) Neglect of Rural Areas

Most of the people contacted were of the view that rural people are discriminated and neglected as compared to the urban population. The Health Department must provide more services to the rural people as they cannot afford to be examined by private physicians. To quote Neutra:

> "We can foresee a time when our technical civilization will keep its promise and serve not only the strictly urban variety of mankind. People who populate vast stretches of the earth, will then no longer feel themselves to be second rate citizens."[22]

(5) More Emphasis on Preventive than Curative Measure

It was observed that most of the members of health team take more interest in curative than preventive measures. The hospital may attend to curative services but its ultimate aim should be preventive and promotive. To quote Mackintosh:

"The appropriate field of study of a hospital is not sickness in the narrow senses but life in the broad sense. Sickness is an incident grave, troublesome or restful—the life of a person, but to the hospital and its staff sickness is a challenge, a focus of enquiry from which prevention should radiate as well as the cure of the Individual."[23]

(6) Lack of Willingness of the Health Experts to Serve in the Villages

Perhaps most formidable obstacle to the setting up of a comprehensive system of medical care in the rural communities of underdeveloped countries is the small number of medical practitioners who will agree to settle in such areas. We have to examine this problem through effective manpower planning. As long as Government cannot offer salaries comparable with the fees paid in the private sector it would be unrealistic and unreasonable to require physicians to accept full-time appointments in public hospitals. Moreover, members of the medical profession in the developing countries prefer to remain in the large towns since the majority of the people can afford to pay higher medical fees.

A questionnaire was issued to employees to understand the process of decision-making. The responses are given in Tables 12.1 and 12.2. The analysis of the tables indicates that there is centralization and no Delegation is given to the employees to take decisions. Besides, there is no participation in decision-making. Speedy and realistic decision-making is one of the essentials of efficient administration. In a big and complex organization, the number of decisions to be taken from time to time is so large and the points at which the decisions are to be implemented are so many that it becomes necessary to distribute decision-making powers among a number of personnel/organs, rather than concentrate in one person/organ. This is expected to prevent the emergence of bottlenecks which bedevil highly centralized power structure.

Besides the respondents were of the view that participation should be encouraged. Participation is an individual's mental and emotional involvement in a group situation that encourages him to contribute to group goals and to share responsibility for them. An employee's participation would build his morale and ultimately his efficiency.[24] An ILO document mentions that the individual worker "is not just a cog in the very big wheel, but that his personal effort is essential for the achievement of the overall production plan."[25]

The research theory in social organizational psychology has also suggested that participation in group decision-making enhances satisfaction among members and removes tensions. Michael R. Cooper and Michael T. Wood have shown that satisfaction is affected by the participation. Satisfaction was greater when participation was complete than where it was partial.[26]

There is a need to practice 'Management Objectives' to ensure fruitful participation. Management by Objectives shifts the focus to goals, to the purpose of the activity rather than the activity itself. It is a process whereby

TABLE 12.1

Patient Opinion Survey in Percentages
(based upon Questionnaire No. 1)

	Service Facility	*Very good*	*Good*	*Satis-factory*	*Bad*	*Hope-less*	*No Reply*
1.	**Service**						
1.1	Medical Treatment	5	50	25	5	5	10
1.2	Dispensary	5	22	53	10	5	5
1.3	Laboratory	10	40	25	15	10	—
1.4	X-Ray	12	23	54	4	—	7
1.5	Physiotherapy	10	20	56	7	4	3
2.	**Behaviour**						
2.1	Receptionists	15	20	32	6	5	22
2.2	Senior Consultants	11	22	44	12	8	3
2.3	Junior Consultants	13	19	51	13	—	4
2.4	House Surgeons	16	21	49	9	3	2
2.5	Registrars	17	24	52	5	2	—
2.6	MRD Staff	7	28	55	8	1	1
2.7	Matrons	9	51	28	7	3	2
2.8	Ward Sisters	6	48	39	6	—	1
2.9	Duty Sisters	12	41	29	11	4	3
2.10	Male Nursing Staff	10	38	47	2	1	2
2.11	Class IV Employees	11	23	56	2	1	7
3.	**Availability of**						
3.1	Medicines	12	55	26	4	3	—
3.2	Injections	8	31	51	3	5	2
3.3	Dressing	11	33	49	5	2	—
3.4	Linen	9	30	41	9	5	6
4.	**Cleanliness**						
4.1	Offices	20	28	43	4	3	2
4.2	Verandahs	7	32	41	11	6	3
4.3	Wards	6	23	48	18	2	3
4.4	Lawns	10	31	40	10	6	3
4.5	Stores	8	32	41	5	6	8
4.6	Bathrooms	9	31	39	11	5	5
4.7	Latrines	11	20	31	20	10	8
4.8	Urinals	10	31	49	5	2	3
4.9	Linen	11	22	51	5	6	5
5.	**Food**						
5.1	Cooking Standard	9	31	50	6	2	2
5.2	Variety	10	24	51	7	4	4
5.3	Quantity	11	25	49	9	6	—
5.4	Service	12	23	48	9	8	2
6.	**Amenities**						
6.1	Light	10	20	55	10	5	—
6.2	Fans	15	22	47	10	6	—
6.3	Drinking Water	8	21	45	15	11	2
6.4	Canteen	9	25	46	12	5	3
6.5	Postal	11	26	47	8	7	1
6.6	Telephone	8	24	45	15	8	—

TABLE 12.2

Hospital Communication and Decision-making Process Employee's Response

Sr. Code	*4*	*3*	*2*	*1*
CD 1	—	—	60	40
CD 2	—	—	80	20
CD 3	—	—	10	90
CD 4	10	30	40	20
CD 5	—	—	40	60
CD 6	—	—	40	60
CD 7	—	—	50	50
CD 8	—	—	20	80
CD 9	—	—	10	90
CD 10	—	—	15	85
CD 11	10	20	40	30
CD 12	—	—	10	90
CD 13	—	—	10	90
CD 14	—	—	40	60
CD 15	—	—	10	90
CD 16	—	20	10	70
CD 17	70	10	10	10
CD 18	—	—	40	40
CD 19	—	20	40	40
CD 20	—	20	40	40

the superior and subordinate personnel of an organization jointly identify its common goals and ensure performance. The Manager must encourage the development of such concepts among employees. The response in Table 3 has been presented to depict the management working environment in the hospital. The respondents were the same as selected in earlier questionnaire. Majority of them rate all activities below average. We must encourage employees' satisfaction to ensure fruitful results. A climate of creativity must be developed and maintained by management. Maier and Hayes say that "the optimal climate for creativity . . . is whatever human conditions' optimal for individual freedom and self-expression in social setting.[27] Most of the respondents were critical of the top persons in the hospital. The success or failure of an organization depends, to a great extent, upon the administrative capability and motivation of its top leadership.

Administrative capability is "the capacity to obtain intended results through organization.[28] Katz says, "Administrative capability for development involves the ability to mobilize, allocate and combine the actions that are technically needed to achieve development objectives.[29]

Leaders must be the persons with vision, initiative and desire to achieve the operational goals with dedication and perseverance. The greatest efficiency and productivity will flow from the efforts of those who find satisfaction in their work and conditions of service, who sense an awareness of usefulness of their function, who feel encouraged to move ahead and to meet new challenges, who perceive their working environment as one in which high standards of performance are maintained and rewarded and not one in which indolence and incompetence can be ignored or even protected and rewarded.

In order to determine personality characteristics of a selected sample of hospital employees, a questionnaire as shown administered to 50 respondents.* [* Physicians (16) , Dentists (2), Pharmacists (3), Nurses (10), Nurse Aides (5), Other staff (14)]. The respondents were asked to rank following six needs in order of priority:

(a) Security of Job,
(b) Salary,
(c) Promotion,
(d) Application and recognition of work,
(e) Power and respect,
(f) Development of personal worth.

TABLE 12.3

Percentage Response Based on Questionnaire 4

Needs	*Priority Ranking*					
	1	*2*	*3*	*4*	*5*	*6*
Security of Job	12	18	30	35	4	1
Salary	50	20	10	5	2	3
Promotion	42	31	14	8	3	2
Appreciation						
Recognition of work						
Power and respect	32	26	16	12	8	6
Development of personal worth	1	4	10	15	30	40

The selection of respondents was based on stratified random sampling where employees belonging to various wards/departments and of different official statuses were chosen. The response in terms of percentages is given in Table 12.3 above.

Analysis of data given in Table 12.3 reveals that maximum number of employees give higher weightage to salary and promotion and their next consideration is security of job/recognition of work. Thus, the management must give due consideration to this aspect.

It is true that the importance of pay or compensation is very great for every employee. The standard of living and the social prestige of an employee depends to a great extent on the pay he draws. Manson Haire remarks, "Pay in one form or another is certainly one of the mainsprings of motivation in our society."[30] Thus, an adequate and sound salary structure, together with other working conditions, is the *sine qua non* for the organizational effectiveness. However, we must be clear that no compensation plan can satisfy all the employees. The true efficiency in an organization can be promoted only through dedication and loyalty of its staff members. We must inculcate pride in the job among the staff members of an organization, i.e., doing job with their best ability to achieve excellence in their own fields. Only such individuals who aspire to fulfil their self-actualization needs can bring about creativity, innovation and development in the structure and functioning of the organization. The administration must provide congenial and creative environment for them as they are the builders of the organization. To quote Nehru, "No administrator, I suppose, or anyone else for the matter of that, can really do first class work without a sense of function, without some measures of a crusading spirit. I am doing this, I have to achieve this, as a part of great movement in a big cause. That gives a sense of function not the sense of individual, narrow approach of doing a job in an office for a salary or a wage, something connected with your life's outlook or anything, perhaps being interested as people inevitably are, on one's personal preferment in that particular work."[31]

Based upon discussion and facts, we maintain here some other areas and their solution.

Escalating Costs

The budgets of hospitals are increasing beyond proportions over the years which is beyond the capacity of poor countries like Thailand. The whole of the health budget is spent in maintaining few hospitals neglecting the vast population needing health and medical care. According to H.A. Goddard,

> "In the management of administration of any enterprise, the quality, quantity, timing and cost of the work necessary to reach the objectives of the enterprise are inter-related factors which must be given constant attention. In the resources for health work in trained persons and in finances were unlimited, the need for constant attention to these factors would not be so great. But the limitation in the number of trained personnel and the lack of adequate financial resources are major obstacles to greatly improved health in the world today. We must, therefore, husband our resources carefully to accomplish as much as possible with what we have available."[32]

Absence of Cost-consciousness among Hospital Staff

A serious problem in health care administration is the absence of cost-consciousness among the staff of public health administrations. All over the world, health, service staff—even of the highest professional cadre—are taught little about the economics of health services and know little about the costs of the equipment and supplies they use. Doctors tend to employ what is new without regard to cost. It is a fashion to prescribe costly drugs. They are also subjected to considerable sales pressure from manufacturing firms. A cheaper drug or cheaper equipment may give just as good a result for the vast majority of patients. Cost-consciousness is not just a matter for central administrators or planners but should be inculcated in all those working in health care. More people can be provided with services if no services cost more than that is a must to provide the necessary level of care. The price paid for high-cost technology for a few is no technology at all for the many. Another aspect of this problem is the use of hospital non-judiciously.

Absence of Co-ordination

At present, all hospitals whether at the state, district or local levels, are working in isolation and their services are not provided in a co-ordinated manner. Most of the patients visit all these hospitals and are examined afresh by all of them resulting in wastage of efforts and resources. The medical staff prescribe medicines to patients without having a proper awareness of his previous treatment.

How can we get out of this chaos to design a system of patient care? The answer is introduction of Regionalization. Regionalization connotes the development of graded patient care within a defined geographical or functional area from lower to higher levels adapting the health services to the characteristics and needs of the area and thus ensuring the optimum utilization of resources. The essential characteristics of regionalization are:[33]

(a) Two-way flow of patients.
(b) Two-way flow of records.
(c) Two-way flow of services.
(d) Two-way flow of personnel.
(e) Mobile units.
(f) Centralized administration and decentralized execution.
(g) Co-ordinating Education Programme for the Region.
(h) Communication and Transport between components.
(i) Co-ordination with other community health services.

Thus, regionalization would ensure the best utilization of time of the specialists and provision of comprehensive health care to the patients nearer their homes with all the benefits of specialities. The regional area should neither be too large nor too small but should be such as to ensure adequate span of attention. It would also automatically develop referral system scientifically.

The referral system presents the following five aspects:[34]

(a) It has to be built into the organizational structure of the medical services of a country. The rule should be that only when one unit cannot provide what a patient needs should the patient be referred for the next higher unit in the chain.
(b) The referral system has to be organized both internally and externally. 'Internally' means that patients in the hospital have to be referred from the inpatients to the outpatients department just as soon as their health situation permits. The 'externally' referred system exists among the several institutions on different levels of the hierarchy.
(c) The referral system, must be established for the purpose of diagnosis and treatments and used for both inpatients and outpatients.
(d) It is a two-way system. Patients should be referred to higher level institutions for diagnosis and treatment when necessary, but they should also be referred to the referring institution as soon as possible.
(e) The referral system concerns not only patients and diagnostic facilities but also the personnel of the medical services. This is also a two-way system, so that human knowledge and skills are utilized fully and are continually developed through consultations and the interchange of ideas and experience.

The specialists from the regional hospital must come to the District hospital and the specialist from the District hospital to the health centre on a regular basis as consultants to hold specialist clinics and give guidance; the medical and para-medical personnel should go to the higher level institution regularly for in-service training.

Lack of Administrative Capability

Hospital administration is a science as well as an art. The hospital administration has become complex and requires administrative capability to solve its managerial problems to provide the optimum care to the patients. It is, therefore, necessary that the persons charged with the efficient running of the hospitals are trained in the managerial techniques and tools which may be applied by them for getting the best out of the resources available.

Lack of Effective Public Relations

Hospitals should try to establish cordial, equitable and, therefore, mutually profitable relations between the hospitals and their beneficiaries. The patients mostly complain of discourteous behaviour of hospital staff especially at the lower level. . . This irritates the patients and their relatives. The test of the efficiency of a hospital is the satisfaction of the beneficiaries.

The sympathetic and courteous behaviour of hospital staff would have a soothing and lasting effect on the patients and their relatives. It is suggested that all hospital personnel must inspire confidence and put the nervous patients and their relatives at ease.

> "The hospital today is more than the combination of medical and therapeutic treatment by specialists, greater and refined medical and surgical knowledge and ever better and more effective facilities and equipment. It includes these factors as the core of its efficient operation but an additional dimension—one which is too often ignored or at least minimized—is the human and social element in the structure of the organization."[35]

Lack of Dedicated Staff and Government Organizational Structure

The ideal of service must be encouraged among the personnel responsible for health care. It is the responsibility of the hospital authorities to set the pattern for the philosophy of patient care. It was rightly mentioned by Gardner:

> "No society can reach heights of greatness unless in all fields critical to its growth and creativity there is an ample supply of dedicated men and women."[36]

The patients also complained of the lack of co-ordination between supportive services and the medical services. Most of the patients complained of the non-availability either of their X-ray report or other laboratory reports. They go on wasting their time in tracing their reports. Besides, many patients complained that preferential treatment is given to friends and relatives of the hospital staff. Many patients complained of the non-availability of medicines. Besides, patients are referred to other departments which results in great delays for the treatment to be given to them because of unsatisfactory co-ordination among the various departments of the hospital. It is suggested that:

(1) To encourage polite and courteous behaviour of the staff towards the patients, orientation and in-service training opportunities should be provided to the staff.
(2) Outpatients should be properly guided by the doctors issuing prescriptions regarding the procedure to be followed to get their blood, urine, stool, etc., samples tested.
(3) Laboratories may be modernized and out-dated equipment replaced as early as possible to improve the accuracy of the test results because these tests form the basis of the medical treatment which the patients are to be imparted.

Further, it is suggested on the basis of the observations by the authority that the patients may be issued the slips on arrival on which may be indicated the probable time of his examination by the doctor.

The following steps could also be taken to improve matters:

(a) Effective co-ordination should be established between the medical services and the supportive services to ensure promptness and clarity.
(b) Effective co-ordination and co-operation must be ensured among the various departments of the hospital to help the patients in diagnosing their ailments. It is suggested that a medical board may meet once a week where all the specialities may be represented and the patients needing the attention of more than one speciality may be asked to attend the board.
(c) A receptionist well-versed with the functioning of hospital system may be appointed to guide the patients to approach the hospital properly.
(d) There is a need of play cards and signboards to guide the patients and their relatives.
(e) Provision of cheap and quality goods to be used by the patients or their relatives.
(f) Arrangement of stay of the relatives in rest houses specially constructed for the purpose.
(g) Hospital beds may be given to patients according to the severity of the diseases rather than other trifle considerations like obliging the VIPs.

In brief, the functioning of the hospital should be organized and re-organized to serve the patients most efficiently. All the personnel engaged in patient care must keep the following definitions of the patient in their minds:

1. The patient is the most important person in the hospital.
2. The patient is not dependent upon us—we are dependent on him.
3. The patient is not an interruption of our work—he is the purpose of it.
4. The patient is not an outsider to our business—he is our business.
5. The patient is a person and not a statistic—he has feelings, emotions, biases and wants.
6. It is our business to satisfy him.

We must attend to all these problems to ensure efficiency of the hospitals. These problems also emanate from a number of constraints on hospital authorities, e.g., shortage of staff at all levels, absence of proper accommodation to provide space to the ever increasing number of patients, shortages of funds, shortages of medicine, shortage of equipment, political and administrative interference, etc. which need to be attended to by the Government to provide satisfactory hospital services. Besides, the patients and their relatives must co-operate with the hospital authorities to make the best use of the available resources. Thus, we shall have to have a three-pronged attack—increasing internal efficiency, mobilizing Government support and enlisting people's co-operation to ensure the reputation, prestige, credibility and viability of the hospital services.

Notes and References

1. Members are elected by People.
2. Ministry of Public Health in Thailand, Bangkok, 1973. This is a piece of doctoral Research by Krienkrai Klimoboul, first Secretary, Thais Embassy, under the guidance of the Author who visited Thailand alongwith the study.
3. Chareon Chittasombat, Presentation of the Government Pharmaceutical Organization, Bangkok, Conference on Health Economics, May 1974
4. Chalad Tirapat, Medical Referral System in CBD Project, Bangkok, Mahidoi University, Public Health Faculty, April, 1977.
5. Uthai Sudsukh, Director of the Rural Health Division, Officer of the Under-Secretary of State MOPH, Personal Interview, Bangkok, November, 1978.
6. Debhanom Maungman, New Approach to Rural Health Care in Thailand and its possible application to other Development Countries, New Delhi, WHO, South-East Regional Schools of Public Health, 1-3, Nov. 1978.
7. WHO: Technical Report Series, 1968, 396, p. 6.
8. Elen, I. Perry: Ward Management and Teaching, Bailliere, Tindall, London, 1978, p. 2.
9. World Health Organization, "Thailand", in Fifth Report on the World Health Situation, 1969-74, Geneva, 1975, p. 151.
10. World Health Organization, Regional Office for South-East Asia, Basic Statistical Information Relating to Health, in WHO South-East Asia Region, New Delhi, July 1978, p. 5.
11. Ministry of Public Health, Division of Public Health Statistics, Public Health Statistics, 1973-74, Bangkok, 1975, pp. 263-67.
12. "Ministry of Public Health", Department of Medical Services, Statistical Report, 1975, Bangkok, 1978, p. 25.
13. Official Records of the Ministry of Public Health, Thailand.
14. Narong Sabudi, Director of Divisions of Provincial Hospitals, Ministry of Public Health, Personal Interview, Nov., 1978.
15. World Bank, Thailand, Appraisal of a Popoulation Project, Report No. 1663 - TH, 18 January, 1978, p. 7.
16. Prawase Wasi, Professor at Siriraj Hospital Medical Faculty, Personal Communication, November, 1978.
17. Narong Sabudi, Director of the Division of Provincial Hospitals, Ministry of Public Health, Communication, November, 1978.
18. *Ibid.*
19. Samboon Vachrotai, Director of the Department of Health, Ministry of Public Health, Personal Communication, November, 1978.
20. South East Asian Medical Information Centre, Seamic Health Statistics, 1978, Tokyo, The rate in the text has been derived from this source.
21. Pravasse Wasi, 9.21.

22. R. Neutra (1948), Architecture of Social Concern in Regions and Mild Climate, Sao Paulo.
23. S.M. Machintosh (1951): What is a Hospital for ? WHO unpublished document, WHO/PHA/4.
24. Keith Davis, "The Case for Participative Management", *Business Horizons*, Vol. 6, No. 3, 1963, p. 141.
25. ILO: International Labour Confernece, 33rd Session, Provisional Records, p. 34.
26. Cooper R. Michael, and Wood, T. Michael, "Member Participation and Commitment in group decision-making on influence satisfaction and decision."
27. Norman R.F. Maier, and John, J. Hayes: Creative Management, New York, John Wiley and Sons, Inc., 1962, p. 36.
28. Saul M. Katz, "A Methodological Note on Appraising Administrative Capability for Development", in Appraising Administrative Capability for Development", (UN Publication Sales No. E.60 11, H.2) p. 8.
29. *Ibid.*, pp. 99-100, 24, Manson Haire, *et. al.*
30. IIPA, Jawaharlal Nehru and Public Administration, New Delhi, 1975, p. 88.
31. H.A. Gaddard, Principles of Administration applied to Nursing Service, World Health Organization, Geneva, 1958, p. 34.
32. Timmappaya, Regionalization of Health Care.
33. WHO, SEARO: SEA/RC 23/1, pp. 39-40.
34. Mary D. Shanks and Dorothy A. Kennedy, The Theory and Practice of Nursing Service Administration, McGraw Hill, London, 1965, p. 95.
35. John W. Gardner, Excellence, New York, 1961, Harner and Brothers, p. 154.
36. Edythe Alexander *et al.* Nursing Service Administration (ed.), New York, C.V. Mosby Co., 1962, p. 63.

Appendix

GUIDANCE NOTES ON THE APPLICATION OF ISO 9001, QUALITY MANAGEMENT SYSTEM IN HOSPITAL AND HEALTH CARE UNITS

Introduction

Quality aspects of health services: Health services include a wide variety of quality aspects all of which are important; indeed, in spite of the long history of health services the concept of "quality" is still not carefully and completely defined. These aspects are outlined below and described in some detail in this chapter. A lack of detailed information about many, if not most, of these aspects simply means that we have not yet faced up to the need for quality control in numerous areas of vital interest to the buyer.

The vital aspects of health service may be described as follows:

1. A seller—doctor, hospital, nursing home, clinic, etc.—offers health services for sale at stipulated prices.
2. A buyer—client, patient, etc.—buys these health services at the stipulated prices, either directly, by means of insurance or subsidies.
3. The buyer wants acceptable quality services which are commensurate with what he or she is paying the seller.
4. Acceptable quality service not only include the quality of direct medical services such as diagnoses, medicines, surgery, and treatments, but indirect operations such as administration, purchasing, etc. whose costs are reflected in what the buyer pays. It also includes the quality of performance that is directly connected and closely related to health care such as food, housing, safety, security, attitude of employees, and other factors which arise in connection with hospital and nursing homes.
5. A major factor of vital importance in much of health service is time—time to appointment, delay time, service time, timing with regard to medicines, treatments and surgery.

The several major aspects and areas of quality control are outlined and described below:

1. Quality of administration and management:
   1.1 In a doctor's office
   1.2 In a hospital

Indian Institution of Quality Management, Ministry of Information Technology, Government of India, Standardisation, Testing and Quality Dte., Malviya Industrial Area, Jaipur-302 017 (Rajasthan).

1.3 In a nursing home
1.4 In a clinic
1.5 In other health offices or institutions

The quality aspects include such operations as the following: staffing, purchasing, supervision, appointments, admissions, discharges, emergency room, physical arrangement, payments and insurance, record-keeping, prescriptions, pharmacy and medicines, linens and laundry, house-keeping, sanitation, operating rooms and laboratories.

2. Time factor in a doctor's office or clinic:
   2.1 Time required to obtain an appointment
   2.2 Waiting time in the office
   2.3 Actual service time
   2.4 Time required for one or more additional visits
3. Quality of a doctor's services:
   3.1 Examination
   3.2 Laboratory tests: blood, urine, other
   3.3 Ofice tests: X-rays, EKG, blood pressule, glaucoma, temperature, pulse weight, other
   3.4 Diagnosis, accuracy of
   3.5 Effectiveness of medicines prescribed
   3.6 Effectiveness of surgery performed
   3.7 Prescriptions: fill and refill
   3.8 Anything unnecessary?
   3.9 Anything important omitted?

The quality of a doctor's service is measured by the accuracy of the diagnosis, the effectiveness of the medicines prescribed, the effectiveness of any surgery performed, the effectiveness of any measures or treatments prescribed, and the effectiveness of any regimen recommended. Is the trouble eliminated? Is the trouble brought under control? Does the medicine control or correct the situation? Does the surgery eliminate the source of trouble? Does the person or patient get well? Considering the situation and conditions, did the doctor do all that could be done?

4. Quality of hospital care:
   4.1 Emergency room
   4.2 Ambulance service
   4.3 Admissions
   4.4 Patient control
   4.5 Patient's room
   4.6 Patient's surroundings
   4.7 Patient's care: food
   4.8 Patient's care: medicines
   4.9 Patient's care: other: personal, batch, attention, cleanliness, security

4.10 Patient's care: monitoring
4.11 Central telephone control
4.12 Visitor control
4.13 Delivery control, mail control
4.14 Discharge control, insurance and billing
4.15 Operating room control
4.16 Nurse performance
4.17 Doctor's care
4.18 House-keeping

Quality enters into every aspect of a hospital directly from the time the patient is admitted until the patient is discharged. One control is simply knowing where the patient is: whether in a certain room in bed, whether preparing for an operation, or whether in the operating room or out of it. Another is keeping a central front office file of patient status, up to the minute literally, so as to handle mail, visitors, and deliveries promptly and accurately—a correct record of the patient's name, when admitted, what room, whether in the hospital, and whether discharged and when.

Consider an example: The key person is the patient, the key characteristic is the health of the patient, and a related characteristic is the cost to the patient. Five areas of quality are of vital interest to the patient:

(1) the location and status of the patient which requires accurate and up-to-the-minute records;
(2) the medical care which includes medicines, nursing care, and doctor's care;
(3) supportive medical care which includes food, housing, personal care, treatment, and security;
(4) financial controls which includes bills, claims, insurance, and medicare; and
(5) unnecessary medical care which includes unnecessary surgery, medicines, tests and medical technology. Control over all of these reflects a concern for the patient's health, welfare, comfort, and pocketbook.

It is asserted by some that patients generally cannot appraise the health services they receive. Except for a very small percentage of patients and for highly specialized illnesses, this simply is not true. Patients are quite competent to pass sound judgments on the food, the medicines, the treatment received, the bills they pay, and on whether the medical services helped them, had no effect, or made them worse. Quality control needs to start with the patient and the quality characteristics associated with the patient.

An example of a proposed quality control system: Although the original quality assurance program was to include the development of several quality control reporting programs, it became evident early in the program that the hospital lacked the necessary resources for this expansion. Seven programs or systems however have been identified:

1. Patient and commodity transportation
2. Material supply and distribution
3. Patient dietary and food services
4. Medication ordering and distribution
5. Ancillary services, e.g., radiology and laboratory
6. Medical chart completion
7. Accounts receivable charge processing

As an example the following specifications were formulated for the first program or system; it should be noted that this specification deals with the very important characteristic of time and the significance of delay time as a quality characteristic.

History of Quality of Health Care

Ever since Hamourabi (3000 B.C.) promulgated his laws for monitoring and controlling goods and bad acts, quality assurance methods have been developing and evolving. History suggest that the first person, who started quality movement in health care was Florence Nightingale back in the mid-1800's. The nurse, Nightingale returned back to England to study this inter-relationship better in English hospitals. She further studied issues related to utilization of care and development process standards for nursing practice.

Dr. Emory W. Groves of the U.K. studied hospital mortality related to surgeries. He recommended the development of a disease classification system and the establishment of a follow-up system early in 1900's. In the US, Dr. Abraham Flexnor in 1910 published his report on the state of medical education. He called for the improvement of standards of education and recommended a set of strict guidelines. Accordingly, his recommendations were adopted by the US government and later forced a number of medical schools to close their doors for inability to need those guidelines. This was followed by the American College of Surgeons initiative to develop the hospital standardization program in 1918 which later evolved in 1952 to create the Joint Commission of Accreditation for Hospitals (JCAHO) (later changed its name to Health Care Organization rather than hospitals).

The date, JCAHO is still very active in surveying thousands health care organizations annually for quality measures. The countries other than US with the most firmly established accreditation systems are Canada and Australia. In the US there were three clear phases in the evolution of the accreditation process: the era of minimal standards 1917-65, the era of optimal achievable standards 1966-87 and the era of performance evaluation and beyond from 1988 (Brooks T., 1990). The performance-based standards, scoring guidelines, aggregation rules, the decision rules are woven together in the Accreditation Manual. The following eligibility requirements are: the Joint Commission and applicable standards for services provided by the organization. The organization is located within the United States or the under a charter of the United States Congress. When applying, the organization identifies all services that it provides and advises the Joint Commission as to whether each of these services is provided directly, under contract, or through some other arrangement.

JCAHO has published its own definition, "Quality of patient care is the degree to which patient care services increases the probability of outcomes, giving the current state of knowledge." The Joint Commissions definitions reflect the view that quality involves at least doing no harm to patients.

QUALITY MANAGEMENT FOR HOSPITALS

Section (A) Outpatient Department (OPD)

1. Planning

(i) Physical facilities for diagnostic, curative, preventive, promotive and rehabilitative.
Emergency for casualty department to provide immediate treatment to patients on arrival.

(ii) Expected workload with regard to number of beds, availability of other health care facility in the vicinity, socio-economic/cultural status, prevalent disease pattern, etc.

(iii) Adequate manpower, equipment, laboratory, etc.

2. Organisational Structure

Well defined organisational structure, including responsibility, authority and job description for medical/paramedical personnel.

3. Functional Management

- Timing of OPD and Emergency
- Entrance and Ambulatory zone
- Enquiry and Registration
- Medical records
- Clinics for various medical disciplines
- Pharmacy (Dispensary)
- Treatment/minor surgical/dressing room/Diagnostic zone (clinics labs/X-ray/ultrasound)
- Health Education
- Family Welfare

The services and facility available at each important point in the flow are as follows:

(A) Emergency Entrance

1. It is easily accessible in terms of time. It takes hardly a minute to reach the department.
2. Two trolleys and a wheel chair are present at the entrance to bring the patient.
3. Door of the entrance of emergency department is double swing, wide enough for two trolleys to pass through it at the same time.

(B) General Entrance

1. General entrance gate is double swing, wide enough for two trolleys to pass through same time.
2. Information counter is staffed by two receptionists during day time and by one staff at night to help and guide the patients.
3. People at the reception were found to be very friendly and courteous in responding to the questions. Their communication was clear and the patients were appropriately directed.
4. On an average the patient has to wait not more than for two minutes for the queries to be answered at the reception.
5. There are four coin telephones available for local call, one STD booth and four intercoms for patients/attendants use.
6. Eatables are available in the shop in the main entrance lobby and in the ICU lobby. Gift shop is also available in the main entrance lobby.
7. Pharmacy, shop for outpatients is also present in the information lobby.

(C) Reception of the OPD Block

1. One receptionist is present for guiding the patients to the particular OPD's and for issuing the ID cards to the Patients who are registering for the first in the hospital. It takes two to three minutes for card to be issued for a patient.
2. Two people are present in the cash counter which is opposite to the reception counter of the OPD block to collect the money of the patients going for investigations.

(D) Respecting of the Particular OPD

1. Two people at the reception are available to guide the patients according to their needs.

Example taken from Documented Procedure of ABC (India) Hospital

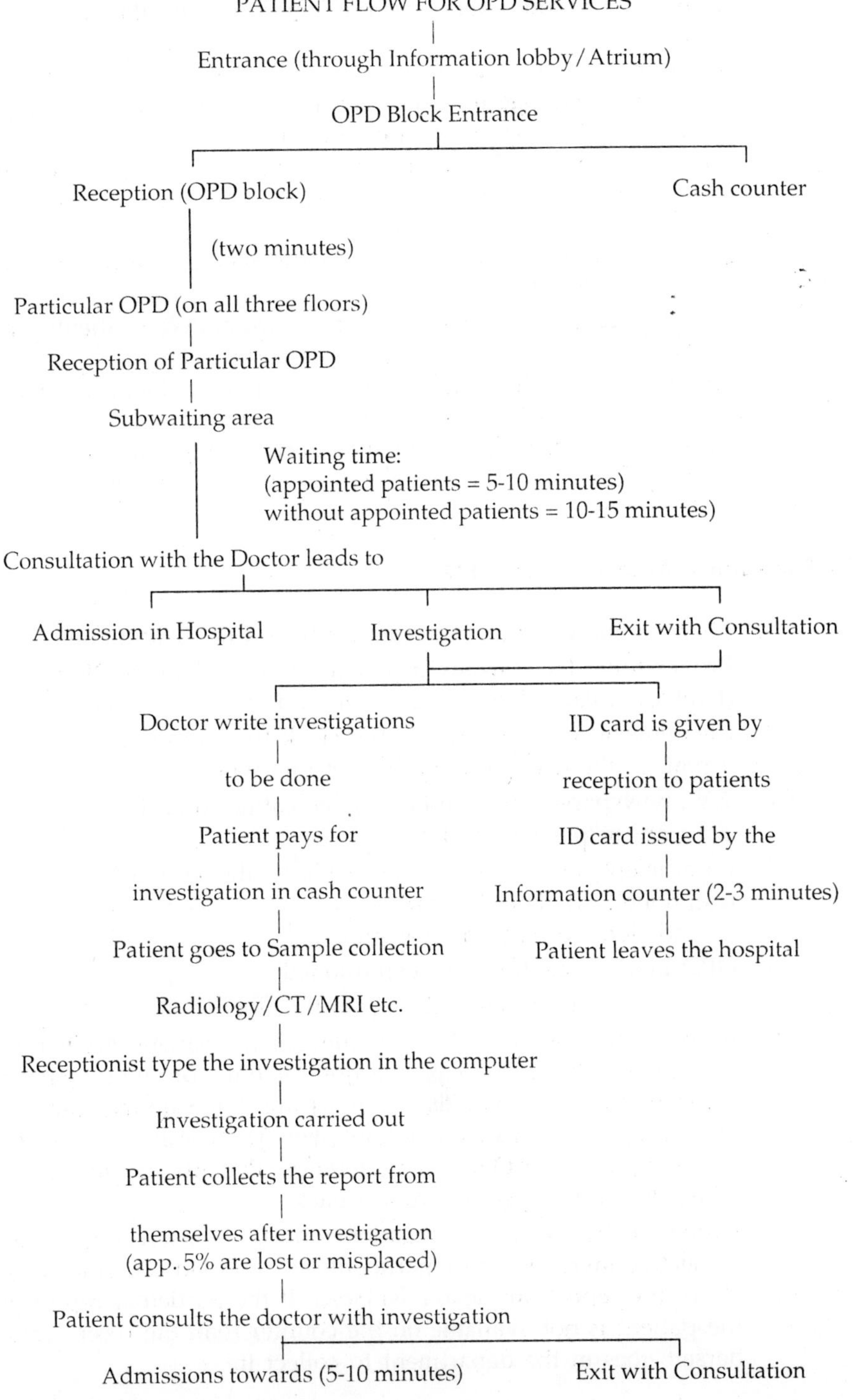

2. New patient has to fill in the registration form (2-3 minutes it takes to fill a form on an average), this information receptionist feed in the computer which is on-line with the admission counter.
3. If the patient has taken appointment, then the patient has to wait on an average for 5-10 minutes. The reported time for the patient who is without appointment has to wait for 15-20 minutes. Approx. 22 minutes is the patient's average waiting time according to the observation made. The reasons found after discussions and observation are:
   (a) File has to be retrieved from the medical records of the unappointed patients.
   (b) Preference is given to the appointed patients for consultation.
4. Medical record file of the appointed patient is already available at reception. Retrieval of files of the appointed patients is done on previous evening from medical records department.
5. Doctors give on an average 15-20 minutes per patient for consultation.

(E) Subwaiting Area of Each OPD

1. There is space for at least thirty patients to sit at a time.
2. Proper toilet facilities are available on each floor of OPD wing (twelve on each floor, six for men and six for women).
3. Cleaning of toilets is around the clock from morning 8 a.m. to 8 p.m. in the evening done by contract workers.
4. T.V., newspapers are present for recreation in each OPD wing. Toys are in paedriatic OPD.
5. Local telephone facilities are available on the second floors (coin telephone), so that the patient has not to come down from second floor to make a local phone.
6. OPD block is centrally air conditioned.
7. There is a appropriate lighting on the floors.
8. It takes approximately 10-15 minutes for the patient to given its sample in the Sample Collection Room for investigation, Investigations for other departments line CT, Gamma Camera, DSA, Dialysis are done on appointment. The vacant slot is given to the patients of OPD on preference. Patients are informed, when they can collect the report back.
9. Patients collect their investigation reports themselves from the respective investigation department. As reported on an average 5% of the reports are lost/misplaced. If the particular report of the patient is not available on the counter than the receptionist herself goes in the department to collect it.

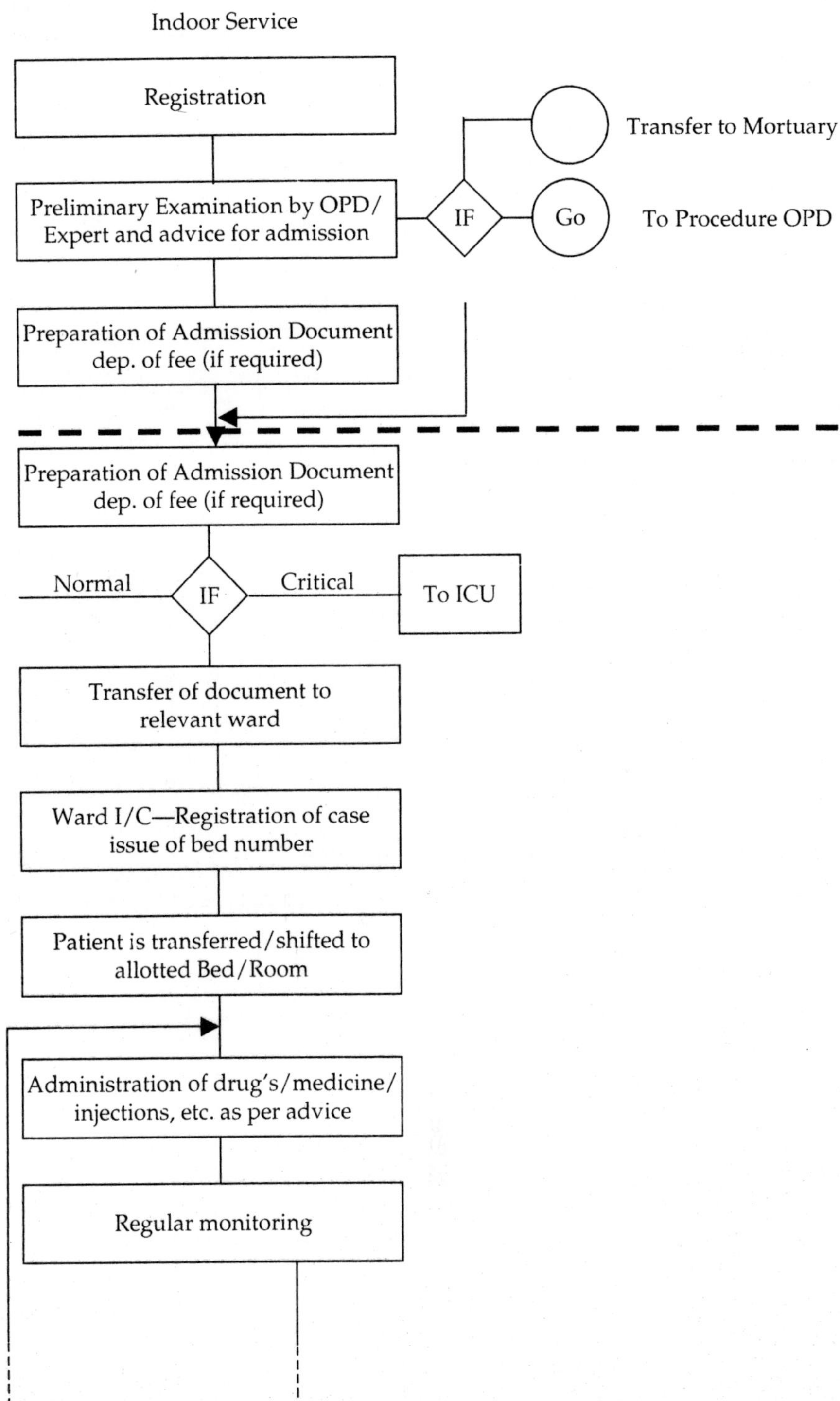
Indoor Service
Registration
Transfer to Mortuary
Preliminary Examination by OPD/ Expert and advice for admission
IF
Go
To Procedure OPD
Preparation of Admission Document dep. of fee (if required)
Preparation of Admission Document dep. of fee (if required)
Normal
IF
Critical
To ICU
Transfer of document to relevant ward
Ward I/C—Registration of case issue of bed number
Patient is transferred/shifted to allotted Bed/Room
Administration of drug's/medicine/ injections, etc. as per advice
Regular monitoring

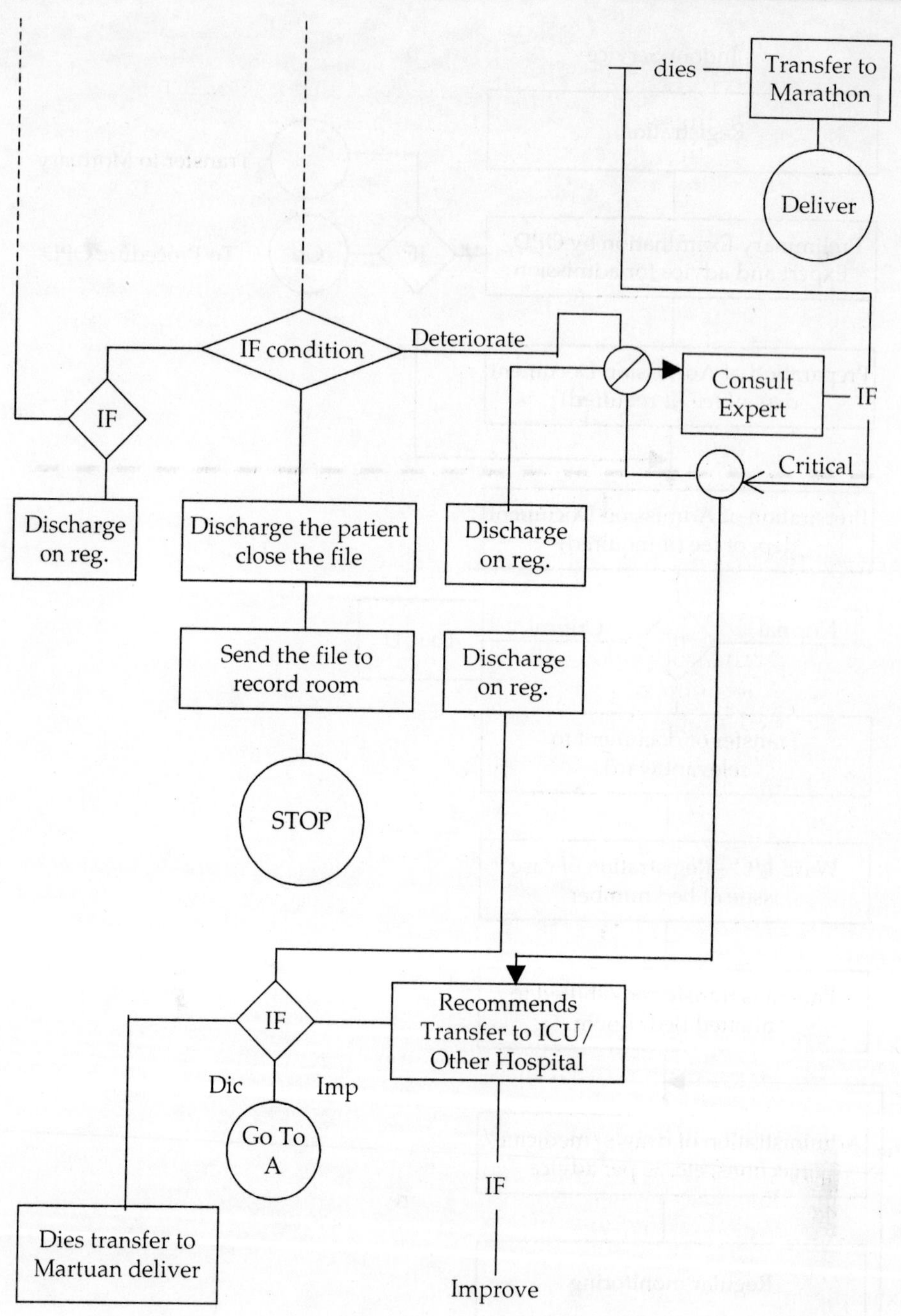
dies
Transfer to Marathon
Deliver
IF condition
Deteriorate
Consult Expert
IF
IF
Critical
Discharge on reg.
Discharge the patient close the file
Discharge on reg.
Send the file to record room
Discharge on reg.
STOP
Recommends Transfer to ICU/ Other Hospital
IF
Dic
Imp
Go To A
IF
Improve
Dies transfer to Martuan deliver

10. Patient Admission Counter:

    1. The patient information from OPD is on line to the admission counter so the patient face sheet is generated within two minutes at the admission counter.
    2. Three persons are always available there. One person takes the face sheet out on computer, other is for giving admissions and passes (putting the face sheet on the file, making IP form filled by the patient/attendant, issuing passes), third person is for the collection of cash (security money has to be deposited before admission). Only money in cash and credit cards are accept.
    3. If the room is not vacant according to the choice of the patient, then there is a provision to admit the patient in Day care or in observation ward. Transfer is given as soon as the room is vacant.

Section [B]: Wards, Nursing Services and Operation Theatre

1. Ward

- ❑ Arrival of patient, Enquiry and Registration
- ❑ Allocation of Bed
- ❑ Bed preparation
- ❑ Nursing records/case sheets
- ❑ Initiation of treatment
- ❑ Medical/Nursing care
- ❑ Investigation
- ❑ Day-to-Day Management
- ❑ Discharge, follow up.

2. Operation Theatre

- ❑ Reception
- ❑ Pre-anaesthetic medication
- ❑ Pre-operative check up
- ❑ Anaesthization
- ❑ Operation theatre check list
- ❑ Operative procedures
- ❑ Recovery and post-operative care
- ❑ Wards/Discharge

Example taken from documented procedure of ABC (India) hospital:

Wards:

1. Ward secretary is the first person receive the patient in the ward, she makes the patient aware about the doctor's timings, investigation's timings and the other facilities like food, house-keeping of the patient room and changing of linen, etc.

2. Inpatient guidelines booklet is given to the patients in the wards. It gives all information about the hospital facilities available to the patients.
3. Rooms are kept ready by house-keeping boys after thorough cleaning before any new patient occupies it.
4. After every consultation/investigation activity card of the inpatient is filled by the ward secretary. It is send for interim billing in the Finance Department, daily for ICU patient and in two days for general ward patient.

(F) Discharge of the Patient

1. If, the patient dues in the hospital then, death drill is followed. All the discharge formalities are carried out urgently without troubling the patient relatives and body its taken to the mortuary immediately.
2. Planned discharges are at 9.00 a.m., in the morning, at 12.00 in the noon and at 5.00 p.m. in the evening. If the discharge is of 9.00 a.m., then the bills and discharge summary is prepared in the night only. Signature on discharge summary is done by the consultant. Activity card of the patients goes for billing at around 10.30 a.m. in the morning for bill preparation.
3. Billing takes on an average one hour to one and a half hour. The prepared bill is audited by the auditors of the finance department, then the patient is informed on telephone that his bill is ready, patient attendant deposit the bill in the admission counter and can also make clarification about the bill from billing department.

Section [C]: Hospital Support Services

1. Hospital Supply System

- Medical and Surgical store
- General store (Linen/furniture, etc.)
- Central sterile supply deptt. (CSSD)

2. Laundry: (5 Kg. Linen/bed/day)

- Patient care linen
- Bed linen
- Body linen
- Operation theatre linen
- Staff linen
- Laundry linen
- Contaminated/Infected linen

- Soiled linen
- Foul linen

3. Hospital Dietary services

- Organisational structure
- Functional activities
- Menu
- Procurement
- Storage/safety/hygienic

4. House-keeping and maintenance

- Waste Management
- Hospital hygiene maintenance
- Infection control/pest control
- Environment control/pest control
- Sanitation

Some typical examples taken from documented procedure on support services of ABC (India) hospital:

Hospital Activities to Ensure High Quality

The hospital has several activities meant primarily for ensuring high quality in services given to the patients. These includes Guest Relations, Post Discharges Contacts, Staff and Team Meetings, Service Manuals and Variety of Training. These are described below:

(i) Guest Relations

There is a department of Guest Relations in the hospital, staffed by two guest relation officers. These people deal with patients' complaints, concerns and problems. This leads to a continual improvement in the services and working of the hospitals.

Main activities of this department are:

(a) Monitoring

Guest relation officers go on rounds every day and ask the patients about the problems they are facing. Each problem is rectified on the same day. Complaints/Problems of the particular department is sent to them, in return they send the response. At the end of the day a monitoring sheet is send to the administrator.

(b) Helpline

This service is from morning 8 a.m. to 7 p.m. in the evening. Any one who is having any problem in the hospital can file its complaint on the phone. Immediate action is taken to solve the problem and complainants are telephoned back with a report on the status of their complaints.

(c) Post-Discharge Contacts

Discharge patients are contacted on phone for information about their health status, to make needed appointments and to remind them about the appointments already made.

(ii) Staff and Team Meetings

Apart from the Guest Relations, it was found that there are Composite team meetings. As observed they are held daily for half an hour on each floor. The team constitutes of one floor doctor on duty (resident), Nurse manager, Sister Incharge, House-keeping Supervisor, Dietitian, Food and Beverage Body, One Ward Secretary. These meetings helps to solve most of the day-to-day operational problems and help, improve the patient care. As discussed by IP executives there are getting minutes of these minutes and they themselves try to be present on all of the floor meetings daily.

All executives of the hospital meet with the Administrator once a day to discuss internal problem and needs. There is a running Trophy for the floor whose complaints in the monitoring sheets by help line are least in the month. All nurse managers and sisters incharges meet every Wednesday with Nursing Superintendent. All the nursing problems are discussed here.

There is a daily meeting at 12.00 in the night. This is attended by Night Manager on duty, Nurse Manager, Billing Supervisor, House-keeping Supervisor, Dietician, Security Supervisor, Ward Secretary, Food and Beverage, IP pharmacy incharge.

Important points/problems are discussed and suggested actions are taken. In the morning, report is given by Night Duty Manager goes to CEO. Other than this, there are frequent meetings of the departmental Heads with the CEO and Managing Director.

(iii) Meetings of the Doctors

(a) As reported by the Secretary of Medical Superintendent there is a weekly meeting of all Senior Registrars headed by Medical Superintendent. Discussions are generated and decisions are taken on the issues and the problems raised. This accountability of the implementation of the decisions is on a group leader from each department who is on rotation for one year.

(b) All residents formally meet with the Medical Superintendent every month. During discussion with the doctors it was found that any doctor having any problem can directly meet the Medical Superintendent in morning for the problems related to patients care and in afternoon for personal problems.

Other than these formal meetings, it was observed that on every Saturday all Head of Departments and Consultants, CEO, Managing Director, Director, Medical Services, Director, Nursing Services meet at lunch. This serves as the ground for discussing inter-departmental problems/issues.

(c) *Open Forum*: Open house is called on the first Saturdays of each month from 2 p.m. to 4 p.m. in the board room. The view is to improve the working environment with the continuous channel of communication among all. Such a forum is attended by all Consultants/HOD's/Coordinates or any key Personnel who need to clarify and obtain different views before are taken.

(iv) Hospital Manual

Doctors and nurses have the close links with the patients and bears the responsibility of implementing patient care decisions. Treatment varies from patient to patient. The consultants have a team of residents, Registrars and Senior Registrars along with nurses for treating the patients. To enable doctors to provide appropriate medical care there is a hospital manual for the doctors, particularly the resident staff. This manual is an attempt to aid and streamline patient care activities by providing standardized information about the hospital system of functioning and regulations. This is to increase the efficiency of the doctors and therefore improve the patient care.

This written manual mainly give the guidelines to the doctors regarding their duties, admissions, transfers, discharge procedures. How and when the consent has to be taken by the patient, about the critical ill list, which is sent daily to the Doctor, Medical Services and to the Medical Superintendent.

(v) Continuous Medical Education

Continuous medical education is held daily during lunch hours for doctors according to the speciality. It is mandatory for all doctors. Attendance at the meetings are recorded and is reflected in the Work Experience Certificate and Performance appraisal of the doctors. As reported by the doctors, Registrars and residents are appointed on six months' contract. They are on probation for the first three months and then they are confirmed after 3 months. After every six months the Performance of the individual is appraised by the consultant and Medical Superintendent and the period of contract is extended.

(vi) Training Programs

Provisions are made for the continuous training of the employees working in the hospital so that skill of the employees is enhanced. This in turn increases the quality of patient care. In the month not more than two departments are focused for training. These trainings are conducted by the Training Officer incharge of the personnel department. Some of training programs are:

1. Patient Satisfaction.
2. Induction Program.
3. Communication Skill Program.

4. Language Program.
5. Supervisory Development.
6. Customer Service: For front office staff.
7. Customer Service: For pharmacy boys.
8. Program for house-keeping.

Performance counselling program for all executives.

Section [D]: Hospital Equipment Management

1. Planning

- ❑ Medical and diagnostic equipment
- ❑ Supportive equipment (kitchen, laundry)
- ❑ Trainer manpower

2. Power Supply

- ❑ Availability of standby power/UPS
- ❑ Automatic switch over
- ❑ Voltage regulation
- ❑ Earthing

3. Preventive Maintenance

- ❑ Recruitment of skilled manpower
- ❑ Bank of spare parts and crucial components
- ❑ Maintenance schedule
- ❑ AMC for sophisticated/vital equipment
- ❑ Calibration

GUIDANCE NOTES ON APPLICATION OF TYPICAL ISO 9002 CLAUSES IN HOSPITAL SERVICES

4.1.2.1 Responsibility and Authority (A typical example)

A trained microbiologist shall have the responsibility for all microbiological aspects and control necessary to assure the sterility of all medical devices and surgical products designed to be sterile before and during use and all designated clear room, and/or clean areas including all transport and storage devices designated sterile/clear.

The responsibilities of the microbiologist shall include:

- ❑ the commissioning of sterilizing plant and the defining of effective sterilization and quarantine procedures;
- ❑ the monitoring of the sterilization procedures;
- ❑ the definition and routine monitoring of the performance of all air conditioning and filtration equipment;

- the approval of written hygiene regulations, and the monitoring of their implementation;
- the approval of written cleaning schedules for all areas, and equipment including medical devices;
- the investigation of the level of pre-sterilization microbial contamination of all areas under the control of the microbiologist and the elimination or reduction of the sources of contamination where possible;
- the monitoring and recording of environmental contamination at an appropriate frequency; isolating and identifying unusual contaminator and attempting to determine their sources;
- the microbiological control of materials and fluids; and
- the specification, control and monitoring of all sub-contracted precleaning and sterilization.

Question: Who carries out the pre-cleaning and sterilization process required by the hospitals?

Should a sub-contractor be used for any pre-cleaning and/or sterilization activities, then the sub-contractor should be also audited for technical/system suitability, unless he is already accredited by the recognised authority.

If accredited, then point 9 above should be assessed as working in accordance with paragraph 4.3 contract review ISO 9002.

Note: For microbiological work, laboratory staff should be capable of carrying out routines using aseptic procedures.

Question: Do the hospitals have access to, or arrange the calling of an Ethics committee?

If the answer is YES then paragraph 4.1.2.1—ISO 9002 is also applicable.

4.1.2.2 Verification Resources and Personnel

(a) *Question*: Who carries out the maintenance, calibrations and repair of Major Surgical and Diagnostic medical devices, i.e., 'X'-Ray, CT, MR., Diathermy, Lasers and Ultrasound.

If the answer to (a) is, an in-house Physical Department, then the paragraph 4.1.2.2 shall apply. The product Electrical Safety Standard IEC 601-1 should be understood and applied. Where relevant the appropriate specific part 2's are to ICE-601-1 should also be applied, there should be evidence of equipment repair, history/test records and signed prior to release for hospital use.

If the answer to (a) is, sub-contract then the sub-contractor shall be audited as being in compliance with ISO 9002 or meeting the requirements of the Mount Elizabeth/Eash Shore Quality Management System, or is independently accredited by a recognised authority. The use of IEC 601-1 and the equipment specific part 2's are applicable as above.

such personnel can adversely effect the quality of patient treatment/care of medical devices sterile or non-sterile.

(D) Environmental Control

The hospital shall establish, document and maintain requirements for the environment to which the patient and or medical devices are directly or indirectly exposed.

If appropriate, the environmental conditions shall be controlled and/ or monitored.

(E) Cleanliness

The Hospital shall establish, document and maintain requirements for cleanliness of premises, medical devices, surgical products and materials if:

The medical devices, surgical procedures and materials are cleaned by the hospital prior to sterilization and/or its use; or

The medical devices, surgical products prior to sterilization and/or its use; or the medical devices, surgical products and materials are supplied non-sterile and its cleanliness is of significance in its use.

Premises, Ref: point 1 above: areas under the specific control of the microbiologist including all non-clinical areas, for example: staff accommodation and recreation areas, laboratories, laundry, food preparation, Hospital waste disposal and incinerating areas.

Note: All microbiological aspects necessary to assure sterility and reduce the microbial contamination shall be controlled, and reduce the microbial contamination shall be controlled, Ref: 4.1.2.1: Responsibility and Authority (Microbiologist).

(F) Maintenance and Repair

The hospital shall establish and document requirements for a routine maintenance, calibration programme and repair activities, when the lack of such activities may affect the quality of patient treatment/care, recorded and archived data, medical devices including test runs on inbuilt software and the efficient running of the hospital clinical and non-clinical services.

(G) Installation

If appropriate, the hospital shall establish and document both instructions and acceptance for installing and checking any medical or non-medical device.

Records of installation and checking performed by the hospital or his authorized representative shall be retained.

4.9.2 Special Processes and Procedures

The hospitals shall ensure that the quality/data records identify:

- ❑ the work instruction used including special clinical/surgical procedures;

- ❑ the date the special process/procedures was performed; and
- ❑ the identity of the operator of the special process.

This procedure should be maintained for both clinical and non-clinical special processes.

Note: Ask an appropriate senior member of the clinical/surgical staff their understanding of a special process and tailor 4.8.2 above to that. Do not accept the statement, "there are no special processes, everything is routine."

Other special processes for example are the method sterilization, the use, storage and analysis of blood products, the means of disposal of radioactive materials, toxic substances, single use sterile medical devices and surgical products for which procedures shall be in place and seen to the working.

Audit of Kitchens and Distribution of Food and Drink

For Food and Drink refer the Guidance Notes for the Application of ISO 9002 for The Food and Drink Industry QCN/41/42/390: Issue 1.

4.10 Inspection and Testing

4.10.1 Receiving Inspection and Testing

(a) Sensitive supplies/products, i.e.: drugs, radioactive materials, sterile devices and toxic substances shall be held in suitable quarantine conditions until released by the person(s) defined by the management structure.

(b) Supplies/products shall be correctly identified at all times. Unauthorised descriptions shall not be permitted.

(c) Each delivery or batch or supplies/products shall have or be allocated an identifying storage and processing through the hospital and any satellite establishments.

4.10.3 Final Inspection and Testing

No product labelled as "sterile" shall be released for distribution until any prescribed microbiological control have been satisfactorily completed, and so approved by the Microbiologist.

The hospital should ensure that supplies/products and devices which do not meet their inspection/test and purchase specifications are investigated. A report should be written, including conclusions and follow up procedures.

4.11 Inspection, Measuring, Test Equipment

This paragraph has particular importance to all research analytical and medical device maintenance, calibration, test and repair laboratories/departments.

Hospitals needs to specifically document control procedures for equipment used in the clinical laboratories, i.e.

(a) Basis for selecting appropriate equipment.
(b) Determine interval for the checking/calibrating the equipment.
(c) Define the process for these calibration and identification.
(d) Define their handling, storage and maintenance.

Typical suggested period between successive calibration for some and the clinical equipment is as follows:

(i)	Autoclaves	Monthly
(ii)	Blanches and scales	Yearly
(iii)	Biological Safety Cabinets	Yearly
(iv)	Manometers (working)	Yearly
	Manometer (Ref.)	Once in 5-years
(v)	Thermometers (working)	Half yearly
	Thermometers (Ref.)	Once in 5-years

In case and analytical instruments, i.e. pH meters, spectrophotometers, chromatographs, etc., these are checked on regular basis (in-house) by use of reference materials.

In case general equipment used in medical and forensic labs, i.e. DNA sizing equipment, electrophoresis, microscopes, temp controlled equipment (water baths Incubators, ovens), etc., these are monitored regularly with known control samples and recorded in the log books

4.14 Corrective and Preventive Action

(A) Complaints and Complaint Files

The hospitals should establish and maintain procedures to ensure that any complaint involving the possible failure of a clinical or non-clinical procedure to meet any of its performance criteria is reviewed, evaluated and investigated.

The procedure should ensure that any complaint relating to injury, death or hazard to health and safety, is immediately reviewed, evaluated and investigated by all relevant staff, and the record of the complaint and the investigation is maintained in a separate portion of the complaint file.

The hospital should ensure that records of the investigation are maintained and that such records include the name of the complaint, any control number used, the nature of the complaint and the reply to the complaint.

(B) Recall and Advisory Notices

The hospital should establish and maintain a documented recall and advisory notice procedure, which should be approved by a designated individual(s) and known to all staff concerned.

It should be capable of being put into operation at all times, 24 hours a day/265 days a year. An individual should be formally designated to initiate and coordinate the procedure and monitor its progress.

4.15 Storage

If special environmental storage conditions are required at any stage, such conditions should be controlled and monitored.

The hospital shall establish and maintain documented procedures for the control of stock with limited shelf life or requiring special storage.

Storage conditions should be orderly to facilitate rotation of stock, batch difference and cleaning.

Access to stock in quarantine areas shall be restricted to authorized persons.

4.16 Control of Quality Records

Quality records in Hospital: Patient records are kept undefinitely (achieved). Lab records are kept for 2-years and some records are microfiched for longer.

4.18 Training

The hospital shall ensure that all personnel who are required to work under special environmental conditions or perform special processes or functions, are appropriately trained or supervised by a trained person.

Education

Education refers to key posts being held by people with the appropriate qualifications.

Training

Training refers to the need for a program of courses to ensure staff have the necessary know-how, on the equipment with which they will be associated. This means both regarding technical and procedural knowledge. A requirement to demonstrate that such ongoing training is carried out, is often a feature of the Medical profession in many countries.

4.20 Statistical Techniques

Where sampling is carried out it shall be based on established statistical techniques. Sampling procedures shall be documented.

Biomed, Radiology and respiratory care, all can use variety of statistical techniques. Some hospitals do measure administrative functions (Nursing functions), customer surveys, etc. SPC could also be used in trend analysis, i.e. complaints, which could be sent to managers and nursing congress.

SPC can also be used to gather data on, percentage utilization of important and costly equipment, i.e. MRI, CT scan, X-rays, Gamma Camera, Dialysis, X-knife, etc. Similarly, down time for these equipment due to break down can help it know effectiveness of the maintenance procedure. Other useful data could be: (a) Average Length and stay of indoor patients, *vis-a-vis* available capacity, (b) Gross death rate, (c) Average Number and OPD cases daily, (d) Average number of IPD cases daily, (e) Surgery, and (g) Employee Satisfaction survey.

Extra Notes

Safety

The application of medical electrical equipment may introduce hazards due to a number of causes including the following:

(a) failure of a device on perform its intended function, (e.g. failure of a lung ventilator to ventilate the patient, failure of an apnoea monitor to given an alarm);
(b) incorrect function, (e.g. excessive drug delivery by an infusion pump, excessive temperature in a baby incubator, inaccurate measurement of a physiological parameter); and
(c) energies delivered when functioning normally, e.g.:
  - ❑ leakage current or functional current flowing from a cardiac defibrillator or from high frequency surgical equipment unit through unintended pathways in the patient or operator;
  - ❑ exposure of the radiation of an unintended part of the patient or operator;
  - ❑ exposure of the patient or operator to ultrasonic energy or accelerated elementary particles; and
  - ❑ excessive heating or cooling of the patient;
(d) equipment faults, e.g.:
  - ❑ fire, electric shock, explosion, expelled parts;
  - ❑ excessive ionizing or non-ionizing radiation resulting from equipment malfunction, leakage or over exposure; and
  - ❑ excessive temperatures of accessible surfaces leading to burns;
(e) fire or explosion from ignition of flammable material within the vicinity of the medical electrical equipment;
(f) mechanical failures in normal and fault conditions;
(g) incorrect installation of medical electrical equipment, e.g.:
  - ❑ inadequate earthing of an item of Class I medical electrical equipment
  - ❑ dangerous surfaces, corners or edges; and
  - ❑ physical instability;
(h) incorrect of medical electrical equipment, (e.g. the use of medical electrical equipment having a Type BF or Type B applied part to carry out an intracardiac procedure);
(i) incorrect use of medical electrical equipment (e.g. selection of an incorrect energy scale while using an internal cardiac defibrillator);

(j) electromagnetic interfaces, (e.g. interference of an ECG display by high frequency surgical equipment, generation of interference with adjacent medical electrical equipment by strong magnetic fields emanating from a display); and

(k) release of corrosive, poisonous or hot liquids or gases, or contact with biologically unsafe materials.

Regulatory Aspects

Radiation Protection (X-Rays and Radioactive Sources)

Publication 26 of the International Commission on Radiation Protection (Ref. 4) provides the basis for Radiation Protection Standards.

The key principles are Justification and Optimisation.

These principles are summarised as ALARA (As Low As Responsibly Achievable).

In the case of Radioactive Sources, special precautions must be in place regarding both their use and disposal.

There may be local (as well as International) regulations on radiation safety.

It is important the Hospital knows what these are and that they follow them.

A Radiation Protection Supervisor with responsibility for the maintenance of Radiation Protection, may be already present.

Lasers

Where LASERS are in use for medical applications, rules should be present to ensure the safe use of these devices

VDUs

If VDUs are in use, guidelines should be considered in the cases of pregnant staff.

Ultra-Violet Radiation

If Ultra-Violet equipment is in use, procedures to ensure protection to eyes and skit of operators (and patients) should be followed.

Magnetic Resonance Imaging (MRI)

The special needs associated with the use of MRI, if present, must be understood. The equipment involves the use of high magnetic fields, making the following precautions necessary:

- ❑ Small metal objects must not come near the equipment.
- ❑ Persons with pacemakers must not be exposed.
- ❑ Pregnant females should avoid exposure.
- ❑ Patients with metal prostheses should have only limited exposure.

This type of imaging equipment may utilise a super-conducting magnet. Procedures to store and handle the coolants are essential.

Electrical and Mechanical Safety

The most appropriate International Regulation on Electrical aspects remains IEC 601-2-9.

The standards developed for Quality Systems are BS 5750, Parts 1-6 and ISO 9000

The British Standard for Medical Equipment is BS 5724, Specification for the safety of Medical Electrical Equipment.

Chemical Safety

The use of Medical Imaging equipment involves the use of Chemical Agents, for example, the use of Contrast Media.

Procedures to store and handle these Chemical Agents is essential.

Index